Lippincott's
CONCISE ILLUSTRATED ANATOMY:

Head & Neck

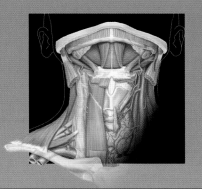
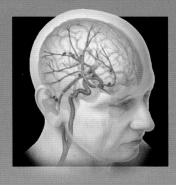

Lippincott's
CONCISE ILLUSTRATED ANATOMY:

Head & Neck

VOLUME 3

Ben Pansky, PhD, MD

Professor Emeritus
Department of Surgery
University of Toledo College of Medicine
and Life Sciences
Toledo, Ohio

Thomas R. Gest, PhD

Professor of Anatomy
Division of Clinical Anatomy
Department of Radiology
University of South Florida Morsani College of Medicine
Tampa, Florida

Wolters Kluwer | Lippincott Williams & Wilkins
Health

Philadelphia · Baltimore · New York · London
Buenos Aires · Hong Kong · Sydney · Tokyo

Acquisitions Editor: Crystal Taylor
Product Manager: Julie Montalbano
Production Project Manager: Marian Bellus
Marketing Manager: Joy Fisher Williams
Designer: Steve Druding
Compositor: SPi Global

351 West Camden Street   Two Commerce Square
Baltimore, MD 21201   2001 Market Street
                                Philadelphia, PA 19103

Printed in China

Library of Congress Cataloging-in-Publication Data
Pansky, Ben.
   Lippincott's concise illustrated anatomy. Vol. 3, Head & neck / Ben Pansky, Thomas R. Gest.
      p. ; cm.
   Concise illustrated anatomy
   Head & neck
   Includes index.
   ISBN 978-1-60913-027-5
   I. Gest, Thomas R. II. Title. III. Title: Concise illustrated anatomy. IV. Title: Head & neck.
   [DNLM: 1. Head—anatomy & histology—Atlases. 2. Brain—anatomy & histology—Atlases. 3. Cranial Nerves—anatomy & histology—Atlases. 4. Neck—anatomy & histology—Atlases. WE 17]
   QM535
   611'.910222—dc23

                                                                              2013003249

9 8 7 6 5 4 3 2 1

RRS1303

I dedicate this new endeavor to my dearly beloved wife **JULIE**, who will live in my loving memory forever, after our more than 50 years together, whose love, patience, understanding, encouragement and constant inspiration, supported me through the seasons of my maturation and productive life.

And to my loving son, **JONATHAN,** who grew up and matured along with me, my writings, illustrations, and stories. He is ever present by my side with love and encouragement helping me maintain the "Spark of Life and Creativity," which has forever glowed brightly within me.

—BEN PANSKY

For my students, past, present, and future, who make teaching so enjoyable, and to all of the courageous body donors, past, present, and future, who teach me and my students so much more than gross anatomy through their amazingly brave and charitable gift.

To the memory of Patrick Tank, colleague and friend, whose legacy as an anatomist and medical educator endures in his published works and in the skills and knowledge of countless former students.

—TOM GEST

Medical education continues to be in a constant state of change. Dedicated teachers experiment with teaching methods and curricula, always striving to refine, to define, to update, and to narrow the gap between the what, the how, and the why of what is being taught and the state of our present knowledge. Academic traditions are often quite rigid, cemented into place by a "yardstick of established time (hours)," so any effort to change becomes formidable and medical, clinical, and scientific relevance may receive secondary consideration. What the art of medicine always requires, no matter how much manipulating is done, is a strong foundation in the basic sciences. To fully appreciate and understand the complexities and nuances of variation in us all, Anatomy is the keystone in that foundation.

Lippincott's Concise Illustrated Anatomy series presents human gross anatomy in more than a synopsis form and far less than one encounters in a massive traditional text. Each title in the series is a highly illustrated, complete, functionally oriented, clinically informative text, concerned with "living" anatomy and stressing the importance of the relationship between structure and function. Repetition only occurs as needed to emphasize particular points or to demonstrate continuity between regions.

Terminology adheres to the *Terminologia Anatomica* (1998) approved by the Federative Committee on Anatomical Nomenclature (FCAT) of the International Federation of Associations of Anatomists (IFAA). Official English-equivalent terms are used throughout this edition.

Anatomy requires one to think three-dimensionally, which is often a new concept for students and a difficult one for practitioners desiring to review. Studying and palpating a body at a dissection table may be the best way to comprehend the three-dimensional fundamentals of anatomy and the relationships of many of its parts. However, lacking the physical body, this text maintains a tradition utilized in six editions of *Review of Gross Anatomy* by Ben Pansky of being planned and written around its illustrations, which come predominantly from the highly acclaimed *Lippincott Williams & Wilkins Atlas of Anatomy* by Drs. Tank and Gest, together with a reworking of a number of illustrations from Dr. Pansky's 6th edition of *Review of Gross Anatomy* into beautiful, full-colored illustrations closely coordinated with those of the *Atlas*.

The illustrations present anatomical images concisely in a logical sequence, making them easier and faster to use, a critical and essential need in this era of compressed anatomical curricula.

The hundreds of illustrations in full color combined with an abbreviated, outlined, but comprehensive and detailed text convey a simplified, multi-faceted, three-dimensional aspect of the beauty and function of the human body not found in other texts.

Because the overall volume of material (in text and illustration) needed to present the true, complete reality of the human body is so massive, many texts have become larger and larger over the years. It was felt that a huge "tome" of 1,000 or more pages would be too overwhelming and formidable as well as difficult for students to tackle without great trepidation. Thus, we have decided to present 3 volumes for the 7 chapters or units of associated areas of the body—namely, Volume 1: Back, Upper Limb & Lower Limb; Volume 2: Thorax, Abdomen, & Pelvis; and Volume 3: Head & Neck. Each volume is approximately 300 pages. Thus, as one studies a respective body region, one needs to essentially carry, transport, and study from a single volume at a time. Furthermore, if a student or practitioner is predominantly involved only in one or two major body areas, he or she may be able to concentrate on the essentials of his or her study or review (i.e., general practitioner, psychologist, neurologist, medical student, physical therapy, occupational therapy, nursing, orthopedics, dentistry, ophthalmology, surgery, etc.) without carrying around a large tome. He or she would still have the other volume(s) for reference since the body functions as a unit and one part depends on or is related to the other.

Progression from region to region, from the Back to the Upper and Lower Limbs, to the Thorax, Abdomen, and Pelvis, and to the Head and Neck, allows one to fully appreciate the continuity between the regions. The regional approach duplicates that used in many human anatomy courses and laboratories of dissection as well as in surgical areas of concentration. However, the illustrations show some overlapping of structures to allow the student to move easily from one region to the next.

The body is discussed from its superficial layers to its deep structures, except for the osteology. Because the bones form the framework of the body and lend themselves to the attachment of soft parts, they tend to appear early in the text and are also to be studied early in most courses. This makes understanding of the relationships of the soft body parts more easy and clear.

By extracting information from within the living organism, the student and practitioner are better able to describe and define both normal and abnormal states. Increasingly, sophisticated tools help them understand that continuum. At first, students of the medical arts used only observations and palpation, then they undertook dissection, and now "tools" have gained momentum, moving quickly from the stethoscopes and ophthalmoscopes to powerful X-rays and imaging technologies. To put this in perspective, X-rays were discovered at the close of the 19th century; nuclear medicine and ultrasonography were introduced in the 1950s; and computed tomography (CT), digital radiography, and nuclear magnetic resonance (NMR) became available in the 1970s.

Thus, an anatomy text would be incomplete without some discussion and illustration of radiography, CT, NMR, and cross-sectional anatomy, which provide a good clinical introduction to the current state of the patient's health. This has been included in our books since the sooner one learns to identify normal anatomy on X-ray film and computer imaging, the easier it becomes to locate and understand the changes brought on by genetics, disease, or trauma and thus, anatomy becomes a "keystone" to all of medicine and its many related fields.

Although much basic and essential clinical consideration has been presented in many areas of our texts, all clinically relevant material cannot be fully discussed for each anatomical region. However, its importance in one's understanding of basic anatomy and how that can be altered is essential for truly appreciating what is generally "normal" before it becomes altered and creates clinical signs and symptoms.

The functional anatomy of the Neck, the Head (including the sense organs), and the Brain and Cranial Nerves are presented in a concise manner, together with correlated clinical material, so that the student can appreciate the relevance of the anatomy to clinical practice. Special functional summaries—especially those for the cranial nerves, arteries of the head and neck, and the autonomic innervation—should help the student to grasp this difficult material.

The average student, clinician, investigator, and instructor are often overwhelmed by the amount of material necessary to be learned for a basic understanding of the very complex anatomy of the neck, the head, and its sense organs, as well as the central nervous system with the brain and cranial nerves. Those seeking to review are often astounded by progress in the field of neuroscience, the overwhelming excess of explanations, references and minute detail, and the amount of time it takes to really study and comprehend the mass of material that is available and still not lose sight of the real essentials.

We, as educators in the Anatomical Sciences, are aware of the fact that gross anatomy and associated neuroscientific material are subjects quickly memorized and just as easily forgotten, unless the student or practitioner constantly reviews the material. Time can be an adversary and multiple duties are often overwhelming. It is our hope that in this volume we have presented information that is relatively simplified, concise, direct, and meaningful in a semi-outlined form that is complete, functionally oriented, and clinically informative without "running on and on" with excessive nonessentials. We believe we have been able to create a volume of basic thoughts and ideas along with many full-colored illustrations for visualizing the regions described that will guide the reader easily and thoughtfully through the very complex detail that makes up the head and neck and its many parts.

ACKNOWLEDGMENTS

Many thanks to those at Lippincott Williams and Wilkins who participated in the development of this textbook, including Acquisitions Editor Crystal Taylor, Product Manager Julie Montalbano, Art Director Jennifer Clements, and Designer Steve Druding. Additional thanks goes to Kelly Horvath for her editorial guidance and copyediting.

Marcelo Oliver and Body Scientific International did a superb job of converting many of Dr. Pansky's original black-and-white illustrations into full color, managing to duplicate the tone, color, and beauty of the illustrations from the *Lippincott Williams & Wilkins Atlas of Anatomy* by Drs. Tank and Gest.

Much gratitude is extended to Danelle Mooi, Secretary, Department of Surgery, and Nick Andrew Bell, Secretary, Departments of Nursing, Emergency Medicine and Staff Development, both at The University of Toledo Medical Center for their persistent encouragement, understanding, and great help to Dr. Pansky with their knowledge of the computer and digital world, which made his transgression into the realm of computers and wireless connections possible and a great learning experience.

And special thanks goes to Patrick Tank, PhD, Professor of Neurobiology and Developmental Sciences, University of Arkansas for Medical Sciences. His inspiration and hard work on the initial chapter of the initial volume of this series helped to get this project underway.

Ben Pansky
Thomas Gest

CONTENTS

Chapter 3: Brain and Cranial Nerves

Neck

Surface Anatomy of the Neck

I. Palpable Features of the Neck

A. Anteriorly (Fig. 1.1A)
   1. Lower margin of mandible
   2. Body of hyoid bone: in midline about 2 cm above laryngeal prominence in line with lower border of 3rd cervical vertebra
   3. Upper margin and lamina of thyroid cartilage
      a. **Laryngeal prominence** (Adam's apple) protrudes anteriorly in males (resulting in deeper voice)
      b. Upper margin lies at level of common carotid bifurcation
   4. Arch of cricoid cartilage: found just below thyroid cartilage at level of 6th cervical vertebra
   5. Trachea
   6. Jugular (suprasternal) notch of sternum
   7. Clavicle
   8. Sternocleidomastoid (SCM) muscle
      a. Passes from sternum and medial clavicle up to mastoid process
      b. Subdivides neck into anterior and posterior cervical triangles
B. Laterally (Fig. 1.1B)
   1. Mastoid process
   2. Transverse processes of cervical vertebrae
   3. **Greater horn of hyoid bone**: tip lies midway between laryngeal prominence and mastoid process (surgical landmark to locate lingual artery)
   4. Carotid pulse: at anterior margin of SCM muscle, midway between angle of jaw and jugular fossa; pulse can be felt in common carotid artery
   5. Acromion

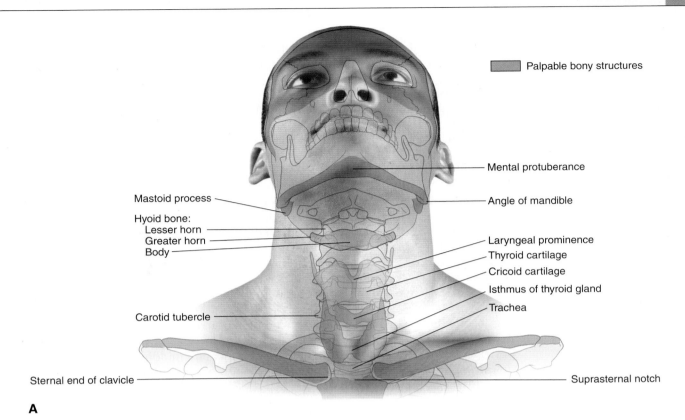

Palpable bony structures

Mental protuberance

Angle of mandible

Mastoid process

Hyoid bone:
  Lesser horn
  Greater horn
  Body

Laryngeal prominence
Thyroid cartilage
Cricoid cartilage
Isthmus of thyroid gland
Trachea

Carotid tubercle

Sternal end of clavicle

Suprasternal notch

A

Zygoma and zygomatic arch

Superior nuchal line

External occipital protuberance

Mastoid process

Inferior border of mandible

Hyoid bone

Lamina of thyroid cartilage

Cricoid cartilage

1st tracheal ring

Spinous process of C7 vertebra

B

Figure 1.1 A,B. Palpable Features and Landmarks of the Neck. **A.** Anterior View. **B.** Lateral View.

C. Posteriorly (**Fig. 1.1C**)

1. External occipital protuberance and superior nuchal line
2. Posterior arch and posterior tubercle of atlas and spine of axis palpable with deep pressure
3. Vertebra (spina) prominens
    a. Tip of spinous process of C7 felt in posterior midline; may be visible, especially with flexion
    b. Typically, most readily palpable cervical spine, although tip of C6 may be felt above

II. Approximate Locations of Neck Structures

A. Vessels

1. Common carotid artery: on line from upper border of sternal end of clavicle to point midway between mastoid process and angle of mandible
2. Subclavian artery: indicated by arch with medial end at sternoclavicular joint and lateral end at middle of clavicle
3. Carotid sinus: pressure near carotid bifurcation can stimulate baroreceptors to elicit vagal reflex that will slow heartbeat and lower blood pressure, causing fainting
4. Internal jugular vein: follows same line as internal/common carotid artery

B. Nerves

1. Vagus: same line as internal jugular vein and internal/common carotid artery
2. Accessory: passes under SCM 3.75 cm (1.5 in) below tip of mastoid; emerges from posterior border of that muscle at junction of upper and middle 2/3; passes obliquely downward and backward across posterior triangle to pass under anterior border of trapezius 5 cm (2 in) above clavicle
3. Phrenic: begins at level of middle of lamina of thyroid cartilage; its caudal course is indicated by line down middle of SCM, parallel to direction of muscle

C. Thyroid gland: upper pole contacts lower portion of lamina of thyroid cartilage, inferolateral to prominence; lower pole may reach level of 5th or 6th tracheal ring; isthmus crosses tracheal rings 2–3

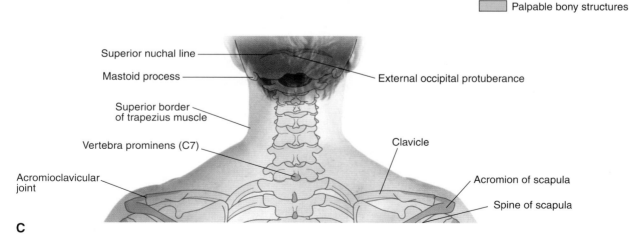

Palpable bony structures

Superior nuchal line

Mastoid process

External occipital protuberance

Superior border of trapezius muscle

Vertebra prominens (C7)

Clavicle

Acromioclavicular joint

Acromion of scapula

Spine of scapula

C

Figure 1.1C. Palpable Features and Landmarks of the Neck, Posterior View.

III. Clinical Considerations

A. **Goiter** (see Section 1.5)
   1. Thyroid gland produces no conspicuous thickening in neck when not enlarged
   2. In goiter, thyroid gland may bulge out, depending on degree of enlargement

B. **Central venous catheterization** (**central line**)
   1. Large vein used: subclavian, internal jugular, or femoral
   2. Internal jugular vein
      a. Reduces risk of pneumothorax
      b. Needle or catheter may be inserted for diagnostic or therapeutic purposes
      c. Right vein preferable due to slightly larger caliber and straighter course
      d. Clinician palpates common carotid artery and locates vein just lateral
      e. Needle is inserted at 30° angle between sternal and clavicular heads of SCM muscle

C. **Carotid (neck) pulse**
   1. Felt by palpating common carotid artery between trachea and infrahyoid muscles
   2. Easily palpated just deep to anterior border of SCM at level of superior border of thyroid cartilage
   3. Absence of pulse indicates cardiac arrest

D. **Pulsation of internal jugular vein**
   1. Can relate information regarding heart activity (i.e., right atrial pressure and mitral valve disease)
   2. Pulsations may be seen deep to SCM, superior to medial end of clavicle
   3. A contraction wave passes up through brachiocephalic vein and superior vena cava (because they have no valves) to inferior jugular vein; pulses are more visible when patient's head is inferior to his or her feet (Trendelenberg position)
   4. Pulses increase in conditions of mitral valve disease because this increases pressure in pulmonary circulation and right side of the heart

Cervical Triangles and Fascia

I. Cervical Triangles

A. Anterior triangle (Fig. 1.2A)
1. Boundaries
   a. Midline
   b. SCM muscle
   c. Body of mandible
2. Subdivisions
   a. **Submandibular triangle**: body of mandible, anterior and posterior bellies of digastric muscle
   b. **Submental triangle**: anterior belly of digastric muscle, body of hyoid bone, midline
   c. **Carotid triangle**: posterior belly of digastric muscle, superior belly of omohyoid muscle, SCM muscle
   d. **Muscular triangle**: SCM muscle, superior belly of omohyoid muscle, midline

B. Posterior triangle (Fig. 1.2B)
1. Boundaries
   a. SCM muscle
   b. Trapezius muscle
   c. Clavicle
2. Subdivisions
   a. **Occipital triangle**: SCM muscle, trapezius muscle, inferior belly of omohyoid
   b. **Omoclavicular (subclavian) triangle**: SCM muscle, inferior belly of omohyoid muscle, clavicle

II. Skin and Superficial Fascia

A. Skin of neck: fibers of dermis (so-called "Langer's lines") run in transverse direction; incisions made accordingly
B. Superficial fascia of neck: loose areolar connective tissue containing platysma muscle, superficial blood vessels, cutaneous nerves, and superficial lymph nodes
1. Platysma muscle
   a. Origin: investing fascia covering pectoralis major and deltoid muscles
   b. Insertion: inferior border of mandible and skin of lower face, decussating with facial muscles
   c. Action: draws corners of mouth down; aids in depression of mandible
   d. Innervation: cervical branch of facial nerve (cranial nerve [CN] VII); emerges from parotid gland near angle of mandible
2. Superficial vessels and cutaneous nerves found primarily beneath platysma

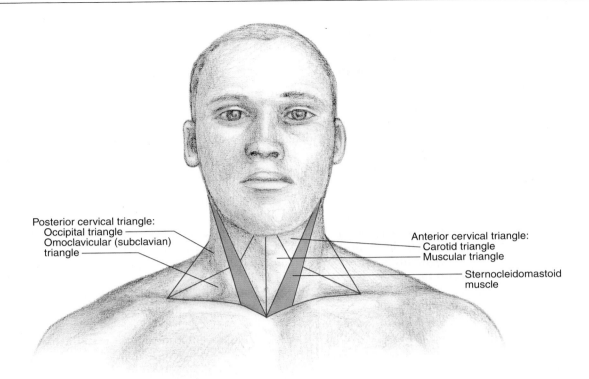

Posterior cervical triangle:
  Occipital triangle
  Omoclavicular (subclavian)
  triangle

Anterior cervical triangle:
  Carotid triangle
  Muscular triangle

Sternocleidomastoid
muscle

A

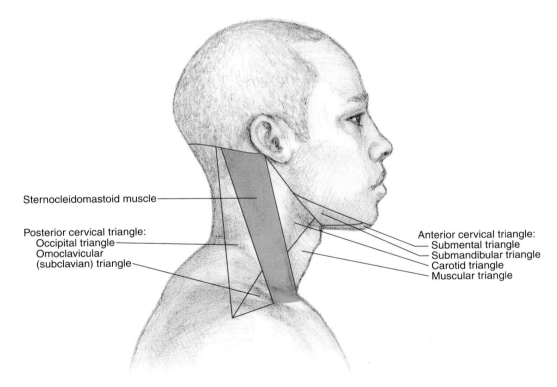

Sternocleidomastoid muscle

Posterior cervical triangle:
  Occipital triangle
  Omoclavicular
  (subclavian) triangle

Anterior cervical triangle:
  Submental triangle
  Submandibular triangle
  Carotid triangle
  Muscular triangle

B

Figure 1.2A,B. Triangles of the Neck. **A.** Anterior View. **B.** Lateral View.

III. Deep Cervical Fascia (Fig. 1.2C,D)

A. **Superficial layer of deep cervical fascia**
   1. Completely encircles neck
      a. Covers anterior and posterior triangles
      b. Splits to enclose SCM and trapezius muscles
   2. Attachments
      a. Posteriorly: external occipital protuberance, ligamentum nuchae, spine of C7
      b. Superiorly: superior nuchal line, mastoid process, mandible; invests parotid and submandibular glands
      c. Inferiorly: clavicle, manubrium of sternum, acromion, and spine of scapula

B. **Infrahyoid fascia**
   1. Investing fascia of infrahyoid muscles (omohyoid, sternohyoid, sternothyroid, thyrohyoid)
   2. Consists of 2 layers
      a. Superficial encloses omohyoid and sternohyoid muscles
      b. Deep invests sternothyroid and thyrohyoid muscles

C. **Visceral fascia**
   1. Encloses viscera of neck: larynx, trachea, thyroid, pharynx, and esophagus
   2. 2 subdivisions
      a. **Pretracheal fascia**
         i. Covers larynx and trachea; splits to enclose thyroid gland (forming false or surgical capsule)
         ii. Attached superiorly to hyoid bone and thyroid cartilage; posterolaterally continuous as buccopharyngeal fascia; inferiorly enters thorax to join fascia of aorta and pericardium
         iii. **Suspensory ligaments of thyroid gland**: thickenings run from upper inner part of thyroid gland to cricoid cartilage, anchoring gland to larynx; must be cut before thyroid gland can be properly mobilized
      b. **Buccopharyngeal fascia**
         i. Covers buccinator muscle and posterior surface of pharynx and esophagus
         ii. Attached superiorly to pharyngeal tubercle and medial pterygoid plates

D. **Prevertebral fascia**
   1. Forms tubular investment of vertebral column and its muscles; covers prevertebral muscles and forms floor of posterior triangle; thicker than visceral fascia
   2. Attachments
      a. Laterally: transverse processes of cervical vertebrae
      b. Superiorly: occipital bone near jugular foramen, superior nuchal line, and mastoid process
      c. Inferiorly: continues into mediastinum; forms 2 structures
         i. **Suprapleural membrane** (Sibson's fascia): scalene muscle fascia covering cervical pleura
         ii. **Axillary sheath**: scalene fascia covering axillary vessels and brachial plexus as they pass through interscalene triangle

E. **Carotid sheath**
   1. Adjacent deep fascial layers blend to form investment of carotid arteries (internal and common) medially, internal jugular vein laterally, and vagus nerve between
   2. Adherent to visceral fascia on thyroid and superficial layer of deep cervical fascia under SCM
   3. Attached superiorly to margins of jugular foramen and carotid canal; continues inferiorly into thorax

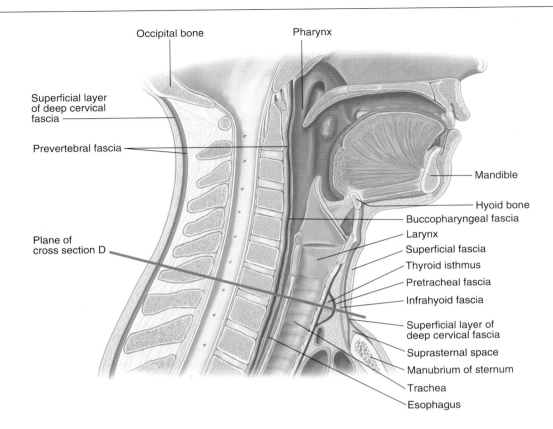

Occipital bone

Pharynx

Superficial layer of deep cervical fascia

Prevertebral fascia

Mandible

Hyoid bone

Buccopharyngeal fascia

Larynx

Superficial fascia

Plane of cross section D

Thyroid isthmus

Pretracheal fascia

Infrahyoid fascia

Superficial layer of deep cervical fascia

Suprasternal space

Manubrium of sternum

Trachea

Esophagus

C

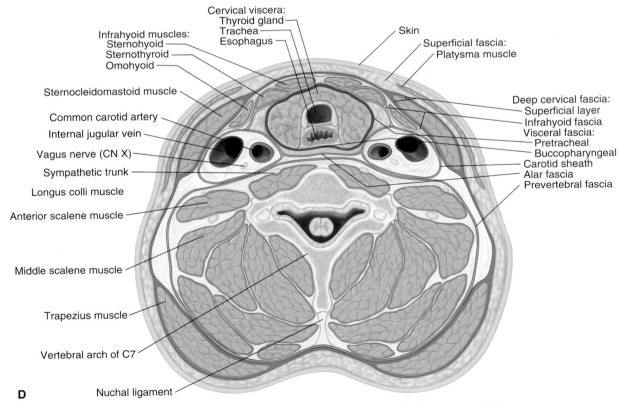

Cervical viscera:
Thyroid gland
Trachea
Esophagus

Skin

Superficial fascia:
Platysma muscle

Infrahyoid muscles:
Sternohyoid
Sternothyroid
Omohyoid

Sternocleidomastoid muscle

Common carotid artery

Deep cervical fascia:
Superficial layer
Infrahyoid fascia
Visceral fascia:
Pretracheal
Buccopharyngeal
Carotid sheath
Alar fascia
Prevertebral fascia

Internal jugular vein

Vagus nerve (CN X)

Sympathetic trunk

Longus colli muscle

Anterior scalene muscle

Middle scalene muscle

Trapezius muscle

Vertebral arch of C7

D

Nuchal ligament

Figure 1.2C,D. Deep Cervical Fascia. **C.** Midsagittal View. **D.** Cross-sectional View.

IV. Fascial Spaces

A. **Retropharyngeal space**
   1. Between buccopharyngeal and prevertebral fascia
   2. Extends from skull into mediastinum; major pathway for infection from neck into thorax
      a. Alar fascia: thin layer of fascia subdivides this space; attached in midline to buccopharyngeal fascia; laterally, joins carotid sheath
      b. Retropharyngeal abscess can cause dysphagia, dysarthria, and mediastinitis
B. **Suprasternal space (of Burns)**
   1. Between layers of superficial layer of deep cervical fascia, which splits at jugular notch to attach to posterior and anterior sides of manubrium
   2. Contains jugular venous arch
C. **Pretracheal space**
   1. Potential space in front of trachea and behind infrahyoid muscles and pretracheal fascia
   2. Limited above by attachment of pretracheal fascia to thyroid cartilage, but continues into mediastinum to level of pericardium
D. **Parapharyngeal (lateral pharyngeal) space**
   1. Lateral to pharynx
   2. Limited laterally by connective tissue capsule of parotid gland and pterygoid muscles, posteriorly by prevertebral fascia, superiorly extends to skull base, and inferiorly continues with connective tissue layer of carotid triangle

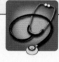

V. Clinical Considerations

A. Infection between superficial layer of deep cervical fascia and infrahyoid fascia: infection will usually stop at superior edge of sternum and clavicle
B. Infection between infrahyoid fascia and pretracheal fascia: can spread into thoracic cavity to position anterior to pericardium
C. Infection deep to pretracheal fascia: can follow trachea and esophagus to thoracic cavity and terminate in posterior mediastinum
D. Infection in retropharyngeal space: can spread into thoracic cavity into mediastinum in plane anterior to vertebral column and posterior to esophagus

Superficial Veins and Cutaneous Nerves of the Neck

I. Superficial Veins (Fig. 1.3A–C)

A. Location: within superficial fascia covered by platysma muscle

B. Major superficial veins

   1. **External jugular vein**

     a. Formed by union of **posterior division of the retromandibular vein** with posterior auricular (which can unite with the occipital vein)

     b. Descends vertically beneath platysma

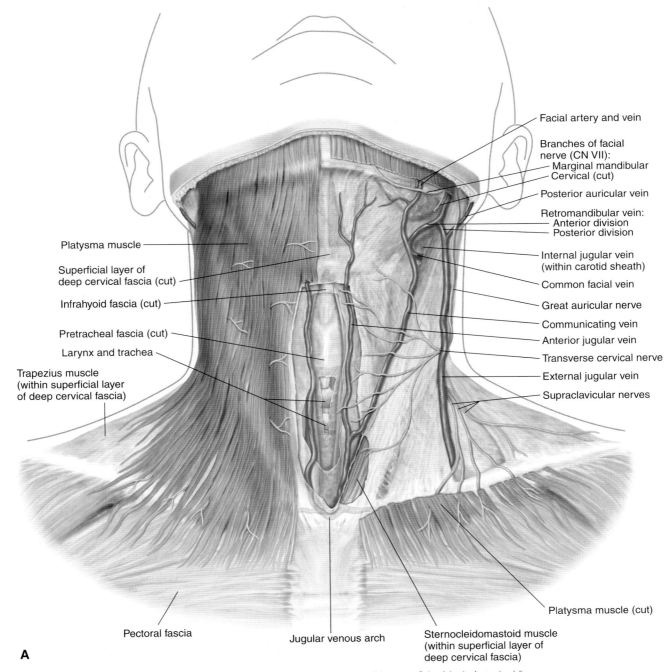

Facial artery and vein

Branches of facial
nerve (CN VII):
Marginal mandibular
Cervical (cut)

Posterior auricular vein

Retromandibular vein:
Anterior division
Posterior division

Internal jugular vein
(within carotid sheath)

Common facial vein

Great auricular nerve

Communicating vein

Anterior jugular vein

Transverse cervical nerve

External jugular vein

Supraclavicular nerves

Platysma muscle

Superficial layer of
deep cervical fascia (cut)

Infrahyoid fascia (cut)

Pretracheal fascia (cut)

Larynx and trachea

Trapezius muscle
(within superficial layer
of deep cervical fascia)

Platysma muscle (cut)

Pectoral fascia

Jugular venous arch

Sternocleidomastoid muscle
(within superficial layer of
deep cervical fascia)

A

Figure 1.3A. Superficial Veins and Cutaneous Nerves of the Neck, Anterior View.

      c. Lies anterior to and roughly parallels great auricular nerve; obliquely crossing SCM muscle

      d. Pierces deep cervical fascia in posterior triangle and drains into subclavian vein; venous valve located at termination

      e. Near termination, receives anterior jugular, transverse cervical, and suprascapular veins

  2. **Anterior jugular vein**

      a. Begins as union of small cutaneous veins in submental triangle; may receive connections with external jugular or facial veins

      b. Descends near midline, parallel with its opposite partner; may be unilateral or absent

      c. Pierces superficial layer of deep cervical fascia above jugular notch of manubrium

      d. **Jugular venous arch** may unite paired anterior jugular veins across midline within suprasternal space

      e. Each vein passes deep to SCM muscle to empty into external jugular

  3. **Common facial (facial) vein**

      a. Union of **facial vein** with **anterior division of retromandibular vein**; often referred to as *facial vein*

      b. Pierces deep fascia to drain to internal jugular vein within upper part of carotid triangle

  4. **Communicating vein (of Kocher)**

      a. Frequent branch of common facial that descends along anterior border of SCM muscle

      b. Drains into anterior jugular vein

C. Other superficial veins

  1. **Posterior auricular vein**

      a. Originates as small vein behind ear

      b. Joins posterior division of retromandibular to form external jugular vein

  2. **Transverse cervical vein**

      a. Drains trapezius muscle and posterior triangle region

      b. May unite with suprascapular before draining into external jugular vein

  3. **Suprascapular vein**

      a. Drains posterior shoulder region

      b. Drains to external jugular vein

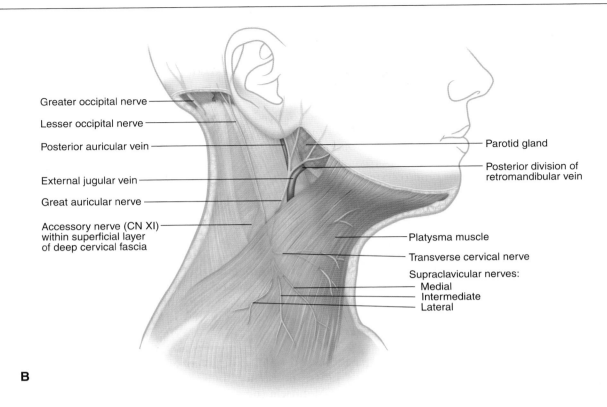

Greater occipital nerve

Lesser occipital nerve

Posterior auricular vein

External jugular vein

Great auricular nerve

Accessory nerve (CN XI) within superficial layer of deep cervical fascia

Parotid gland

Posterior division of retromandibular vein

Platysma muscle

Transverse cervical nerve

Supraclavicular nerves:
Medial
Intermediate
Lateral

B

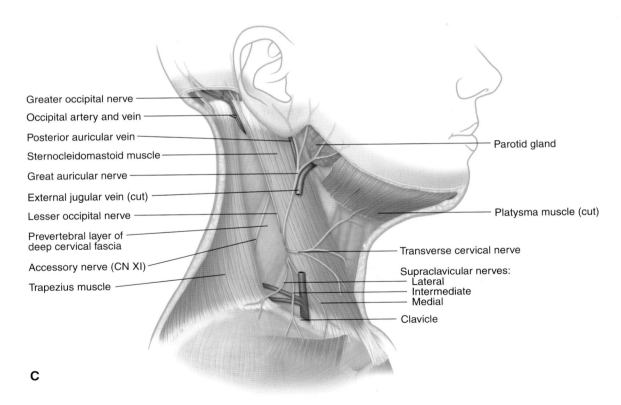

Greater occipital nerve

Occipital artery and vein

Posterior auricular vein

Sternocleidomastoid muscle

Great auricular nerve

External jugular vein (cut)

Lesser occipital nerve

Prevertebral layer of deep cervical fascia

Accessory nerve (CN XI)

Trapezius muscle

Parotid gland

Platysma muscle (cut)

Transverse cervical nerve

Supraclavicular nerves:
Lateral
Intermediate
Medial
Clavicle

C

Figure 1.3B,C. Superficial Veins and Cutaneous Nerves of the Neck. **B.** Superficial Dissection, Lateral View.
C. Intermediate Dissection, Lateral View.

II. Cutaneous Nerves (Fig. 1.3D–F)

A. Posterior rami
1. **Greater occipital nerve** (posterior ramus of C2)
   a. Passes below obliquus capitis inferior to penetrate semispinalis capitis and reach skin
   b. Distributes to skin on back of head up to vertex
2. **Occipitalis tertius** (posterior ramus of C3): to skin of upper posterior neck
3. Cutaneous branches of posterior rami of C4–C8: posterior neck and upper back laterally to rib angles approximately
B. Anterior rami (cervical plexus, C1–C4)
1. Cervical plexus is represented by multiple looping connections between adjacent anterior rami
2. Cutaneous branches of cervical plexus
   a. Segmental distribution
      i. C1 has no cutaneous sensory distribution
      ii. C2: borders on sensory area of trigeminal nerve (CN V) and is limited mainly to cutaneous area behind pinna of ear up to vertex of head
      iii. C3: passes cranially up to margin of mandible; extends over entire anterior cervical triangle and spreads out laterally beyond SCM muscle area into posterior cervical triangle
      iv. C4: supplies root of neck and cutaneous area of thoracic wall to level of 1st intercostal space (borders on distribution of anterior ramus of T1)
   b. Specific cutaneous nerves of cervical plexus: 4 cutaneous branches emerge at posterior margin of SCM muscle (near its midpoint)
      i. **Lesser occipital nerve** (C2): hooks around spinal accessory nerve, ascends along posterior border of SCM muscle, and ends behind ear
      ii. **Great auricular nerve** (C2–C3): exits from under middle of posterior border of SCM muscle; branches pass to skin of ear and adjacent areas
      iii. **Transverse cervical nerve** (C2–C3): exits below great auricular nerve, crosses SCM muscle transversely to reach anterior triangle (crossing under external jugular vein), and supply skin between sternum and chin
      iv. **Supraclavicular nerves**: (C3–C4): exit from posterior middle border of SCM muscle and divides into 3 terminal branches
         a) Medial: innervates skin as far as 2nd intercostal space and sternoclavicular joint
         b) Intermediate (middle): descends over middle 1/3 of clavicle, may pierce bone resulting in persistent neuralgia if involved in callus following bone fracture
         c) Lateral: distributed to skin over point of shoulder and acromioclavicular joint

III. Clinical Considerations

A. External jugular vein
1. When venous pressure is normal, can be seen above clavicle for short distance
2. If venous pressure rises (i.e., in heart failure, obstruction of superior vena cava, enlargement of supraclavicular lymph nodes, or increased intrathoracic pressure), becomes prominent throughout its course along side of neck
B. **Erb's point**: point along posterior border of SCM muscle where anterior rami of C5–C6 meet; also marks approximate point at which cutaneous branches of cervical plexus emerge along posterior border of SCM

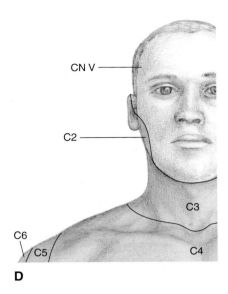

D

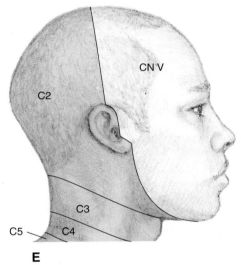

E

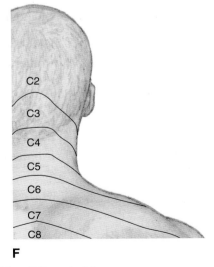

F

Figure 1.3D–F. Dermatomes of the Neck. **D.** Anterior View. **E.** Lateral View. **F.** Posterior View.

Anterior Triangle of the Neck

I. Boundaries of Anterior Triangle (Fig. 1.4A,B)

A. Medially: midline
B. Posterolaterally: anterior border of SCM muscle
C. Superiorly: inferior border of mandible
D. Roof: skin, superficial fascia, platysma muscle

II. Subdivisions

A. **Carotid triangle** (Fig. 1.4C)
   1. Boundaries: posterior belly of digastric, superior belly of omohyoid, and anterior border of SCM muscle
   2. Floor: thyrohyoid, lowest portion of hyoglossus, and middle and inferior pharyngeal constrictor muscles
   3. Contents: bifurcation of common carotid artery; origins of external carotid artery and its 1st 5 branches; hypoglossal and superior laryngeal nerves; superior root of ansa cervicalis
      a. Carotid sinus (see Section 1.6)
      b. Carotid body (see Section 1.6)
      c. Branches of external carotid artery within carotid triangle (see Section 1.6)
         i. Superior thyroid artery
         ii. Lingual artery
         iii. Facial artery
         iv. Ascending pharyngeal artery
         v. Occipital artery
      d. **Hypoglossal nerve (CN XII)**
         i. Swings forward below lower border of posterior belly of digastric muscle
         ii. Crossed by occipital artery and its SCM branch
         iii. Gives off superior root of ansa cervicalis (C1–C2 fibers)
         iv. Lies on hyoglossus muscle; passes forward into genioglossus muscle
B. **Muscular triangle** (Fig. 1.4D,E)
   1. Boundaries: superior belly of omohyoid muscle, anterior border of SCM muscle, midline
   2. Contents: sternohyoid, sternothyroid, and thyrohyoid muscles; thyroid and parathyroid glands; larynx; and trachea
C. **Submandibular triangle**
   1. Boundaries: mandible and both bellies of digastric muscle
   2. Floor: mylohyoid muscle
   3. Contents: superficial portion of submandibular gland, facial vessels (vein crosses superficial to gland, artery lies deep), mylohyoid vessels and nerve
D. **Submental triangle**
   1. Boundaries: body of hyoid bone, anterior belly of digastric muscle, and midline
   2. Floor: mylohyoid muscle
   3. Contents: submental lymph nodes, submental branch of facial artery, and small tributaries of anterior jugular vein

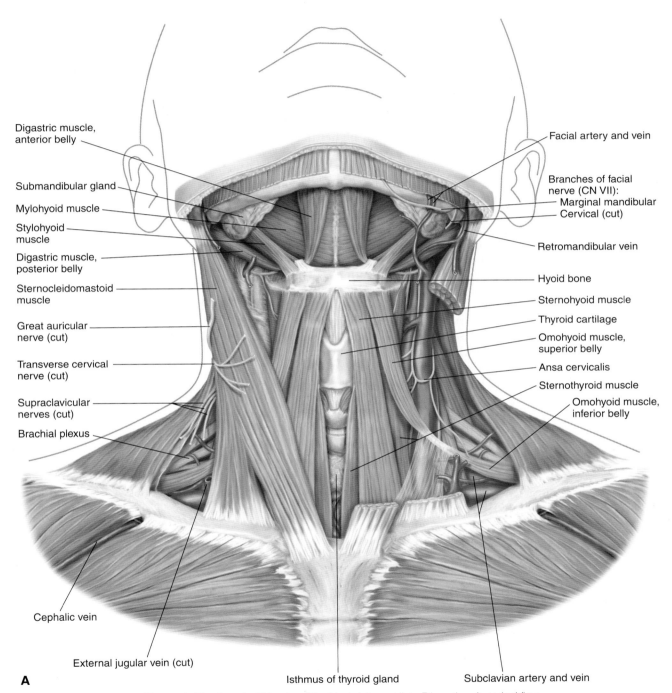

Digastric muscle, anterior belly

Submandibular gland

Mylohyoid muscle

Stylohyoid muscle

Digastric muscle, posterior belly

Sternocleidomastoid muscle

Great auricular nerve (cut)

Transverse cervical nerve (cut)

Supraclavicular nerves (cut)

Brachial plexus

Cephalic vein

External jugular vein (cut)

Facial artery and vein

Branches of facial nerve (CN VII):
Marginal mandibular
Cervical (cut)

Retromandibular vein

Hyoid bone

Sternohyoid muscle

Thyroid cartilage

Omohyoid muscle, superior belly

Ansa cervicalis

Sternothyroid muscle

Omohyoid muscle, inferior belly

Isthmus of thyroid gland

Subclavian artery and vein

A

Figure 1.4A. Anterior Triangle of the Neck, Intermediate Dissection, Anterior View.

III. Hyoid Bone

A. Location
   1. Body lies at level of body of 3rd cervical vertebra behind lower border of mandible
   2. Suspended below skull and mandible by muscles and ligaments
   3. Serves as important landmark for neck, support structure for neck viscera, and platform for muscle actions in neck
B. Features
   1. U shaped
   2. **Body**
      a. Anterior portion, somewhat flattened anteroposteriorly
      b. Ends laterally where it meets greater and lesser horns bilaterally
   3. **Greater horns**
      a. Extend posteriorly toward C3 vertebra
      b. Posterior ends slightly higher than anterior ends, which meet body
   4. **Lesser horns**
      a. Short superior projections from point at which greater horns meet body
      b. Serve as attachment points for stylohyoid ligament
C. Ligaments and membrane attachments
   1. Stylohyoid ligament: suspends hyoid bone from styloid process of temporal bone; attached at lesser horn
   2. Thyrohyoid membrane: attaches along lower border of hyoid, suspending thyroid cartilage; thickened as median and lateral thyrohyoid ligaments
   3. Hyoepiglottic ligament: tethers epiglottis to posterior surface of body
D. Muscle attachments
   1. Suprahyoid muscles attaching to hyoid (see Chapter 2)
      a. Digastric muscles, anterior and posterior bellies via intermediate tendon tethered by fascial sling to body near lesser horns
      b. Stylohyoid muscles: body near lesser horns
      c. Mylohyoid muscles: body
      d. Geniohyoid muscles: body
      e. Hyoglossus muscles: greater horn
   2. Infrahyoid muscles attaching to hyoid (strap muscles)
      a. Sternohyoid muscles: body
      b. Omohyoid muscles: body
      c. Thyrohyoid muscles: greater horn
      d. *Note*: sternothyroid muscle is only strap muscle that does not attach to hyoid bone
   3. Middle pharyngeal constrictor muscle: arises from greater and lesser horns and lower portion of stylohyoid ligament

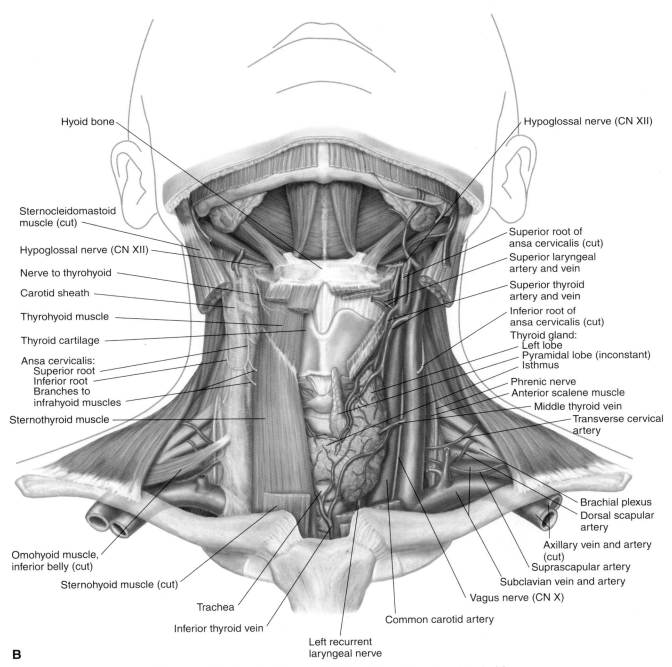

Hyoid bone

Hypoglossal nerve (CN XII)

Sternocleidomastoid muscle (cut)

Hypoglossal nerve (CN XII)

Nerve to thyrohyoid

Carotid sheath

Thyrohyoid muscle

Thyroid cartilage

Ansa cervicalis:
Superior root
Inferior root
Branches to
infrahyoid muscles

Sternothyroid muscle

Superior root of
ansa cervicalis (cut)

Superior laryngeal
artery and vein

Superior thyroid
artery and vein

Inferior root of
ansa cervicalis (cut)

Thyroid gland:
Left lobe
Pyramidal lobe (inconstant)
Isthmus

Phrenic nerve

Anterior scalene muscle

Middle thyroid vein

Transverse cervical
artery

Omohyoid muscle,
inferior belly (cut)

Sternohyoid muscle (cut)

Trachea

Inferior thyroid vein

Left recurrent
laryngeal nerve

Common carotid artery

Vagus nerve (CN X)

Subclavian vein and artery

Suprascapular artery

Axillary vein and artery
(cut)

Dorsal scapular
artery

Brachial plexus

B

Figure 1.4B. Anterior Triangle of the Neck, Deep Dissection, Anterior View.

IV. Muscles of Anterior Triangle

Muscle	Origin	Insertion	Action	Nerve
Platysma	Deltoid and pectoral fascia	Inferior border of mandible, skin, and subcutaneous tissue of lower face	Depresses angle of mouth, opens mouth, draws skin of neck superiorly when clenching teeth	Cervical branch of facial nerve (CN VII)
Sternocleidomastoid	Upper anterior surface of manubrium of sternum; upper border of medial third of clavicle	Lateral surface of mastoid process; lateral half of superior nuchal line	Bends head to same side, rotates head, raises chin to opposite side; together bend head forward and elevate chin	Accessory nerve (CN XI), C2 and C3 (pain and proprioception)
Anterior belly of digastric	Digastric fossa of lower border of mandible	Intermediate tendon to body and greater horn of hyoid	Opens mouth, draws hyoid forward	Nerve to mylohyoid, from trigeminal nerve (CN V$_3$)
Posterior belly of digastric	Mastoid notch of temporal bone	Intermediate tendon to body and greater horn of hyoid	Draws hyoid back, together raise hyoid	Facial nerve (CN VII)
Stylohyoid	Styloid process of temporal bone	Body of hyoid	Draws hyoid up and back	Facial nerve (CN VII)
Sternohyoid	Medial end of clavicle, posterior surface of manubrium	Body of hyoid	Depresses hyoid	C1–C3 via ansa cervicalis
Sternothyroid	Posterior surface of manubrium	Oblique line of thyroid cartilage	Depresses thyroid cartilage	C1–C3 via ansa cervicalis
Thyrohyoid	Oblique line of thyroid cartilage	Lateral side of greater horn of hyoid	Depresses hyoid, elevates larynx	Superior root of ansa cervicalis (C1–C2) via hypoglossal nerve
Inferior belly of omohyoid	Superior border of scapula, transverse scapular ligament	Intermediate tendon to clavicle	Depresses hyoid	C1–C3 via ansa cervicalis
Superior belly of omohyoid	Intermediate tendon tethered to clavicle	Body of hyoid bone	Depresses hyoid	C1–C3 via ansa cervicalis

V. Clinical Considerations

A. **Branchial cleft sinuses and cysts**

1. Common in posterior part of submandibular region and result from remnants of upper 2–3 original pharyngeal (branchial) clefts, which normally completely disappear, but instead sometimes keep their connection with the lateral surface of neck; opening can be anywhere along anterior border of SCM muscle

2. If sinus remnant does not connect to surface, it can form lateral cervical cyst (branchial cyst), which is usually found just inferior to angle of mandible; can be present in infants and children, but usually do not enlarge until early adulthood

3. Cysts may lie close to CNs IX, XI, and XII; avoid these nerves when removing cysts

(Continued)

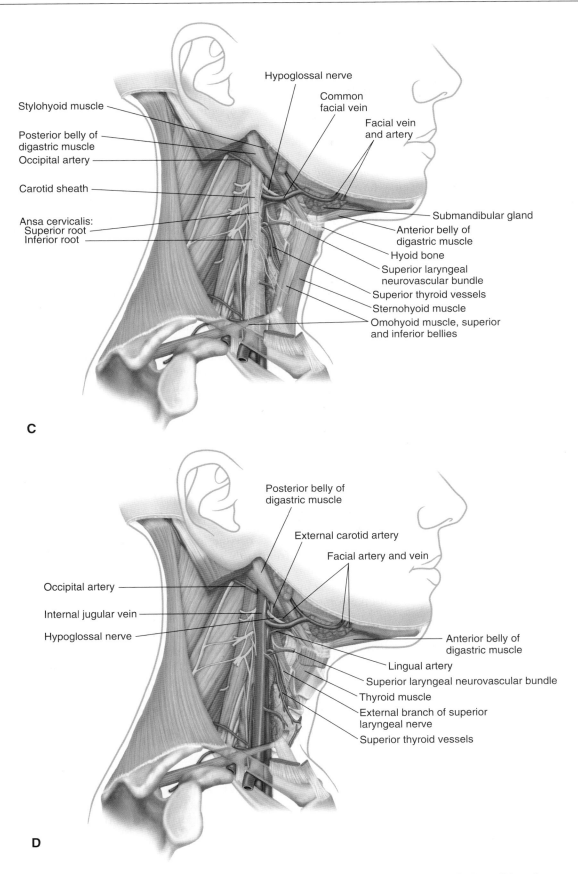

Hypoglossal nerve

Common facial vein

Facial vein and artery

Stylohyoid muscle

Posterior belly of digastric muscle

Occipital artery

Carotid sheath

Ansa cervicalis:
Superior root
Inferior root

Submandibular gland

Anterior belly of digastric muscle

Hyoid bone

Superior laryngeal neurovascular bundle

Superior thyroid vessels

Sternohyoid muscle

Omohyoid muscle, superior and inferior bellies

C

Posterior belly of digastric muscle

External carotid artery

Facial artery and vein

Occipital artery

Internal jugular vein

Hypoglossal nerve

Anterior belly of digastric muscle

Lingual artery

Superior laryngeal neurovascular bundle

Thyroid muscle

External branch of superior laryngeal nerve

Superior thyroid vessels

D

Figure 1.4C,D. Anterior Triangle of the Neck, Lateral View. **C.** Intermediate Dissection. **D.** Deep Dissection.

B. **Branchial fistula**
1. Uncommon abnormal canal that opens internally into tonsillar fossa and externally into neck
2. Saliva can drip from it and can become infected
3. Due to persistence of remnant of 2nd pharyngeal pouch and groove, ascends from its cervical opening along anterior border of SCM muscle in inferior 1/3 of neck, through subcutaneous tissue, platysma, and neck fascia to enter carotid sheath; passes between external and internal carotid arteries to open in tonsillar fossa

C. Cervical fascial spaces: any form of fluid accumulation (blood, pus, etc.) may have great clinical significance because various layers of cervical fascia constitute confined spaces with strong fascial coverings; thus, postoperative bleeding in pretracheal area can be confined by pretracheal fascia and place pressure on trachea, hindering breathing

D. Carotid thrombosis and embolism
1. Internal carotid artery is common site for thrombi formation, particularly at bifurcation of common carotid due to arteriosclerosis
2. Clots may produce emboli that go to lungs or brain

E. External carotid artery injury
1. Because external carotid artery supplies most of blood to extracranial structures in head, injury may have widespread implications
2. Maxillary branch supplies nose and nasopharynx; oral cavity supplied by branches of facial, lingual, and maxillary arteries; only orbit and bridge of nose supplied by vessels from internal carotid artery

F. **Torticollis**
1. Deformity of neck, which generally includes elements of rotation (twisting) and flexion (tilting) of cervical muscles; in most cases, 1 SCM muscle is shortened, resulting in head tilted toward affected side and chin rotated toward opposite side; more common in females than males
2. Congenital: deformity evident at birth due to a variety of causes, such as abnormal position of head in uterus, prenatal injury and interference with vascular supply to SCM, fibroma (fibrous tissue tumor, or fibromatosis colli) in SCM developing before or after birth, rupture or tearing of muscle fibers with hematoma and scar tissue formation, or a primary congenital defect in cervical spine frequently seen after difficult deliveries with abnormal presentation and in primiparas; prognosis is poor without treatment
3. Acquired: occurs in 1st 10 years of life and often accompanied by pain (unlike congenital type)
   a. Acute: due to direct irritation of muscles from injury or inflammatory reaction (myositis) or cervical lymphadenitis
   b. Spasmotic: rhythmic convulsive spasms of muscles occur due to organic disorder of central nervous system (CNS); seen in adulthood and may involve bilateral contraction of lateral muscles, especially SCM and trapezius muscles
      i. **Cervical dystonia**: abnormal contraction of cervical muscles (also known as *spasmotic torticollis*)
      ii. **Hysterical**: due to psychogenic inability of patient to control neck muscles

G. **Fracture of hyoid bone**: seen in people who are manually strangled by throat compression; body of hyoid bone is compressed onto thyroid cartilage; results in inability to elevate hyoid, making it difficult to swallow and maintain separation of alimentary and respiratory tracts and resulting in **aspiration pneumonia**

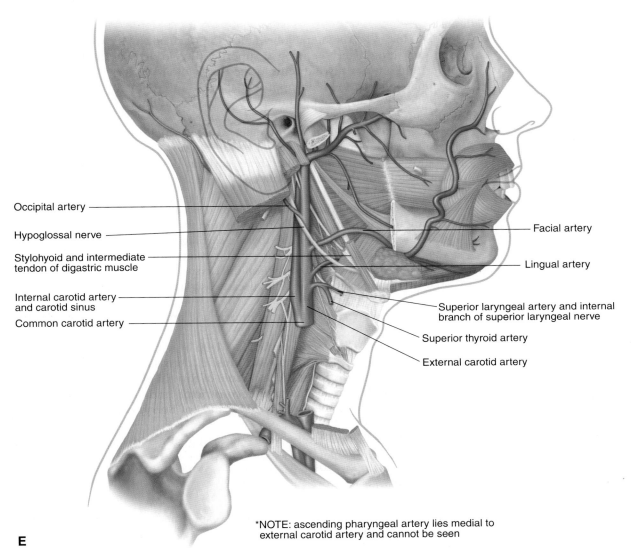

Occipital artery

Hypoglossal nerve

Stylohyoid and intermediate
tendon of digastric muscle

Internal carotid artery
and carotid sinus

Common carotid artery

Facial artery

Lingual artery

Superior laryngeal artery and internal
branch of superior laryngeal nerve

Superior thyroid artery

External carotid artery

*NOTE: ascending pharyngeal artery lies medial to
external carotid artery and cannot be seen

E

Figure 1.4E. Carotid Triangle of the Neck, Deep Dissection, Lateral View.

Thyroid and Parathyroid Glands

I. Thyroid Gland (Fig. 1.5A)

A. Location, parts, and development
  1. In muscular triangle, on either side of larynx and trachea
  2. Soft, reddish-brown, U-shaped organ; weighs about 25 g (18–60 g)
  3. 2 lateral lobes connected by isthmus
  4. **Lateral lobes** lie against lower 1/3 of thyroid cartilage; base lies at level of 5th or 6th tracheal ring
  5. **Isthmus**
      a. Connects lower 1/3 of lateral lobes at level of tracheal rings 2 and 3
      b. Communicating artery between 2 superior thyroid arteries runs on its cephalic border, and inferior thyroid veins located at its lower border
      c. **Pyramidal lobe** (present in approximately 50%): remnant of thyroglossal duct extending superiorly from isthmus slightly left of midline
  6. Development
      a. Thyroid gland develops from **thyroglossal duct** which grows down from floor of pharynx in region in which tongue later develops
      b. Thyroglossal duct normally disappears early in development, but may persist as pyramidal lobe or thyroglossal duct cyst
      c. Accessory thyroid tissue
          i. Can be found anywhere along path of descent of developing gland but most commonly found in base of tongue behind foramen cecum
          ii. Can develop in neck lateral to thyroid cartilage lying on thyrohyoid muscle
          iii. Can be functional, but often too small to maintain normal function of gland
          iv. May be associated with thyroglossal duct cysts
          v. Accessory tissue subject to same diseases as gland itself
B. Relations (Fig. 1.5B)
  1. Anteriorly and superiorly: sternothyroid muscle and infrahyoid fascia; superior thyroid vessels
  2. Laterally: convex; covered from superficial to deep by skin, superficial and deep fascia, SCM muscle, superior belly of omohyoid muscle, pretracheal layer of visceral fascia, which forms capsular investment (false capsule of thyroid gland)
  3. Medially: trachea, inferior pharyngeal constrictor muscle, cricothyroid muscle, esophagus; suspensory ligament of thyroid gland (of Berry) connect gland to cricoid and upper trachea
  4. Posteriorly: inferior thyroid artery, recurrent laryngeal nerve, common carotid artery and superior parathyroid glands
C. Arteries
  1. **Superior thyroid artery**
      a. 1st branch of external carotid artery
      b. Descends deep to sternothyroid muscle to reach gland
  2. **Inferior thyroid artery**
      a. From thyrocervical trunk
      b. Passes superiorly, then turns medially to run deep to carotid sheath; branches closely associated with recurrent laryngeal nerve
  3. **Thyroidea ima** (up to 10%)
      a. Small, unpaired; usually from aortic arch or brachiocephalic trunk
      b. Passes superiorly near midline to reach isthmus
D. Veins
  1. **Superior and middle thyroid veins**: end in internal jugular vein
  2. **Inferior thyroid veins**: often unite to drain inferiorly into left brachiocephalic vein or stay separate to drain into both brachiocephalic veins

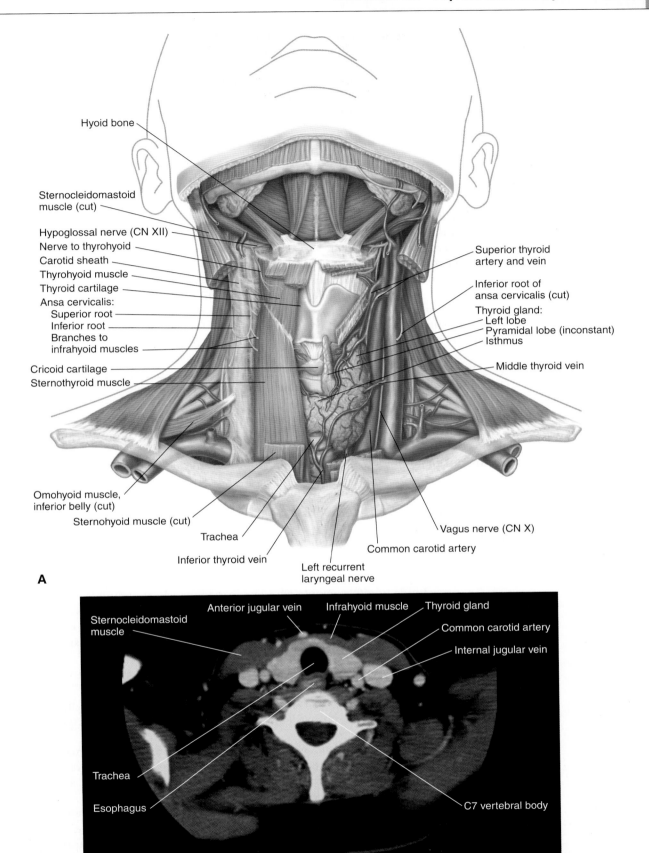

Hyoid bone

Sternocleidomastoid muscle (cut)

Hypoglossal nerve (CN XII)
Nerve to thyrohyoid
Carotid sheath
Thyrohyoid muscle
Thyroid cartilage
Ansa cervicalis:
    Superior root
    Inferior root
    Branches to infrahyoid muscles
Cricoid cartilage
Sternothyroid muscle

Omohyoid muscle, inferior belly (cut)
Sternohyoid muscle (cut)
Trachea
Inferior thyroid vein
Left recurrent laryngeal nerve

Superior thyroid artery and vein

Inferior root of ansa cervicalis (cut)
Thyroid gland:
    Left lobe
    Pyramidal lobe (inconstant)
    Isthmus
Middle thyroid vein

Vagus nerve (CN X)
Common carotid artery

A

Anterior jugular vein   Infrahyoid muscle   Thyroid gland

Sternocleidomastoid muscle

Common carotid artery

Internal jugular vein

Trachea

Esophagus

C7 vertebral body

B

Figure 1.5A,B. Thyroid Gland. **A.** Intermediate Dissection, Anterior View. **B.** Computed Tomography Image, Transverse View.

E. Lymphatic drainage: from subcapsular plexus to superior and inferior deep cervical, pretracheal, paratracheal, and retropharyngeal lymph nodes

F. Nerves
1. Sympathetic fibers: from superior, middle, and inferior cervical ganglia; vasomotor
2. Parasympathetic fibers: from cardiac and laryngeal branches of vagus (CN X) nerve
3. Neither thyroid nor parathyroid glands depend on CNS to control secretory activity

II. Parathyroids (Fig. 1.5C)

A. Parts
1. 4 glands, arranged into superior and inferior pairs
2. Supernumerary parathyroid glands occur in 5%

B. Location
1. Usually found external to fibrous capsule of posterior or inferior surface of thyroid gland lobes
2. Superior parathyroid usually lies posterior to thyroid gland at level of lower cricoid cartilage, often just superior to inferior thyroid artery
3. Inferior parathyroid usually lies below or near lower end of lateral lobes

C. Arteries: both are usually supplied from inferior thyroid artery although branches of superior thyroid artery may reach superior parathyroid

D. Veins and lymphatics: inferior thyroid veins usually drain parathyroid glands; lymphatics are similar to thyroid gland

III. Special Features

A. Thyroid gland secretes thyroid hormones, thyroxine (T_4) and triiodothyronine (T_3), and peptide called *calcitonin*

B. Superior thyroid artery accompanies superior thyroid vein, but inferior thyroid artery passes posterior to middle thyroid vein; thyroidea ima, present in nearly 10%, is accompanied by inferior thyroid vein

C. Parathyroid glands secrete parathormone, important in calcium metabolism

IV. Clinical Considerations

A. **Goiter**
1. Pathologic enlargement of thyroid gland, causing swelling in anterior neck that may compress trachea to point of hindering respiration; may also displace trachea, esophagus, and carotid sheath
2. Tends to affect people who live in regions where iodine is lacking in soil and drinking water
3. Nonneoplastic, non-inflammatory enlargement, not to be confused with variable normal enlargement of thyroid gland during menstruation and pregnancy
4. Enlargement does not usually extend superiorly due to attachments of sternothyroid muscles; substernal extension is also common
5. Patient's hormone status may be hypothyroid (underactive), hyperthyroid (overactive), or euthyroid (normal), which cannot be predicted by size of gland
    a. **Hypothyroidism**: adult hypothyroidism leads to **myxedema** (also used specifically to refer to skin changes in syndrome), thyroid follicles storing non-iodinated colloid; condition is end result of a number of thyroid diseases or secondary to pituitary failure
        i. In adult, symptoms often seen are: very low metabolic rate; abnormal sensitivity to cold; physical sluggishness; poor appetite, but patient gains weight; apathetic and lethargic attitude giving appearance of mental dullness; puffy, thick, and leathery skin, yet dry, cool, and keratotic; dry, brittle hair that breaks easily; lowered blood pressure

(Continued)

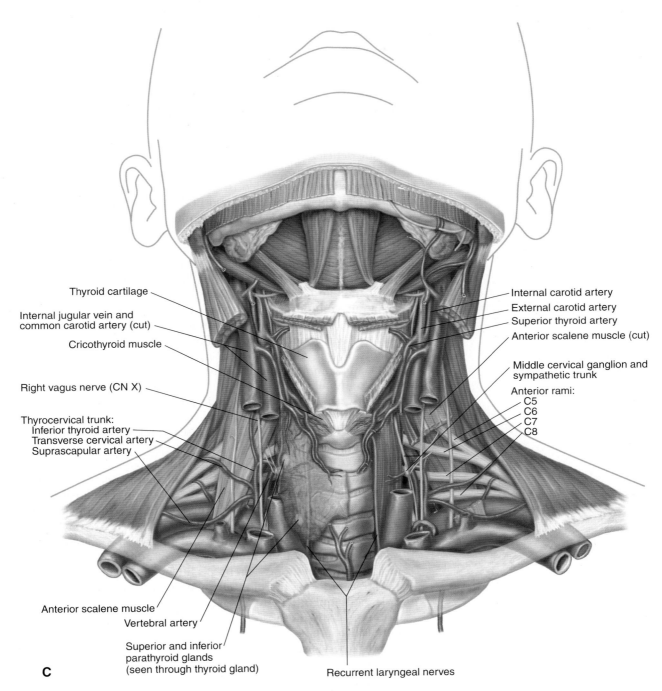

Thyroid cartilage

Internal jugular vein and
common carotid artery (cut)

Cricothyroid muscle

Right vagus nerve (CN X)

Thyrocervical trunk:
Inferior thyroid artery
Transverse cervical artery
Suprascapular artery

Anterior scalene muscle

Vertebral artery

Superior and inferior
parathyroid glands
(seen through thyroid gland)

Internal carotid artery
External carotid artery
Superior thyroid artery
Anterior scalene muscle (cut)

Middle cervical ganglion and
sympathetic trunk

Anterior rami:
C5
C6
C7
C8

Recurrent laryngeal nerves

C

Figure 1.5C. Thyroid Gland, Deep Dissection, Anterior View.

with low heart and respiratory rates; and swollen tissues due to fluid accumulation

 ii. **Cretinism**: hypothyroidism in infants; child appears normal at birth (received hormones from mother in utero), but own gland fails to produce sufficient amounts of hormones, and child develops stunted growth, abnormal bone formation, retarded mental development (within a month or following birth), low body temperature, and sluggishness from birth; born with dwarfism, mental retardation, and with enlarged protruding tongue and pot-belly

 iii. Chronic thyroiditis (Hashimoto's struma): lymphadenoid goiter or thyroiditis

 iv. Riedel's struma (ligneous thyroiditis): chronic, stony-hard fibrosing gland

 v. Familial goiter

 vi. Iodide deficiency

 vii. Ingestion of goitrogens (iodides; thiouracil-like drugs)

b. **Hyperthyroidism** (thyrotoxicosis): variety of disorders, in rare instances may be due to benign or malignant nodular tumors as well as thyroid-stimulating hormone (TSH)-secreting pituitary tumors

 i. Usually seen in patients over age 40 years (general range is ages 12–50 years)

 ii. Classical: middle-aged female with cardiac symptoms (i.e., rapid pulse (palpitations), marked shortness of breath (dyspnea), to fibrillation and frank heart failure)

 iii. General symptoms frequently seen are: nervousness, weight loss, hyperphagia, heat intolerance, increased pulse rate, fine tremor of outstretched fingers, shortness of breath, marked tachycardia, ankle edema, warm, soft skin, a basal metabolic rate from +10 to high of +100, and commonly heart failure

 iv. No exophthalmos

c. **Grave's disease** (**exophthalmic toxic goiter**): most common form of hyperthyroidism (diffuse hyperplasia of gland); should be noted that exophthalmos is common in Grave's disease, but it is not an invariable concomitant

 i. Symptoms: exophthalmos, warm and velvety skin, tachycardia, palpitations with poor response to digitalis, increased appetite, occasional diarrhea, tremors, finger clubbing, muscle weakness and fatigability, muscle wasting, shortness of breath (dyspnea), weight loss, rapid pulse, localized myxedemia in lower extremity, nervous excitability, restlessness, insomnia and emotional instability

 ii. May be seen in young women as type of autoimmune disease, in which body's immune system produces antibodies that bind to TSH receptors of thyroid cell membranes and mimic action of TSH; consequently, gland's cells are stimulated to secrete excessive amounts of thyroid hormone; treated with surgery or exposure to radioactive iodine

 iii. Other causes: benign or malignant tumors or TSH-secreting pituitary tumors

d. Other hyperthyroid conditions with goiter

 i. Plummer's disease: toxic nodular goiter

 ii. DeQuervain's disease: subacute thyroiditis

 iii. Chronic thyroiditis

 iv. Thyroid carcinoma

e. Other simple goiter with euthyroid conditions
  i. Colloid and nodular goiter
  ii. Chronic and subacute thyroiditis
  iii. Adenomas and carcinoma of thyroid
  iv. Iodide deficiency or ingestion of goitrogens

B. **Thyroglossal duct cyst**: remnant of thyroglossal duct, which forms thyroid gland, persisting between foramen cecum and pyramidal lobe; usually slightly left of midline

C. Accessory thyroid tissue
  1. Due to remnants of thyroglossal duct
  2. Usually found on thyrohyoid muscle or base of tongue (lingual thyroid)

D. **Thyroidectomy**
  1. Neoplastic growth may require removal of all or part of gland
  2. Recurrent laryngeal nerves: at risk of lesion; causes hoarseness or inability to speak
  3. Parathyroid glands: must be preserved
  4. Postoperative hemorrhage after thyroid surgery may compress trachea and lead to difficulty in breathing or even suffocation due to possible containment of hemorrhage by pretracheal fascia

E. Parathyroid atrophy or removal leads to severe convulsive disorder called **tetany**, which is life threatening due to fall in serum calcium levels

F. **Parathyroid tumors:** may lead to increased secretion of parathormone, resulting in hypercalcemia, hypophosphatemia, demineralization of bones (soften and deform when calcium plasma levels reach 16 mg/1mL and calcium begins to deposit in unusual places (i.e., kidneys, causing kidney stones; hypercalciuria; and bone disease caused by hyperparathyroid function [ostitis fibrosa cystica with multiple bone cysts])

Carotid Sheath and Sympathetic Trunk

I. Structures Beneath Sternocleidomastoid Muscle (Fig. 1.6A,B)

A. **Ansa cervicalis**
  1. Embedded in surface of carotid sheath
  2. Inferior root of ansa (from C2–C3) usually passes anteromedially to join superior root (C1–C2), although may pass medial to internal jugular vein

B. **Carotid sheath**
  1. Formed by local deep fascia, including superficial layer of deep cervical fascia, infrahyoid fascia, visceral fascia, and prevertebral fascia
  2. Extends from base of skull surrounding jugular foramen and carotid canal to root of neck
  3. Contains internal jugular vein laterally, common and internal carotid arteries medially, and vagus nerve behind and between the vessels

II. Contents of Carotid Sheath

A. Carotid arteries (Fig. 1.6C)
  1. **Common carotid**
    a. Right: from brachiocephalic trunk
    b. Left: arises as second branch of aortic arch
    c. Both: course superiorly in carotid sheath with internal jugular vein laterally and vagus nerve posterolaterally
    d. 2 terminal branches at superior border of thyroid cartilage: internal and external carotid arteries
    e. **Carotid body**
      i. Small, flattened, ovoid nodule of specialized cells (0.5 cm) in outer connective tissue of bifurcation of common carotid artery
      ii. Functions as chemoreceptor that monitors oxygen content of blood before it reaches brain, such that a decrease in partial pressure of oxygen, which can occur at high altitudes or in pulmonary disease, activates aortic and carotid chemoreceptors, increasing alveolar ventilation; also sensitive to changes in blood acidity (relative amount of carbon dioxide)
      iii. Innervated by **carotid sinus nerve (Hering's nerve)** of glossopharyngeal (CN IX), vagus (CN X), and sympathetics

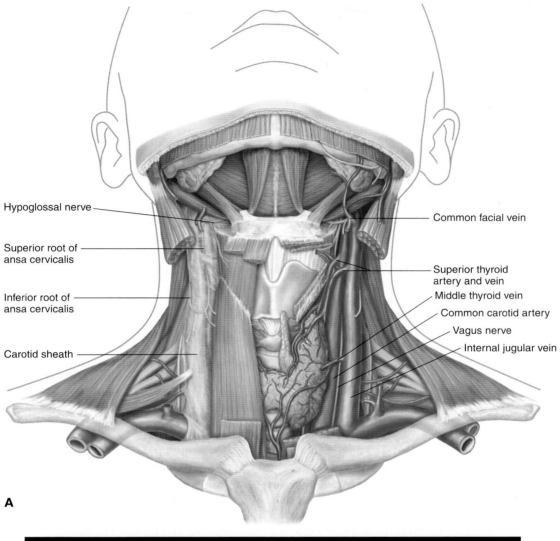

Hypoglossal nerve

Superior root of
ansa cervicalis

Inferior root of
ansa cervicalis

Carotid sheath

Common facial vein

Superior thyroid
artery and vein

Middle thyroid vein

Common carotid artery

Vagus nerve

Internal jugular vein

A

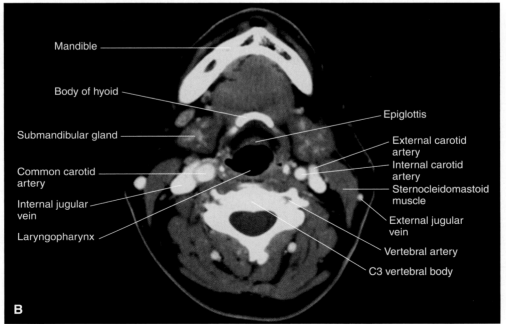

Mandible

Body of hyoid

Submandibular gland

Common carotid
artery

Internal jugular
vein

Laryngopharynx

Epiglottis

External carotid
artery

Internal carotid
artery

Sternocleidomastoid
muscle

External jugular
vein

Vertebral artery

C3 vertebral body

B

Figure 1.6A,B. A. Carotid Sheath and its Contents. **B.** Neck, Computed Tomography Image, Transverse View.

2. **Internal carotid artery**
   a. Continues in carotid sheath to enter carotid canal in base of skull
   b. No branches in neck; supplies brain and orbit; further course and branches are discussed in Chapter 2
   c. **Carotid sinus**
      i. Slight dilation of terminal portion of common carotid and proximal part of internal carotid artery
      ii. Functions as baroreceptor important in regulating arterial blood pressure
      iii. Innervated mainly by carotid sinus nerve from glossopharyngeal (CN IX); also supplied by vagus (CN X) and sympathetic fibers

3. **External carotid artery**
   a. Leaves carotid sheath by passing anterosuperiorly within carotid triangle
   b. 8 branches: 5 below posterior belly of digastric within carotid triangle, 3 above
      i. **Superior thyroid artery**: 1st branch; passes anteromedially to supply infrahyoid muscles, thyroid gland, larynx, and laryngopharynx; gives off **superior laryngeal artery** that passes through thyrohyoid membrane with internal branch of superior laryngeal nerve
      ii. **Ascending pharyngeal artery**: often 2nd branch; arises from medial surface to pass superiorly to supply oro- and nasopharynx, prevertebral muscles, palatine branch to soft palate
      iii. **Lingual artery**: 2nd anteromedially directed branch; passes above greater horn of hyoid to supply tongue, suprahyoid region, sublingual gland, and palatine tonsils
      iv. **Facial artery**: 3rd anteromedial branch; passes deep to posterior belly of digastric and stylohyoid muscles and superficial portion of submandibular gland to reach mandibular margin and enter face anterior to masseter insertion; supplies submandibular gland and face up to orbit
      v. **Occipital artery**: arises posteriorly near lower border of posterior belly of digastric muscle, crosses hypoglossal nerve superiorly; passes posterosuperiorly roughly medial to posterior belly of digastric to eventually distribute on head posteriorly; supplies SCM muscle, meningeal branches, and scalp posteriorly
      vi. **Posterior auricular artery**: posteriorly directed branch arising between posterior belly of digastric and stylohyoid muscles; ends in occipital and auricular branches; branches to parotid gland; enters stylomastoid foramen to medial wall of middle ear, mastoid air cells, stapedius muscle, and middle ear bones
      vii. **Maxillary artery**: anteromedially directed terminal branch; supplies muscles of mastication, meninges, midface including upper teeth, nasal cavity, and hard and soft palates
      viii. **Superficial temporal artery**: superiorly directed terminal branch; supplies scalp laterally

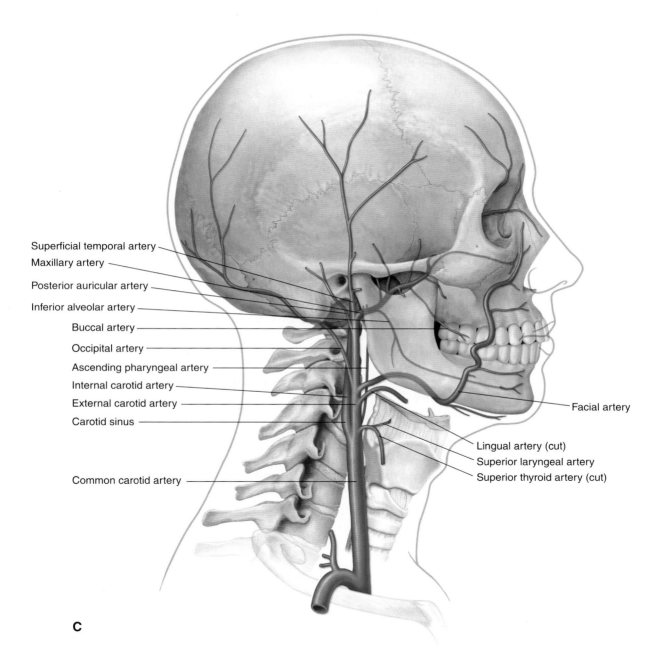

Superficial temporal artery

Maxillary artery

Posterior auricular artery

Inferior alveolar artery

Buccal artery

Occipital artery

Ascending pharyngeal artery

Internal carotid artery

External carotid artery

Carotid sinus

Common carotid artery

Facial artery

Lingual artery (cut)

Superior laryngeal artery

Superior thyroid artery (cut)

C

Figure 1.6C. Carotid Arteries.

B. **Internal jugular vein** (Fig. 1.6D)
   1. Origin: in jugular fossa, as continuation of sigmoid sinus
   2. Course: in carotid sheath, first with internal and then common carotid artery
   3. Termination: joins subclavian vein just lateral to sternoclavicular joint to form brachiocephalic vein
      a. Superior bulb: dilation at its origin
      b. Inferior bulb: dilation 1 in above termination, below pair of valves
   4. Tributaries (variable)
      a. At origin: inferior petrosal sinus and a meningeal vein
      b. Pharyngeal plexus, near angle of jaw
      c. Common facial (formed from anterior division of retromandibular and facial vein) enters at level of hyoid bone
      d. Lingual, from tongue, may enter with or just below common facial, drains tongue and sublingual area
      e. Superior thyroid, from upper thyroid gland, enters with or just below common facial vein
      f. Middle thyroid vein, from the lateral portion of gland

C. Vagus nerve (CN X) in neck
   1. Exits skull at jugular foramen to enter carotid sheath and lie between and behind internal jugular vein and internal and common carotid arteries
   2. Gives off superior laryngeal nerve and superior cardiac branch below base of skull
   3. Gives multiple small branches to pharynx
   4. Gives off inferior cardiac branch in root of neck
   5. Passes anterior to right subclavian artery or lateral to left common carotid to enter thorax

D. Other contents of carotid sheath
   1. Superior laryngeal nerve (from CN X): passes medial to internal carotid artery to leave sheath and pass to larynx
   2. Accessory nerve (CN XI): leaves sheath near base of skull to pass laterally toward SCM muscle
   3. Glossopharyngeal nerve (CN IX): leaves sheath to pass inferoanteriorly onto posterior wall of pharynx
   4. Hypoglossal nerve (CN XII): passes inferoanteriorly between internal jugular vein and internal carotid artery to reach tongue
   5. Deep cervical lymph nodes: lie along internal jugular vein and between it and common carotid artery; not always easily visible, being small and scattered, but are important in carcinoma of mouth, larynx, or other head and neck structures

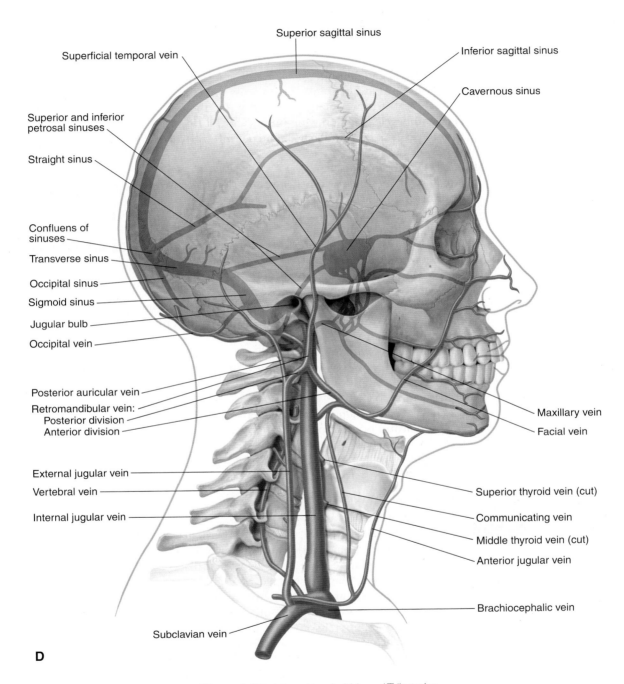

Figure 1.6D. Internal Jugular Vein and Tributaries.

III. Cervical Sympathetic Trunk (Fig. 1.6E)

A. Location: anterior to transverse processes of vertebrae, embedded in prevertebral fascia medial to carotid sheath

B. Composition: pre- and postsynaptic sympathetic fibers; 3 ganglia connected by interganglionic rami

C. Origin of preganglionic fibers: from intermediolateral gray column of spinal cord segments Tl–T5; white rami communicantes leave anterior roots of corresponding thoracic nerves and ascend in trunk

D. Ganglia

  1. Inferior cervical ganglion

    a. Lies between base of transverse process of C7 and neck of 1st rib, posteromedial to vertebral artery, usually fused with 1st thoracic ganglion to form **stellate or cervicothoracic ganglion** lying on neck of 1st rib

    b. Branches: gray rami to C7, C8, and Tl; inferior cardiac nerve; and vertebral nerve along vertebral artery

  2. Middle cervical ganglion

    a. Smallest (sometimes absent); lies anterior to transverse process of C6 at level of inferior thyroid artery and vertebral artery entering 6th transverse foramen

    b. Branches: gray rami to C5 and C6; middle cardiac nerve; thyroid nerves to form plexus on inferior thyroid artery

    c. Ansa subclavia: connects inferior and middle ganglia anterior to subclavian artery

  3. Superior cervical ganglion

    a. Largest; lies on transverse process of C2 (and C3)

    b. Branches (all postsynaptic)

      i. Internal carotid nerve to form internal carotid plexus

      ii. External carotid nerve to form external carotid plexus

      iii. Branches to CNs IX–XII

      iv. Branches to tympanic plexus

      v. Deep petrosal nerve, which unites with greater petrosal nerve to form nerve of pterygoid canal

      vi. Gray rami to Cl–C4

      vii. Pharyngeal branch to pharyngeal plexus

      viii. Intercarotid branch to carotid body and sinus

      ix. Superior cardiac nerve

      x. Branches to larynx and thyroid

IV. Clinical Considerations

A. Common carotid artery

  1. Found on line drawn from sternoclavicular joint to point of its bifurcation, which lies 1 cm inferior and posterior to tip of greater horn of hyoid bone at level of upper border of thyroid cartilage

  2. Blood flow may be stopped by digital compression at anterior border of SCM muscle at level of cricoid cartilage, with pressure exerted posteriorly against carotid tubercle on the transverse process of the 6th cervical vertebra (tubercle of Chassaignac)

B. Carotid arteriography

  1. Used for X-ray localization of extracranial arterial obstruction and intracranial lesions (vascular and non-vascular)

  2. Radiopaque dye injected via needle into common carotid artery anywhere along its course

  3. Artery best approached in carotid triangle, where it is covered by skin and deep fascia and overlapped slightly laterally by anterior border of SCM muscle

  4. Artery can be fixed between thumb and index finger, with thumb acting to retract muscle more laterally

(Continued)

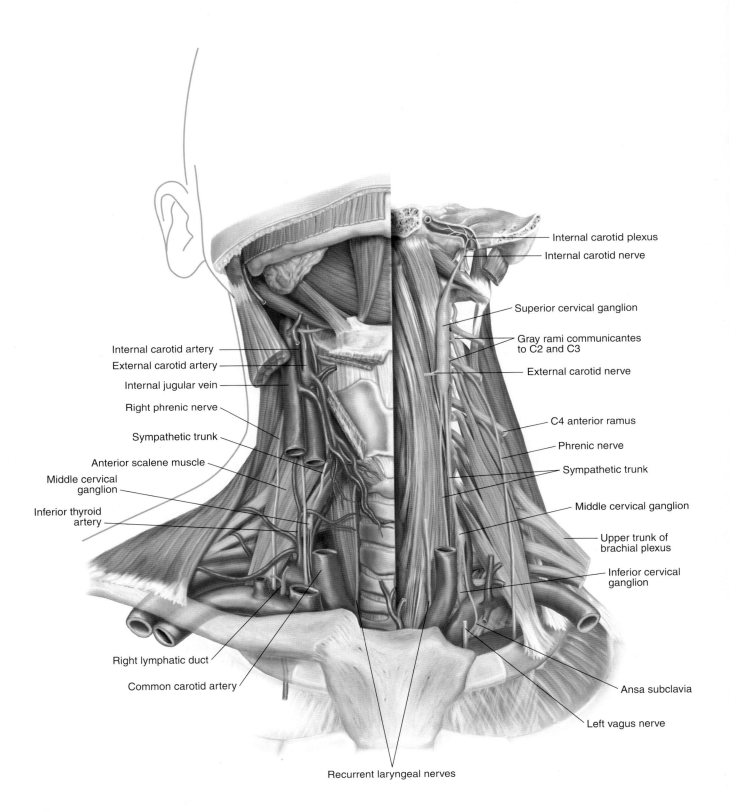

Internal carotid plexus

Internal carotid nerve

Superior cervical ganglion

Gray rami communicantes
to C2 and C3

External carotid nerve

C4 anterior ramus

Phrenic nerve

Sympathetic trunk

Middle cervical ganglion

Upper trunk of
brachial plexus

Inferior cervical
ganglion

Ansa subclavia

Left vagus nerve

Internal carotid artery

External carotid artery

Internal jugular vein

Right phrenic nerve

Sympathetic trunk

Anterior scalene muscle

Middle cervical
ganglion

Inferior thyroid
artery

Right lymphatic duct

Common carotid artery

Recurrent laryngeal nerves

E

Figure 1.6E. Cervical Sympathetic Trunk.

C. **Carotid endarterectomy**
1. Thickening of intima of common and internal carotid arteries may be due to atherosclerosis and may obstruct blood flow
2. Symptoms depend on degree of obstruction and amount of collateral blood flow to brain and eye structures from other arteries
3. Partial occlusion: may cause transient ischemic attack, dizziness, and disorientation that can disappear in 24 hours
4. Arterial occlusion may cause minor stroke with weakness or sensory loss on 1 side of body that lasts for more than 24 hours, but may disappear within several weeks
5. Obstruction of blood flow can be seen with Doppler ultrasonography
6. Endarterectomy: removal of plaque from carotid arteries, usually near common carotid bifurcation and internal carotid artery

D. **Carotid sinus hypersensitivity**: may occur in various types of vascular disease in which external pressure on carotid artery may cause slowing of heart rate, fall in blood pressure, and cardiac ischemia resulting in fainting (due to sudden decrease in cerebral perfusion)

E. Loss of major vein such as internal jugular is well tolerated because of interconnections between veins of the 2 sides, both within and outside skull

F. Interruption of cervical sympathetic trunk
1. Occurring above C8 or T1, all sympathetic control for head, neck, and upper extremity is lost, resulting in **Horner's syndrome** (narrowed palpebral fissure, constriction of pupil, flushing of skin, and lack of sweating)
2. If bilateral, there is no acceleration of heart rate; thus, when performed for relief of **Raynaud's disease** (involves severe vasospasm of vessels of upper extremity and vascular constriction can lead, if not treated, to ischemia and tissue necrosis) or palmar **hyperhidrosis** (**profuse sweating**), it is preferable to avulse anterior roots of T2 and T3 or, still better, white rami at those levels
3. **Cervicothoracic ganglion block**: anesthesia placed around ganglion to block transmission of stimuli through cervical and 1st thoracic ganglia for relief of vascular spasms involving brain and upper limb in order to decide if surgical resection of ganglion would help with excessive vasoconstriction of ipsilateral limb

Posterior Triangle of the Neck

I. Posterior Triangle (Fig. 1.7A)

A. Boundaries: anterior border of trapezius muscle, posterior border of SCM muscle, and clavicle

B. Subdivided by inferior belly of omohyoid muscle into occipital triangle above and subclavian or omoclavicular triangle below

  1. **Occipital triangle**

    a. Muscles in floor: splenius capitis, levator scapulae, posterior and middle scalene muscles

    b. Structures crossing floor: accessory nerve and cervical and brachial plexus

    c. Structures piercing roof: lesser occipital, great auricular, transverse cervical, and supraclavicular nerves; all emerge just behind posterior border of SCM muscle

  2. **Omoclavicular (subclavian) triangle**

    a. Floor: 1st rib and 1st part of serratus anterior muscle

    b. Structures crossing floor: subclavian artery and vein, part of brachial plexus

    c. Structures crossing through: transverse cervical and suprascapular vessels

    d. Structures piercing roof: external jugular vein

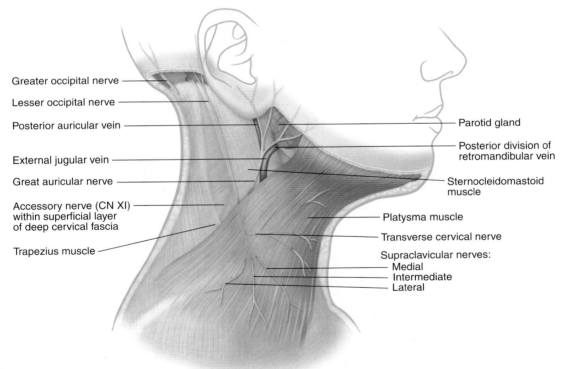

A

Figure 1.7A. Posterior Cervical Triangle, Lateral View, Superficial Dissection.

II. Muscles within Posterior Triangle (Fig. 1.7B)

Muscle	Origin	Insertion	Action	Nerve
Anterior scalene	Anterior tubercle of transverse processes of vertebrae C3–C6	Scalene tubercle on upper surface of 1st rib	Raises 1st rib, bends neck to same side	C4–C6
Middle scalene	Posterior tubercle of transverse processes of vertebrae C3–C7	Upper surface of 1st rib, behind subclavian groove	Raises 1st rib, bends neck to same side	C3–C8
Posterior scalene	Posterior tubercle of transverse processes of vertebrae C4–C6	Outer surface of 2nd rib	Raises 2nd rib, bends neck to same side	C6–C8

III. Vessels within Posterior Cervical Triangle (Fig. 1.7C,D)

A. Inferior thyroid artery
   1. From thyrocervical trunk
   2. Passes superiorly, gives off ascending cervical branch to scalene muscles, then turns medially to pass posterior to carotid sheath
B. Transverse cervical artery
   1. From thyrocervical trunk
   2. Passes posteriorly across scalene muscles to reach trapezius muscle
C. Suprascapular artery
   1. From thyrocervical trunk
   2. Passes over transverse scapular ligament to reach supraspinous fossa
D. Dorsal scapular artery
   1. From 3rd part of subclavian artery
   2. Passes deep within root of neck to reach rhomboid muscles
E. Subclavian vessels: lie on the upper surface of 1st rib; discussed in Section 1.8
F. Lymphatics: thoracic duct and right lymphatic duct; discussed in Section 1.8

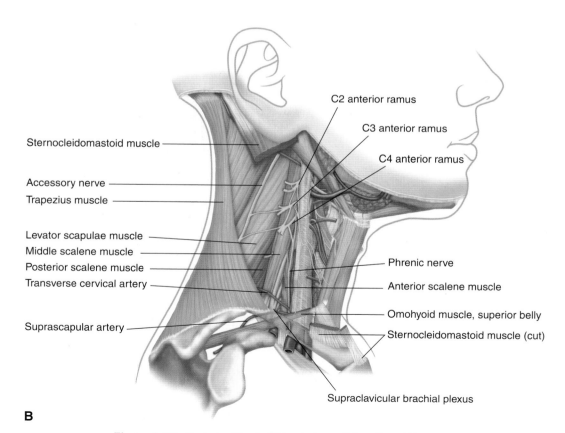

B

Figure 1.7B. Posterior Cervical Triangle, Lateral View, Deep Dissection.

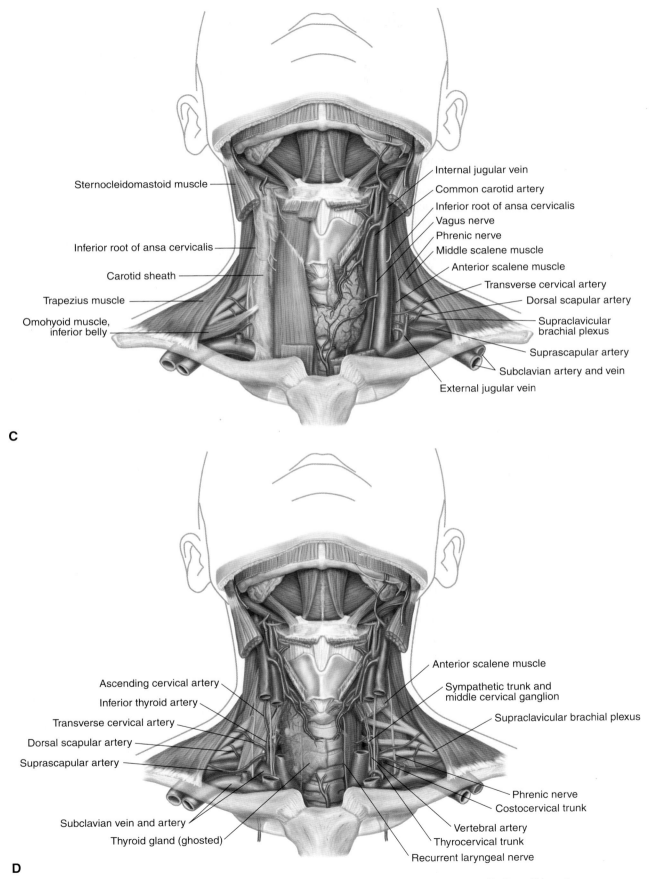

Sternocleidomastoid muscle

Inferior root of ansa cervicalis

Carotid sheath

Trapezius muscle

Omohyoid muscle,
inferior belly

Internal jugular vein

Common carotid artery

Inferior root of ansa cervicalis

Vagus nerve

Phrenic nerve

Middle scalene muscle

Anterior scalene muscle

Transverse cervical artery

Dorsal scapular artery

Supraclavicular
brachial plexus

Suprascapular artery

Subclavian artery and vein

External jugular vein

C

Ascending cervical artery

Inferior thyroid artery

Transverse cervical artery

Dorsal scapular artery

Suprascapular artery

Subclavian vein and artery

Thyroid gland (ghosted)

Anterior scalene muscle

Sympathetic trunk and
middle cervical ganglion

Supraclavicular brachial plexus

Phrenic nerve

Costocervical trunk

Vertebral artery

Thyrocervical trunk

Recurrent laryngeal nerve

D

Figure 1.7C,D. Posterior Cervical Triangle, Anterior View. **C.** Intermediate Dissection. **D.** Deep Dissection.

IV. Nerves within Posterior Triangle (Fig. 1.7E,F)

- **A. Cervical plexus**: anterior rami of cervical nerves 1–4, forming 3 loops
  1. Location: lateral to cervical vertebrae 1–4, anterior and lateral to levator scapulae and middle scalene muscles
  2. Distribution (see Section 1.3)
     a. Cutaneous branches (described earlier)
        i. **Lesser occipital nerve**: from C2 to skin behind ear
        ii. **Great auricular nerve**: from C2–C3 to skin of ear and below
        iii. **Transverse cervical nerve**: from C2–C3 to skin of anterior cervical triangle
        iv. **Supraclavicular nerves**: from C3–C4 to skin of root of neck and upper chest
     b. Muscular branches
        i. Direct branches to rectus capitis anterior and lateralis, longus capitis and cervicis, levator scapulae, and scalene muscles
        ii. **Phrenic nerve**
           a) Union of branches from C3–C5
           b) Passes inferiorly on anterior scalene muscle, covered by scalene or prevertebral fascia; crossed by transverse cervical and suprascapular arteries
           c) Enters chest anterior to subclavian artery to pass through superior and middle mediastinum of thorax to reach and innervate diaphragm
        iii. **Ansa cervicalis**
           a) Embedded in carotid sheath; formed by superior and inferior roots; supplies infrahyoid (strap) muscles (sternohyoid, omohyoid, sternothyroid, and thyrohyoid muscles)
           b) Superior root (descendens hypoglossi) from C1–C2 joins hypoglossal nerve near base of skull; leaves hypoglossal nerve above greater horn of hyoid bone to unite with inferior root, although some fibers continue with hypoglossal nerve to innervate thyrohyoid and geniohyoid muscles
           c) Inferior root (descendens cervicalis) from C2–C3 wraps internal jugular vein laterally to join superior root on carotid sheath
        iv. Sensory branches to SCM muscle from C2 and C3, and trapezius from C3 and C4 distribute with accessory nerve (CN XI)
- **B. Accessory nerve** (**CN XI**)
  1. After passing through posterior fibers of SCM muscle, emerges from between its upper and middle 2/3 to travel obliquely posteroinferiorly across posterior triangle
  2. Passes deep to trapezius at its lower 1/3
  3. Usually joined by branches from anterior rami of C3–C4 (proprioceptive sensory fibers)
  4. Enveloped within superficial layer of deep cervical fascia and accompanied by small lymph nodes (accessory nodes)
- **C.** Phrenic nerve (see "Cervical plexus" above)
- **D.** Supraclavicular brachial plexus (described in Section 1.8)

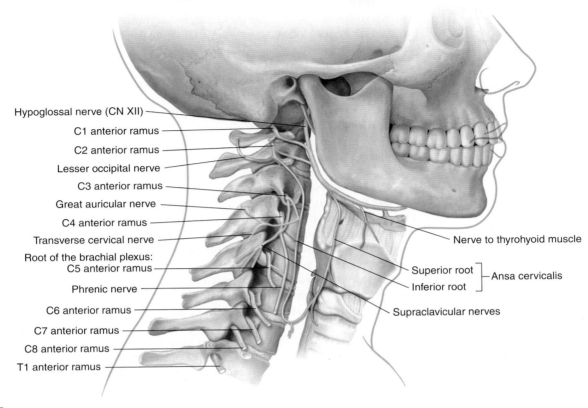

Hypoglossal nerve (CN XII)
C1 anterior ramus
C2 anterior ramus
Lesser occipital nerve
C3 anterior ramus
Great auricular nerve
C4 anterior ramus
Transverse cervical nerve
Root of the brachial plexus:
C5 anterior ramus
Phrenic nerve
C6 anterior ramus
C7 anterior ramus
C8 anterior ramus
T1 anterior ramus

Nerve to thyrohyoid muscle
Superior root
Inferior root
Ansa cervicalis
Supraclavicular nerves

E

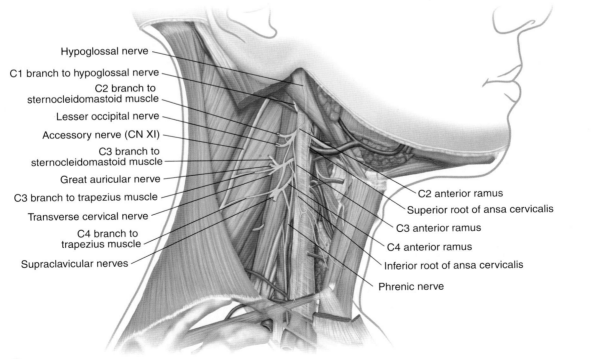

Hypoglossal nerve
C1 branch to hypoglossal nerve
C2 branch to sternocleidomastoid muscle
Lesser occipital nerve
Accessory nerve (CN XI)
C3 branch to sternocleidomastoid muscle
Great auricular nerve
C3 branch to trapezius muscle
Transverse cervical nerve
C4 branch to trapezius muscle
Supraclavicular nerves

C2 anterior ramus
Superior root of ansa cervicalis
C3 anterior ramus
C4 anterior ramus
Inferior root of ansa cervicalis
Phrenic nerve

F

Figure 1.7E,F. E. Cervical Plexus, Lateral View. **F.** Nerves of the Posterior Triangle, Lateral View.

V. Clinical Considerations

A. **Cervical nerve block:** anesthetic agent infiltrated at multiple points along posterior border of SCM muscle, mainly at the junction of its superior and middle 2/3 (nerve point of the neck)

B. Accessory nerve lesion (CN XI)
   1. Can be damaged by trauma (penetrating), surgical procedures, tumors, and fractures of jugular foramen
   2. Lesion results in weakness and atrophy of trapezius, resulting in "drooping of the shoulder"
   3. Unilateral paralysis of trapezius muscle is noticed by patient's inability to elevate and retract shoulder and difficulty in elevating arm above horizontal level
   4. Unilateral lesion does not necessarily result in abnormal head position, but weakness can occur in turning head to side against resistance

C. **Cervical sentinel nodes:** inferior deep cervical lymph nodes often involved in spread of abdominal and/or thoracic cancer; **Virchow's node** is inferior deep cervical lymph node on left that may be first indication of abdominal cancer

D. **Scalenus anticus syndrome**
   1. A cause of **thoracic outlet syndrome**
   2. Spasm or hypertrophy of anterior scalene muscle may lead to circulatory and neurologic symptoms of upper limb
   3. Clinical manifestations similar to cervical rib
   4. Spasm tends to compress brachial plexus and subclavian artery
   5. Treatment consists of transection of muscle at insertion
   6. Care must be taken to avoid subclavian vein and phrenic nerve lying anterior to muscle

E. **Lesion of phrenic nerve (C3–C5):** leads to paralysis of the corresponding half of diaphragm (on 1 side)

Root of the Neck

I. General Features (Fig. 1.8A,B)

A. Connects neck with thoracic cavity and upper limb
   1. Structures connecting thoracic cavity with neck course vertically
   2. Structures connecting thoracic cavity with upper limb course more transversely and laterally as they cross the 1st rib
B. Thoracic inlet: bounded by manubrium of sternum anteriorly, 1st rib laterally, and vertebral column posteriorly
C. Anterior scalene muscle: important landmark; inserts on 1st rib
D. Cupula: dome of cervical pleura extends above 1st rib, well into neck region
E. Esophagus: lies just anterior to vertebral column, in the midline
F. Trachea: lies anterior to esophagus

II. Subclavian Artery (Fig. 1.8C)

A. Origin: right, from brachiocephalic trunk; left, from aoric arch
B. 3 parts: 1st, from origin to medial border of anterior scalene muscle; 2nd, lies behind anterior scalene muscle; 3rd, extends from lateral border of anterior scalene to lateral border of 1st rib
C. Relations and branches
   1. 1st part
      a. Relations
         i. Superiorly: thoracic duct (left), right lymphatic duct (right), vertebral veins
         ii. Anteriorly: beginning of brachiocephalic veins, vertebral veins, vagus, phrenic, and cardiac nerves; ansa subclavia
         iii. Posteriorly: sympathetic trunk and stellate ganglion, recurrent laryngeal nerve
         iv. Inferolaterally: cupula (cervical dome of parietal pleura), recurrent laryngeal nerve (right)

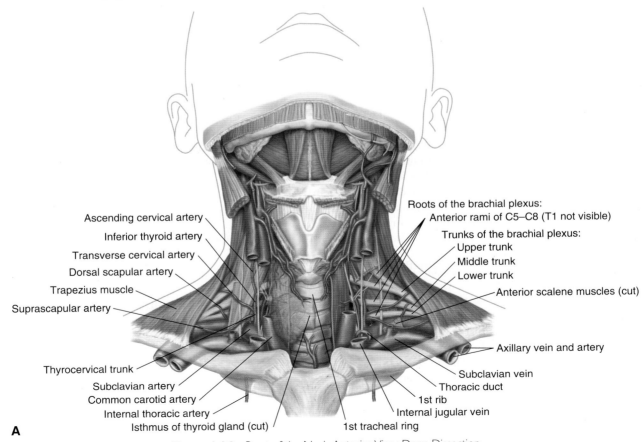

Ascending cervical artery
Inferior thyroid artery
Transverse cervical artery
Dorsal scapular artery
Trapezius muscle
Suprascapular artery

Thyrocervical trunk
Subclavian artery
Common carotid artery
Internal thoracic artery
Isthmus of thyroid gland (cut)

Roots of the brachial plexus:
Anterior rami of C5–C8 (T1 not visible)
Trunks of the brachial plexus:
Upper trunk
Middle trunk
Lower trunk
Anterior scalene muscles (cut)

Axillary vein and artery
Subclavian vein
Thoracic duct
1st rib
Internal jugular vein
1st tracheal ring

A

Figure 1.8A. Root of the Neck, Anterior View, Deep Dissection.

b. Branches
  i. **Vertebral artery**: arises superoposteriorly; ascends to enter transverse foramen of 6th cervical vertebra; supplies cervical spinal cord, vertebral column, brain
  ii. **Thyrocervical trunk**: arises superiorly; 3 branches; suprascapular artery supplies supra- and infraspinatus muscles; transverse cervical artery supplies trapezius and other cervical muscles; inferior thyroid artery supplies thyroid gland, larynx, pharynx, esophagus, and root of neck muscles
  iii. **Internal thoracic artery**: arises inferiorly; supplies anterior chest wall and pericardium
2. 2nd part
  a. Relations
    i. Anteriorly: anterior scalene muscle
    ii. Posteriorly: anterior rami of C8–T1; middle scalene muscle
    iii. Inferiorly: cupula
  b. Branches: **costocervical trunk**, arising posteriorly and supplying posterior neck muscles and upper posterior chest wall
3. 3rd part
  a. Relations
    i. Anteriorly: external jugular vein, subclavian vein
    ii. Posteriorly: inferior trunk of brachial plexus; middle scalene muscle
    iii. Superiorly: upper and middle trunks of plexus
    iv. Inferiorly: upper surface of 1st rib
  b. Branches: **dorsal scapular artery**, arising posteriorly, passing through brachial plexus and supplying levator scapulae and rhomboid muscles

III. Subclavian Vein

A. Begins at lateral border of 1st rib as continuation of axillary vein and ends behind sternoclavicular joint by joining internal jugular vein to form brachiocephalic vein
B. Lies anterior to anterior scalene muscle and subclavian artery
C. Tributaries
  1. External jugular vein: at lateral border of SCM muscle
  2. Transverse cervical and suprascapular veins usually join end of external jugular, although either may join subclavian separately

IV. Lymphatic Vessels

A. **Thoracic duct**
  1. Arches over subclavian artery from groove between esophagus and vertebral column on left
  2. Descends to empty into union of left subclavian and internal jugular veins
  3. Receives **jugular**, **subclavian**, and **bronchomediastinal lymph trunks** near end, although these may drain separately
B. **Right lymphatic duct**
  1. Union of jugular, subclavian, and bronchomediastinal lymph trunks on right, although these may drain separately
  2. Drains into union of right subclavian and internal jugular veins

V. Nerves at the Root of the Neck (Fig. I.8D,E)

A. Supraclavicular brachial plexus
  1. Anterior rami C5–T1 emerge between anterior and middle scalene muscles
  2. Made of 5 roots (rami), 3 trunks, and 6 divisions (posterior to clavicle), which lead to infraclavicular brachial plexus of 3 cords and their branches
  3. Branches from roots
    a. Direct branches to scalene muscles
    b. **Dorsal scapular nerve**
      i. From C5
      ii. Passes posteriorly through middle scalene muscle to reach lower levator scapulae and rhomboid muscles

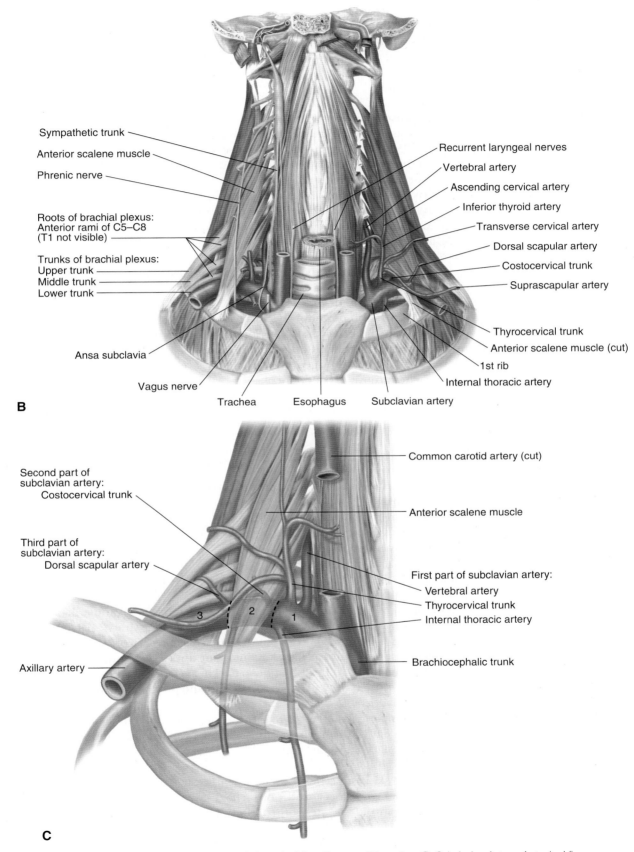

Sympathetic trunk

Anterior scalene muscle

Phrenic nerve

Roots of brachial plexus:
Anterior rami of C5–C8
(T1 not visible)

Trunks of brachial plexus:
Upper trunk
Middle trunk
Lower trunk

Ansa subclavia

Vagus nerve

Trachea   Esophagus   Subclavian artery

Recurrent laryngeal nerves

Vertebral artery

Ascending cervical artery

Inferior thyroid artery

Transverse cervical artery

Dorsal scapular artery

Costocervical trunk

Suprascapular artery

Thyrocervical trunk

Anterior scalene muscle (cut)

1st rib

Internal thoracic artery

B

Second part of
subclavian artery:
Costocervical trunk

Third part of
subclavian artery:
Dorsal scapular artery

Axillary artery

Common carotid artery (cut)

Anterior scalene muscle

First part of subclavian artery:
Vertebral artery
Thyrocervical trunk
Internal thoracic artery

Brachiocephalic trunk

C

Figure 1.8B,C. B. Root of the Neck, Anterior View, Deepest Dissection. **C.** Subclavian Artery, Anterior View.

    c. **Long thoracic nerve**
       i. From C5–C7
       ii. Passes posteroinferiorly within middle scalene muscle to lie on serratus anterior muscle
  4. Trunks
    a. **Upper trunk**
       i. Union of C5 and C6
       ii. **Suprascapular nerve**
         a) Passes posterolaterally across omoclavicular triangle behind clavicle
         b) Passes beneath superior transverse scapular ligament to enter supraspinous fossa
         c) Innervates supraspinatus and infraspinatus muscles
       iii. **Nerve to subclavius**
         a) Passes anteriorly to enter and innervate subclavius muscle
         b) May carry accessory phrenic nerve fibers that descend to join phrenic nerve
       iv. Branches into anterior and posterior divisions
    b. **Middle trunk**
       i. Continuation of C7
       ii. No branches other than anterior and posterior divisions
    c. **Lower trunk**
       i. Union of C8 and T1
       ii. Lies on 1st rib posterior to subclavian artery
       iii. No branches other than anterior and posterior divisions
B. Recurrent laryngeal nerves: different on each side
  1. Left reaches tracheoesophageal groove at lower level due to recurring around aortic arch
  2. Right reaches groove in root of neck
C. Sympathetic trunk and **cervicothoracic (stellate) ganglion**: inferior cervical ganglion usually fuses with 1st thoracic ganglion to form cervicothoracic (stellate) ganglion, posteriorly located on neck of 1st rib

VI. Other Structures at the Root of the Neck

A. Cupula: dome of cervical pleura
  1. Covers apex of lung and extends upward into root of neck about 1.5 in above border of 1st rib anteriorly
  2. Posteriorly, lung reaches neck of 1st rib
  3. Cervical pleura is supported and protected by thickening of scalene fascia called **suprapleural membrane** (Sibson's fascia)
B. Cervical trachea
  1. Features
    a. Mobile, cartilaginous and membranous tube
    b. Supported by C-shaped hyaline cartilages united by elastic anular ligaments
    c. Posterior wall is flattened, membranous and muscular (trachealis muscle)
    d. Suspended from lower border of cricoid cartilage by cricotracheal ligament
    e. Descends superficially in neck midline, but directed slightly posteriorly so that at suprasternal notch, it lies 1.5 in deep to skin surface (extends into thorax to end as 2 main bronchi at level of disc between 4th and 5th thoracic vertebra)
    f. Dimensions
       i. 9–15 cm long from larynx to bifurcation (about half the length of esophagus)
       ii. 2.0–2.5 cm in diameter in adult (larger in male); in child, it is smaller, more deeply placed and more moveable
  2. Relations
    a. Anteriorly: skin; superficial fascia; deep fascia (superficial layer of deep cervical fascia, infrahyoid fascia, and pretracheal layer of visceral fascia); jugular venous arch; sternohyoid and sternothyroid muscles; thyroid isthmus (2nd to 3rd tracheal rings); inferior thyroid veins; thyroidea ima artery (up to 10%)
    b. Posteriorly: recurrent laryngeal nerves (in tracheoesophageal grooves); esophagus; vertebral column
    c. Laterally: thyroid lobes and carotid sheath

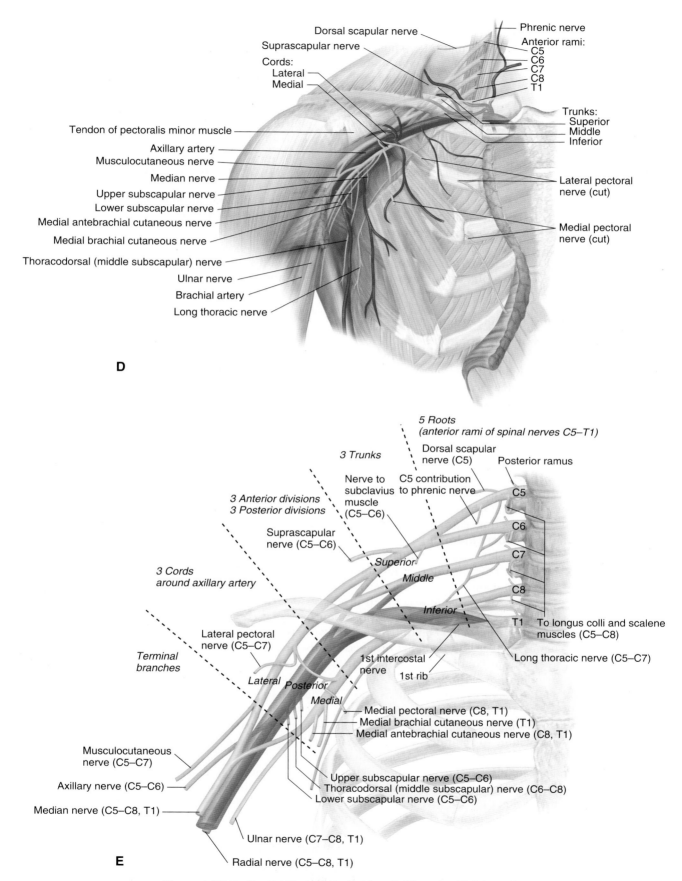

Dorsal scapular nerve

Suprascapular nerve

Cords:
Lateral
Medial

Phrenic nerve

Anterior rami:
C5
C6
C7
C8
T1

Trunks:
Superior
Middle
Inferior

Tendon of pectoralis minor muscle

Axillary artery

Musculocutaneous nerve

Median nerve

Upper subscapular nerve

Lower subscapular nerve

Medial antebrachial cutaneous nerve

Medial brachial cutaneous nerve

Thoracodorsal (middle subscapular) nerve

Ulnar nerve

Brachial artery

Long thoracic nerve

Lateral pectoral nerve (cut)

Medial pectoral nerve (cut)

D

5 Roots
(anterior rami of spinal nerves C5–T1)

3 Trunks

Dorsal scapular nerve (C5)

Posterior ramus

Nerve to subclavius muscle (C5–C6)

C5 contribution to phrenic nerve

C5

3 Anterior divisions
3 Posterior divisions

Suprascapular nerve (C5–C6)

C6

C7

Superior

Middle

C8

3 Cords around axillary artery

T1

To longus colli and scalene muscles (C5–C8)

Inferior

Lateral pectoral nerve (C5–C7)

1st intercostal nerve

1st rib

Long thoracic nerve (C5–C7)

Terminal branches

Lateral   *Posterior*

Medial

Medial pectoral nerve (C8, T1)

Medial brachial cutaneous nerve (T1)

Medial antebrachial cutaneous nerve (C8, T1)

Musculocutaneous nerve (C5–C7)

Axillary nerve (C5–C6)

Median nerve (C5–C8, T1)

Upper subscapular nerve (C5–C6)

Thoracodorsal (middle subscapular) nerve (C6–C8)

Lower subscapular nerve (C5–C6)

Ulnar nerve (C7–C8, T1)

E

Radial nerve (C5–C8, T1)

Figure 1.8D,E. Brachial Plexus, Anterior View. **D.** Dissection. **E.** Schematic.

C. Cervical esophagus

   1. Features

      a. Muscular tube, which begins at level of 6th cervical vertebra (lower border of cricoid cartilage) in continuity with laryngopharynx and extends through thorax to pass through diaphragm and empty to stomach; approximately 23–25 cm long

      b. Primarily midline

      c. Potential weakness in interval between transverse and oblique fibers of lower part of inferior pharyngeal constrictor may result in pharyngoesophageal diverticulum (Zenker's)

   2. Relations

      a. Anteriorly: trachea, recurrent laryngeal nerves anterolaterally

      b. Posteriorly: prevertebral layer of deep cervical fascia; longus colli muscles and vertebral column

      c. Laterally: on each side are lobes of thyroid and carotid sheath; on left, thoracic duct

D. Neurovasculature of cervical trachea and esophagus

   1. Arteries: from inferior thyroid arteries

   2. Veins: drain into inferior thyroid veins

   3. Nerves: from recurrent laryngeal nerves and sympathetic trunks

   4. Lymphatic drainage: into deep cervical nodes

VII. Clinical Considerations

A. **Subclavian steal syndrome**

   1. Rare; caused by narrowing of left subclavian artery near origin

   2. To compensate for decreased flow to arm, blood passes through basilar artery from right to left vertebral artery and into left subclavian

   3. Leads to less blood flow to left arm and brain, causing giddiness and fainting spells

B. Collateral blood flow in posterior triangle: possible to tie off subclavian artery entirely and still maintain blood to upper extremity because there is adequate collateral circulation for upper limb

C. Cervical dome of pleura: pleura and apex of lung protrudes above anterior end of 1st rib into base of posterior triangle and may be injured, particularly when needles are inserted here in an attempt to place catheter, causing pneumothorax

D. **Brachial plexus block**: needle inserted above mid-clavicle and directed medially and downward toward 1st rib; when there is paresthesia in arm, needle is reinserted, directed from above and below; index finger usually placed at upper clavicle border to depress subclavian artery

E. **Thoracic outlet syndrome**

   1. Brachial plexus nerves, usually lower trunk, and subclavian artery may be compressed where they pass between anterior and middle scalene muscles and where they cross 1st rib

   2. Common causes include scalenus anticus syndrome (see Section 1.7) and cervical ribs (1%–2%, often bilateral), which are accessory ribs, fascial band or cord from 7th cervical vertebra to 1st rib that may compress neurovascular components

   3. Condition may also be contributed to by carrying shoulder abnormally low, which results in neurovascular bundle being dragged against or angulated over firm structures

      a. Postural changes result in gradual stretching of the middle and lower parts of brachial plexus over rib

      b. Repeated trauma produces brachial neuritis, followed by weakness and atrophy beginning in intrinsic muscles of hand

   4. Symptoms include: tingling and numbness, perhaps pain, and often obviously disturbed circulation to or innervation of the hand; symptoms may appear in adult life at about age 30 years and are seen more often in women

F. **Tracheostomies**: create opening into trachea through neck, in area between cricoid cartilage and suprasternal notch, with tracheal mucosa being brought into continuity with skin

   1. Usual site: through thyroid isthmus and tracheal rings 2–3

   2. High tracheostomy: above level of thyroid isthmus; must avoid section of cricoid, which leads to laryngeal stenosis

   3. Low tracheostomy: between 3rd and 6th tracheal rings below thyroid gland isthmus; inferior thyroid veins and thyroidea ima artery (up to 10%) may be encountered

G. **Tracheotomy**: incision through skin and muscle to provide airway patency in emergencies or even electively, by patient, whose nasal or oral breathing is not reliable following nerve injury or tumor growth

Cervical Vertebrae and Posterior Neck

I. Cervical Vertebrae (Fig. 1.9A,B)

A. Atlas and axis: 1st and 2nd cervical vertebrae do not resemble any other vertebrae
   1. **Atlas** (**C1**) (Fig. 1.9C,D)
      a. No body and no spinous process
      b. 2 **lateral masses** connected by 2 rather thin arches
         i. **Anterior arch**: smaller and contains small midline **anterior tubercle** and **articular facet** on posterior aspect for articulation with dens of atlas
         ii. **Posterior arch:** has **posterior tubercle** and grooves for vertebral artery and 1st cervical nerve; attached to posterior rim of foramen magnum by **atlanto-occipital membrane**
         iii. Lateral masses have superior facets for articulation with occipital condyles and inferior facets for articulation with axis
      c. Transverse processes
         i. Large and possess a large foramen for vertebral artery and vein
         ii. Vertebral arteries pass posterior to lateral masses to enter skull via foramen magnum
         iii. Vertebral veins do not originate inside skull; arise from vessels of internal vertebral venous plexus; drain inferiorly to brachiocephalic veins
   2. **Axis** (**C2**) (Fig. 1.9E)
      a. Consists of typical cylindrical **body** anteriorly, **transverse processes**, posterior bifid **spinous process**, **arch** and projection extending superiorly from its body, the **dens** (**odontoid process**), which protrudes upward into space left by "missing" body of C1
      b. Transverse processes contain transverse foramina
      c. Spinous process: large and bifid
      d. Superior articular facets of axis articulate with inferior articular facets of atlas and dens of axis articulates with anterior arch of atlas

B. Cervical vertebrae 3–6 (Fig. 1.9F,G)
   1. Bodies: relatively small and approximately rectangular when seen from above; have uncinate processes extending superiorly from lateral edges of bodies
   2. Spinous processes: bifid
   3. Transverse processes have anterior and posterior tubercles and transverse foramina
   4. Vertebral foramina: relatively large and triangular
   5. Articular processes: large and facets face posterosuperiorly and anteroinferiorly

C. Cervical vertebra 7
   1. Spinous process: 1st spine that can be felt in upper back (**vertebra or spina prominens**); not bifid
   2. Vertebral artery and vein do not usually pass through C7 transverse foramina

II. Articulations of Cervical Vertebral Column (Fig. 1.9H,I)

A. **Atlanto-axial and atlanto-occipital joints**
   1. Important in reference to many complaints of pain as result of collisions in cars, namely, a "whiplash condition"
   2. Ligaments
      a. Axis to atlas: anterior longitudinal ligament, ligamenta flava, and ligamentum nuchae
      b. Axis to skull
         i. Ligamentum nuchae
         ii. **Cruciate or cruciform ligament**: transverse ligament of atlas not only extends between the lateral masses, but also has upward and downward extensions, attaching to anterior edge of foramen magnum and body of axis, respectively; these extensions give transverse ligament of atlas a cross appearance

      iii. Apical dental (from apex of dens to anterior margin of foramen magnum) and **alar ligaments** (originate at lateral surfaces of dens and attach at inner surface of occipital condyles and medial margin of adjoining foramen magnum); and **tectorial membrane** (an upward extension of posterior longitudinal ligament, which extends vertically from base of dens across its posterior surface to anterior lip of foramen magnum)

    3. Atlas to skull: anterior and posterior atlanto-occipital membranes from anterior and posterior arches of atlas to anterior and posterior margins of foramen magnum

    4. Ligament functions
      a. All the ligaments help to firmly secure upper cervical vertebral column to base of skull
      b. Dens acts as pivot for rotational movements of head; thus skull and C1 move as unit at atlanto-axial joint with respect to C2
      c. Conversely, flexion and extension of head involve movement of skull with respect to C1 vertebra at atlanto-occipital joint

B. **Ligamentum nuchae**
    1. Supraspinous ligament extends posteriorly, forming large, strong sickle-shaped membrane that separates muscles on 2 sides of neck and provides attachment for them
    2. Attaches to external occipital protuberance and crest
    3. Helps to support weight of head when it is inclined forward
    4. Much stronger in quadrupeds that graze, in whom ligament is very rich in elastic tissue

C. **Ligamenta flava**
    1. Strongest and most important ligament, and composed entirely of elastic tissue
    2. Each is flattened band that stretches from anterior surface of lower edge of 1 lamina to upper part of posterior surface of succeeding lamina
    3. Fill space between 2 adjacent laminae, except for narrow slit in midline
    4. Violent extension (hyperextension) of neck may carry cervical laminae so close together that ligamenta flava bulge forward and may impinge on spinal cord

D. **Posterior longitudinal ligament**
    1. Lies on posterior surfaces of vertebral bodies and intervertebral discs within spinal canal, anterior to spinal cord
    2. Specializations above axis include **tectorial membrane** and cruciform ligament

E. **Anterior longitudinal ligament**
    1. Lies anteriorly on vertebral bodies and intervertebral discs
    2. Ascends as far as atlas and is directly continuous with **anterior atlanto-occipital membrane,** which attaches to occipital bone
    3. If this membrane is removed, tubercle of anterior arch of atlas is seen; dens is posterior to this tubercle, the 2 bones being separated by joint cavity
    4. **Atlanto-axial membrane** extends from anterior arch of C1 to C2

III. Prevertebral Muscles (Fig. I.9J)

A. Associated with anterior surface of cervical vertebrae

B. **Longus colli muscle**
    1. Originates on anterior surface of cervical and upper thoracic vertebrae (C5–T3) and transverse processes of C3–C5
    2. Inserts on vertebral bodies of C1–C3, transverse processes of C3–C6, and anterior tubercle of atlas
    3. Supplied by anterior rami of C2–C6
    4. Major action: flexes and rotates neck to same side

C. **Longus capitis muscle**
    1. Lies on anterior surface of upper cervical vertebrae only
    2. Originates from anterior tubercles of transverse processes of cervical vertebrae 3–6 (Note: this is same as origin of scalenus anterior muscles; 2 muscles form continuity)
    3. Inserts onto basilar portion of occipital bone close to pharyngeal tubercle
    4. Supplied by anterior rami of C1–C3
    5. Major action: flexes neck and turns face slightly to same side

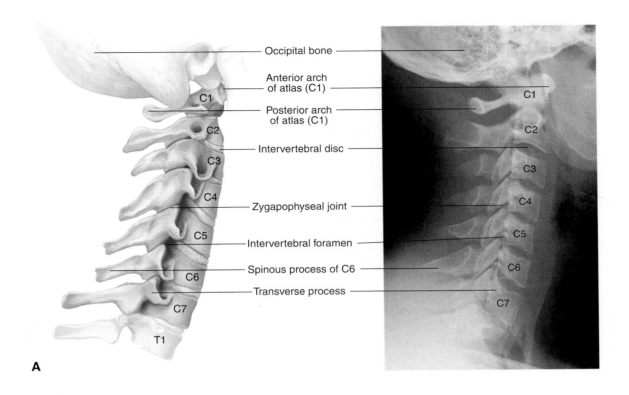

Occipital bone

Anterior arch
of atlas (C1)

Posterior arch
of atlas (C1)

Intervertebral disc

Zygapophyseal joint

Intervertebral foramen

Spinous process of C6

Transverse process

C1
C2
C3
C4
C5
C6
C7
T1

A

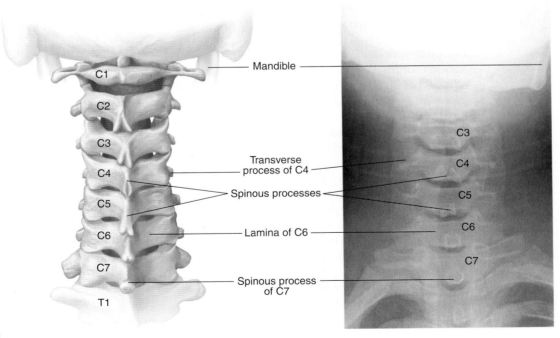

Mandible

Transverse
process of C4

Spinous processes

Lamina of C6

Spinous process
of C7

C1
C2
C3
C4
C5
C6
C7
T1

C3
C4
C5
C6
C7

B

Figure 1.9A,B. Vertebrae of the Neck. **A.** Lateral View. **B.** Posterior View.

D. **Rectus capitis anterior muscle**
  1. Lies deep to longus capitis
  2. Originates from anterior surface of lateral mass of atlas
  3. Inserts onto basilar portion of occipital bone anterior to occipital condyle
  4. Supplied by anterior ramus of C1
  5. Major action: flexes neck

E. **Rectus capitis lateralis muscle**
  1. Lateral in position to rectus capitis anterior
  2. Originates from transverse process of atlas
  3. Inserts onto occipital bone just posterior to jugular fossa
  4. Supplied by anterior ramus of C1
  5. Major action: bends neck to same side

IV. Suboccipital Region (Fig. 1.9K)

A. Important clinically when dealing with "whiplash" injury
B. Muscles overlying suboccipital triangle
  1. Trapezius muscle: most superficial muscle on back of neck
  2. Splenius capitis and cervicis lie beneath trapezius
  3. Semispinalis capitis deep to these and immediately superficial to suboccipital triangle
C. **Suboccipital triangle**
  1. Boundaries
    a. Inferior border: **obliquus capitis inferior muscle**
    b. Lateral border: **obliquus capitis superior**
    c. Medial border: **rectus capitis posterior major**
  2. Contents
    a. Vertebral artery: passes transversely posterior to lateral mass of atlas to penetrate posterior atlanto-occipital membrane and pass superiorly through foramen magnum
    b. 1st cervical nerve: lies between vertebral artery and posterior arch of atlas, where it may be compressed
    c. Plexus of veins
    d. **Rectus capitis posterior minor muscle**: does not take part in formation of triangle, but lies medial to rectus capitis posterior major
    e. **Greater occipital nerve**: crosses triangle on way to scalp; **occipital artery** is lateral to triangle
  3. **Suboccipital muscles**
    a. Actions confined to joints of head, make small, precisely synchronized movements of head possible, independent of position of vertebral column; in contrast, powerful extensive head movements are possible by contraction of long muscles inserting at head
    b. **Obliquus capitis inferior muscle**
      i. Arises from spine of axis
      ii. Inserts on transverse process of atlas
      iii. Major action: turns head toward same side
    c. **Obliquus capitis superior muscle**
      i. Arises from transverse process of atlas
      ii. Inserts on occipital bone on lateral part of region between nuchal lines
      iii. Major action: pulls head posteriorly and turns head toward same side; if muscles on both sides work simultaneously, neck is extended (head is pulled directly posteriorly)
    d. **Rectus capitis posterior major muscle**
      i. Arises from spine of axis
      ii. Inserts on the occipital bone on the middle 1/3 of inferior nuchal line
      iii. Major action: extends neck (pulls head posteriorly) and turns head toward same side; if muscles on both sides work simultaneously, neck is extended

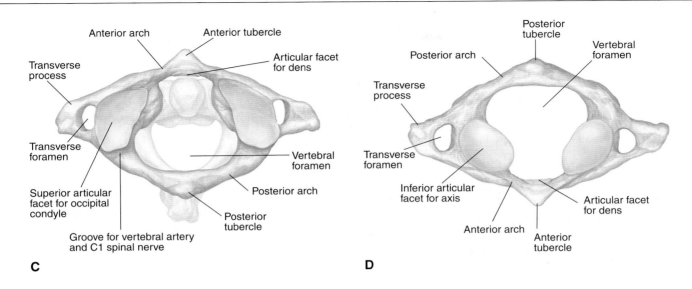

Anterior arch

Anterior tubercle

Articular facet
for dens

Transverse
process

Transverse
foramen

Superior articular
facet for occipital
condyle

Vertebral
foramen

Posterior arch

Posterior
tubercle

Groove for vertebral artery
and C1 spinal nerve

C

Posterior
tubercle

Posterior arch

Vertebral
foramen

Transverse
process

Transverse
foramen

Inferior articular
facet for axis

Anterior arch

Anterior
tubercle

Articular facet
for dens

D

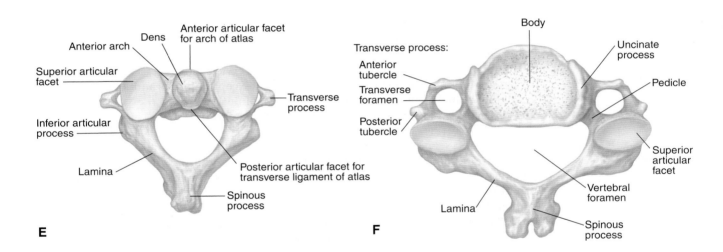

Anterior articular facet
for arch of atlas

Dens

Anterior arch

Superior articular
facet

Inferior articular
process

Lamina

Posterior articular facet for
transverse ligament of atlas

Spinous
process

Transverse
process

E

Body

Uncinate
process

Transverse process:

Anterior
tubercle

Transverse
foramen

Posterior
tubercle

Lamina

Vertebral
foramen

Spinous
process

Pedicle

Superior
articular
facet

F

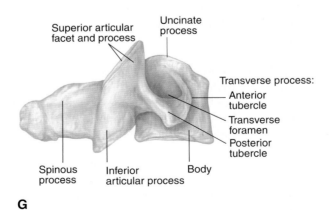

Superior articular
facet and process

Uncinate
process

Transverse process:

Anterior
tubercle

Transverse
foramen

Posterior
tubercle

Spinous
process

Inferior
articular process

Body

G

Figure 1.9C–G. **C.** Atlas (C1), Superior View. **D.** Atlas (C1), Inferior View. **E.** Axis (C2), Superior View. **F.** Cervical
Vertebra (C4), Superior View. **G.** Cervical Vertebra (C4), Lateral View.

e. **Rectus capitis posterior minor muscle**
   i. Arises from posterior tubercle of atlas
   ii. Inserts on occipital bone just medial to insertion of rectus capitis posterior major, below inferior nuchal line
   iii. Major action: extends neck (head is pulled posteriorly) and turns head toward same side; if muscles on both sides work simultaneously, neck is extended
f. Suboccipital muscles all innervated by posterior ramus of C1 (suboccipital nerve)

V. Neurovascular Structures of Posterior Neck

A. Nerves: posterior rami of 1st 4 cervical nerves
   1. Posterior ramus of C1 (**suboccipital nerve**)
      a. No cutaneous sensory component; difficult to find any spinal ganglion on this nerve
      b. Emerges from spinal cord between atlas and occipital bone, passes posteriorly between vertebral artery and posterior arch of atlas; branches immediately to innervate suboccipital muscles and semispinalis capitis
   2. Posterior ramus of C2
      a. Carries both sensory and motor components, as do posterior rami of other spinal nerves
      b. Has both lateral and medial branches
         i. Lateral branch innervates several cervical muscles
         ii. Medial branch, the **greater occipital nerve**, wraps below obliquus capitis inferior and passes superiorly superficial to muscles of suboccipital triangle to ramify on posterior part of head as sensory nerve to scalp up to vertex
   3. Posterior rami of C3 and C4
      a. Between semispinalis cervicis and longissimus cervicis muscles
      b. Lateral branches innervate all muscles in area except trapezius and levator scapulae
      c. Medial branches become cutaneous on back of neck
      d. C3 reaches scalp where it is called **3rd occipital nerve**
B. Arteries
   1. Do not exhibit segmental arrangement of blood vessels in trunk wall
   2. Arise from vertebral and deep cervical arteries; in addition, branches of occipital, transverse cervical, and ascending cervical arteries pass to neck muscles, as well as to skin of region
   3. **Vertebral artery**
      a. 1st branch of subclavian artery; enters transverse foramen of C6 vertebra; passes cranially through transverse foramina of remaining cervical vertebrae
      b. Courses medially in sulcus of vertebral artery behind lateral mass of atlas, pierces posterior atlanto-occipital membrane, dura, and arachnoid to pass into subarachnoid space
      c. Enters skull via foramen magnum
      d. Both vertebral arteries unite on clivus of occipital bone at posterior margin of pons to become basilar artery
      e. Extracranial branches
         i. Spinal, through intervertebral foramina to spinal nerves and ganglia
         ii. Muscular, to deep cervical muscles
         iii. Near anterior and posterior opening of foramen magnum, gives off meningeal branches (anterior and posterior) to dura and diploe of posterior cranial fossa
      f. Intracranial branches: discussed in Chapter 3
   4. **Deep cervical artery**
      a. Branch of costocervical trunk of subclavian artery, enters semispinalis capitis dorsally between transverse process of C7 and neck of 1st rib, lateral to semispinalis cervicis and medial to longissimus capitis muscle; anastomoses with descending branch of occipital
      b. Supplies nuchal muscles and also gives off spinal branches to vertebral canal

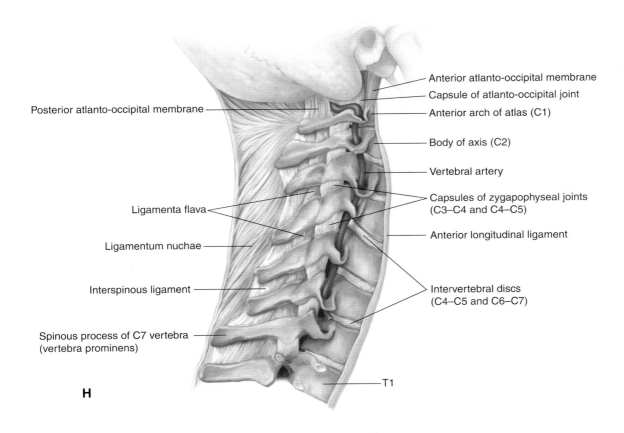

Posterior atlanto-occipital membrane

Ligamenta flava

Ligamentum nuchae

Interspinous ligament

Spinous process of C7 vertebra
(vertebra prominens)

Anterior atlanto-occipital membrane

Capsule of atlanto-occipital joint

Anterior arch of atlas (C1)

Body of axis (C2)

Vertebral artery

Capsules of zygapophyseal joints
(C3–C4 and C4–C5)

Anterior longitudinal ligament

Intervertebral discs
(C4–C5 and C6–C7)

T1

H

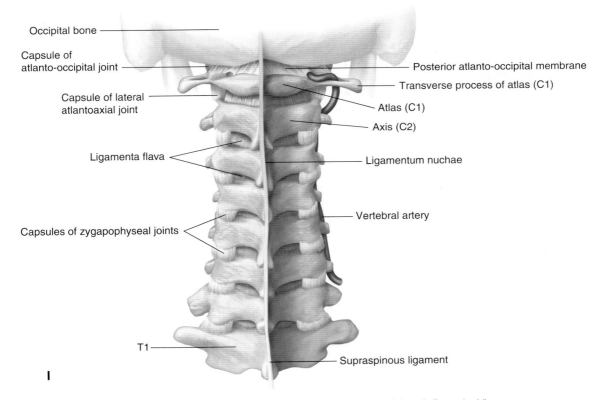

Occipital bone

Capsule of
atlanto-occipital joint

Capsule of lateral
atlantoaxial joint

Ligamenta flava

Capsules of zygapophyseal joints

T1

Posterior atlanto-occipital membrane

Transverse process of atlas (C1)

Atlas (C1)

Axis (C2)

Ligamentum nuchae

Vertebral artery

Supraspinous ligament

I

Figure I.9H,I. Articulations of Cervical Vertebrae. **H.** Lateral View. **I.** Posterior View.

5. **Occipital artery**
   a. Arises from external carotid artery in anterior neck and passes posterosuperiorly
   b. Sends branch to SCM muscle that crosses superior to hypoglossal nerve
   c. Passes in groove just deep to mastoid process of temporal bone, gives off mastoid branch to diploe and dura of posterior cranial fossa and auricular branch to posterior surface of pinna of ear
   d. Continues posteriorly between obliquus capitis superior and splenius capitis, close to skull
   e. Becomes superficial to semispinalis capitis and trapezius muscles, or pierces latter and ramifies on posterior surface of head to anastomose with branches of superficial temporal and posterior auricular arteries
   f. Major source of blood for scalp
   g. Descending branch passes across obliquus capitis inferior muscle and anastomoses with deep cervical artery

C. Veins
   1. Tend to form plexus of vessels called **suboccipital plexus**, the superior limit of a similar plexus of veins that is located throughout entire length of vertebral column, the vertebral plexus
   2. Branches make important communication via emissary veins with dural venous sinuses within cranial cavity via condyloid canal
   3. **Vertebral vein** begins in plexus; accompanies vertebral artery as plexus of communicating veins and receives segmental, intervertebral, and tributaries from vertebral canal; exits from C6 transverse foramen and receives deep cervical vein just before emptying into brachiocephalic vein
   4. Blood from nuchal region passes into external jugular vein by superficial veins and flows into brachiocephalic vein via vertebral vein and **deep cervical vein** (carries blood from posterior external vertebral venous plexus); both anastomose with occipital vein and suboccipital venous plexus

VI. Clinical Considerations

A. "Whiplash" injury of cervical spine
   1. Forceful extension then flexion of cervical spine
   2. Often involves no permanent displacement of vertebral structures, but muscles and ligaments injured usually followed by inflammation and muscle spasm
   3. Occurs during rapid decelerations (i.e., car hitting tree), in which driver's head and neck snap forward, then backward forcefully
   4. Generally treated by immobilization and rest

B. Cervical spinal cord injury
   1. Fractures of cervical region, especially those consequent to whip-like action that is common in automobile accidents, particularly likely to cause death
   2. Injury to spinal cord in cervical region above origin of brachial plexus could result in quadriplegia
   3. Compression of cervical cord rarely occurs without evidence of nerve root compression
   4. Transverse ligament of atlas protects and secures dens, preventing crushing of spinal cord; in hanging, this ligament is often torn, allowing cord to be crushed, leading to death

C. **Cervical spondylosis**: degenerative, arthritic disease involving cervical spine and may result in compression of cervical cord, cervical nerves, and/or vertebral arteries

(Continued)

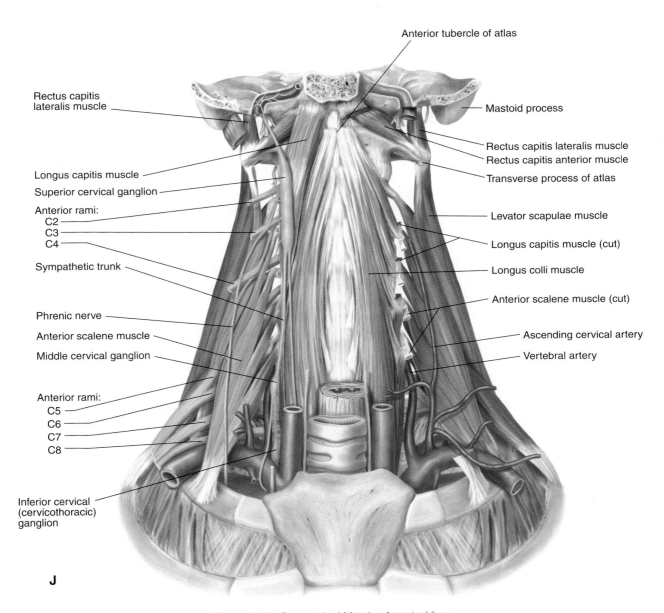

Anterior tubercle of atlas

Rectus capitis
lateralis muscle

Mastoid process

Rectus capitis lateralis muscle
Rectus capitis anterior muscle

Longus capitis muscle

Transverse process of atlas

Superior cervical ganglion

Anterior rami:
C2
C3
C4

Levator scapulae muscle

Longus capitis muscle (cut)

Longus colli muscle

Sympathetic trunk

Phrenic nerve

Anterior scalene muscle (cut)

Anterior scalene muscle

Ascending cervical artery

Middle cervical ganglion

Vertebral artery

Anterior rami:
C5
C6
C7
C8

Inferior cervical
(cervicothoracic)
ganglion

J

Figure 1.9J. Prevertebral Muscles, Anterior View.

D. Cervical disc herniation: location of pain, peripheral numbness, muscular weakness and wasting, and reflex changes due to cervical herniated discs and nerve root involvement will depend on specific disc involved, but usually affects nerve below disc (C4–C5 disc usually compresses C5)

E. **Cervical root syndrome**: describes signs and symptoms produced by irritation or compression of cervical nerve roots, in or near intervertebral foramina, before they divide into anterior and posterior rami

   1. Predisposing causes of cervical root irritation include swelling of roots after traumatic intervertebral compression, congenital anomalies, postinflammatory adhesions, and rheumatoid arthritis

   2. Persistent cervical root irritation may produce reflex stimulation of cervical sympathetic system, causing symptoms (i.e., vision blurring, pupil dilation, loss of balance, headache, swelling and stiffness of fingers, tendonitis, and capsulitis)

   3. Causes: degenerative disc disease without trauma; neck sprains in accidents, neck injuries in contact sports, neck twisting in sleep or while anesthetized; and certain postural abnormalities (hemorrhage, edema, and local inflammation can be superimposed on compression)

   4. Posterior subluxations: incomplete dislocation of cervical vertebrae produced by hyperextension of cervical spine, which can compress nerve roots by narrowing vertebral diameter of foramina anteriorly; flexing neck increases vertical diameter of foramina and does not lead to nerve compression

F. **Suboccipital puncture**

   1. Needle inserted between occipital bone and posterior arch of atlas through posterior atlanto-occipital membrane (palpable with some resistance), dura, and arachnoid, into subarachnoid space, enlarged here to form cerebellomedullary cistern

   2. Cerebrospinal fluid can be removed or air injected for filling of ventricular system (via openings of 4th ventricle)

   3. Care must be taken to place puncture as close to median plane as possible to avoid injury to vertebral artery

G. Movements of cervical vertebrae

   1. Full flexion of cervical spine and atlanto-occipital joints should put chin on chest with mouth closed; full extension of same joints, catches examiner's finger between occiput and C7, but doesn't "trap" it

   2. In lateral bending of head and neck, when shoulders are steadied, approximating ear to shoulder should provide total range of movement between right and left sides that is a little less than 90° (Note: lateral flexion is always accompanied by some rotation)

   3. With shoulders steadied, rotation of head and neck normally brings chin level with shoulders (2/3 of this action takes place at atlanto-axial joints)

   4. Combined extension and rotation of head and neck compresses intervertebral foramina and provokes or exaggerates symptoms caused by nerve compression in these foramina

H. Injury to or blockage of the vertebral arteries

   1. If vertebral artery injured, site of injury must always be ligated proximally and distally because of intracranial and extracranial connections of right and left vertebral arteries (basilar artery, spinal arteries)

   2. May result in ischemia of brainstem; in most cases, recovery occurs without neurologic sequelae, but a minority of cases show evidence of brainstem involvement with ataxia and asymmetry of stretch reflexes; tends to occur in older patients with some degree of atherosclerosis, but can be demonstrated in younger patients

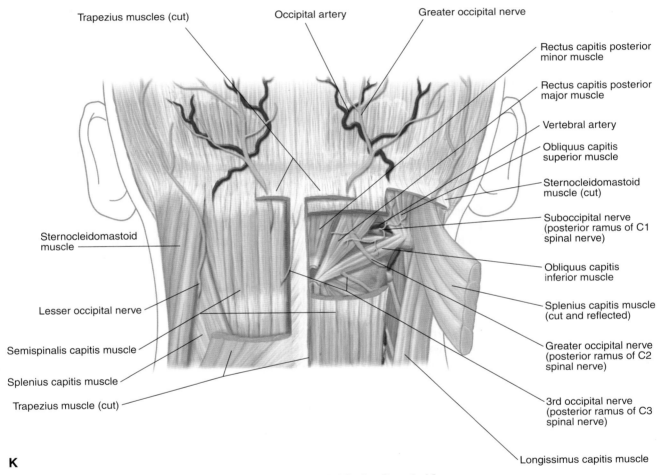

Trapezius muscles (cut)

Occipital artery

Greater occipital nerve

Rectus capitis posterior minor muscle

Rectus capitis posterior major muscle

Vertebral artery

Obliquus capitis superior muscle

Sternocleidomastoid muscle (cut)

Suboccipital nerve (posterior ramus of C1 spinal nerve)

Obliquus capitis inferior muscle

Splenius capitis muscle (cut and reflected)

Greater occipital nerve (posterior ramus of C2 spinal nerve)

3rd occipital nerve (posterior ramus of C3 spinal nerve)

Longissimus capitis muscle

Sternocleidomastoid muscle

Lesser occipital nerve

Semispinalis capitis muscle

Splenius capitis muscle

Trapezius muscle (cut)

K

Figure 1.9K Suboccipital Region, Posterior View.

Larynx: Parts and Relations

I. Location and Size (Fig. 1.10A,B)

A. Opposite 3rd to 6th cervical vertebrae
B. Female larynx lies slightly higher than male (about ½ vertebra higher)
C. Newborn larynx is 1–2 vertebrae higher
D. **Thyrohyoid membrane**
1. Suspends thyroid cartilage from hyoid bone
2. **Median thyrohyoid ligament**: thickened midline portion
3. **Lateral thyrohyoid ligament**: thickened posterolateral edge; often contains a small cartilage, the **triticeal cartilage**
4. Pierced by internal branch of superior laryngeal nerve (from vagus, CN X) and by superior laryngeal blood vessels
E. Size: 44 mm long, 43 mm wide, 36 mm deep

II. Cartilages (Fig. 1.10C–E)

A. 9 (3 unpaired, 3 paired)
B. **Thyroid cartilage**
1. Largest and single; suspended from hyoid bone by thyrohyoid membrane
2. Parts
   a. **Laminae**: bilateral, meeting at acute angle in midline of neck; angle formed by laminae is approximately 90° in adult males and usually >120° in females
   b. **Superior horn**: directed superiorly from posterior border of each lamina
   c. **Inferior horn**: directed inferiorly from posterior border of each lamina
   d. **Superior tubercle**: at root of superior horn
   e. **Inferior tubercle**: on lower border
   f. **Oblique line**: on lateral surface of lamina; attachment for thyrohoid, sternothyroid, and inferior pharyngeal constrictor muscles
   g. **Laryngeal prominence** ("Adam's apple")
      i. Anterior midline projection of upper border
      ii. Sexually dimorphic: more prominent in males, causing longer vocal ligaments and lower voice
      iii. **Thyroid notch**: variable notch in laryngeal prominence
C. **Cricoid cartilage**
1. Single; only complete cartilaginous ring in respiratory tract
2. Parts
   a. **Lamina**: posteriorly, 2–3 cm long
   b. **Arch**: narrow, convex ring of cartilage anteriorly
   c. Articular facets
      i. Lateral: at junction of lamina and arch, for articulation with inferior horns of thyroid cartilage
      ii. Superior: on superior border of lamina laterally, for articulation with arytenoid cartilages
D. **Epiglottis**
1. Single, leaf shaped
2. Yellow elastic cartilage
E. **Arytenoid cartilage**
1. Paired
2. Each consists of a pyramidal piece with 3 surfaces, a base, and an apex
3. Inferior surface of base is the articular surface
4. Muscular process projects posterolaterally and vocal process projects anteriorly from base
F. **Corniculate cartilage**
1. Small paired pieces of yellow elastic cartilage
2. Contact apices of arytenoid cartilages, extending posteriorly

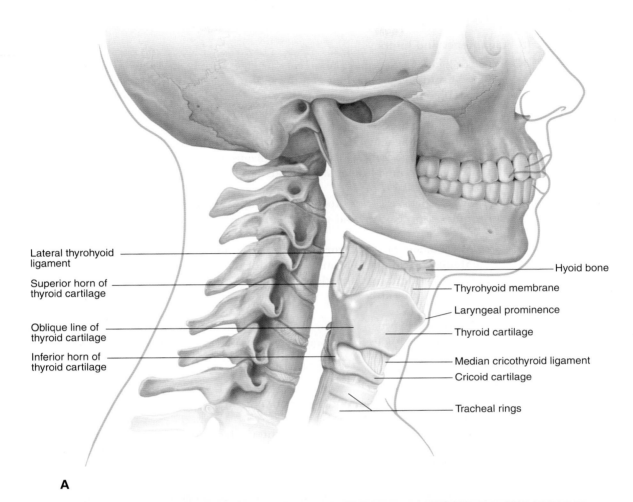

Lateral thyrohyoid ligament

Superior horn of thyroid cartilage

Oblique line of thyroid cartilage

Inferior horn of thyroid cartilage

Hyoid bone

Thyrohyoid membrane

Laryngeal prominence

Thyroid cartilage

Median cricothyroid ligament

Cricoid cartilage

Tracheal rings

A

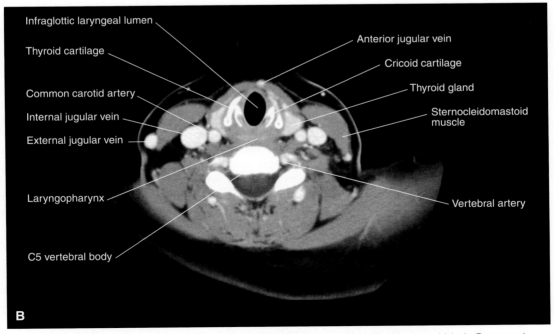

Infraglottic laryngeal lumen

Thyroid cartilage

Common carotid artery

Internal jugular vein

External jugular vein

Laryngopharynx

C5 vertebral body

Anterior jugular vein

Cricoid cartilage

Thyroid gland

Sternocleidomastoid muscle

Vertebral artery

B

Figure 1.10A,B. A. Location of the Laryngeal Cartilages, Lateral View. **B.** Larynx and Neck, Computed Tomography Images, Transverse View.

G. **Cuneiform cartilage**
1. Small paired pieces of yellow elastic cartilage
2. Lie within the aryepiglottic folds

III. Ligaments and Joints

A. Extrinsic ligaments: connect laryngeal cartilages with hyoid bone or trachea
   1. **Thyrohyoid membrane**: between thyroid cartilage and hyoid bone
      a. **Median thyrohyoid ligament**: thickened middle part of membrane
      b. **Lateral thyrohyoid ligaments**: thickened, cordlike posterior edge of membrane
   2. **Hyoepiglottic ligament**: from epiglottis to hyoid bone
   3. **Cricotracheal ligament**: from cricoid cartilage to 1st tracheal ring
B. Intrinsic ligaments: connect laryngeal cartilages together
   1. **Quadrangular membrane**: submucous layer between arytenoid and lateral edges of epiglottic cartilages
   2. **Conus elasticus**: extends superiorly from upper edge of cricoid ring to attach anteriorly on inner aspect of thyroid where lamina unite and posteriorly on vocal processes of arytenoid cartilages
      a. **Vocal ligament** (**vocal cord**): thickened upper edge
      b. **Median cricothyroid ligament**: anterior part of the conus
   3. Thyroepiglottic and hyoepiglottic ligaments: attach epiglottis to thyroid cartilage and hyoid bone anteriorly
C. Synovial joints
   1. Cricothyroid: between inferior horn of thyroid and lateral facet of cricoid cartilage
   2. Cricoarytenoid: between superior border of cricoid lamina and base of arytenoid cartilage

IV. Interior of Larynx (Fig. 1.10F)

A. Extends from entrance to lower border of cricoid cartilage
B. **Vestibule**
   1. **Laryngeal inlet** (aditus): bounded anteriorly by epiglottis, posteriorly by apices of arytenoid cartilages and corniculate cartilages, and laterally by **aryepiglottic folds**
   2. Lies behind epiglottis and between mucous membranes covering **quadrangular membrane** (submucosa)
   3. Ends inferiorly at the vestibular or **false vocal folds**, formed by inferior borders of quadrangular membrane
C. **Ventricle**
   1. Laterally extending space between false and true vocal folds
   2. Serves as resonance chamber for vibrating vocal ligaments
D. **True vocal folds**
   1. Formed by mucous membrane lining conus elasticus, with thyroarytenoideus muscle lying laterally
   2. Serve to divide larynx into supraglottic and infraglottic portions, with separate sensory supply
   3. **Vocal cord**: thickened upper edge of conus elasticus, attaching specifically to vocal process of arytentoid cartilage and junction of thyroid laminae anteriorly; also known as **vocal ligament**; pearly white with covering of fine blood vessels when seen via laryngoscope (Note: the terms "vocal folds" and "vocal cords" are often used interchangeably, because movement of 1 means movement of the other; however, cord is the part of the fold which is most involved in vibrating to create sound waves)
   4. **Rima glottidis**
      a. Fissure between true vocal folds, including vocal processes
      b. 2 parts
         i. Intramembranous: anterior 3/5 between folds
         ii. Intercartilaginous: posterior 2/5 between arytenoid cartilages
E. Inferior border of larynx
   1. Inferior edge of cricoid cartilage
   2. Connected to 1st tracheal ring (actually C shaped, not ring) by cricotracheal ligament

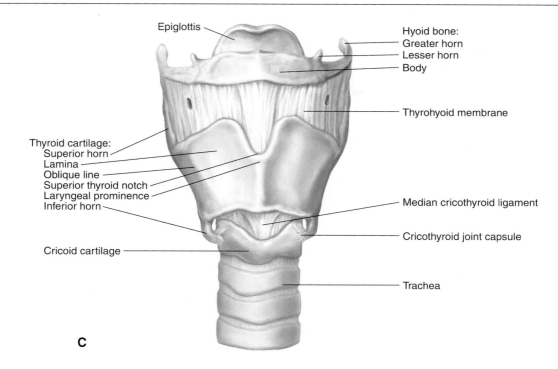

Epiglottis

Hyoid bone:
Greater horn
Lesser horn
Body

Thyrohyoid membrane

Thyroid cartilage:
Superior horn
Lamina
Oblique line
Superior thyroid notch
Laryngeal prominence
Inferior horn

Cricoid cartilage

Median cricothyroid ligament

Cricothyroid joint capsule

Trachea

C

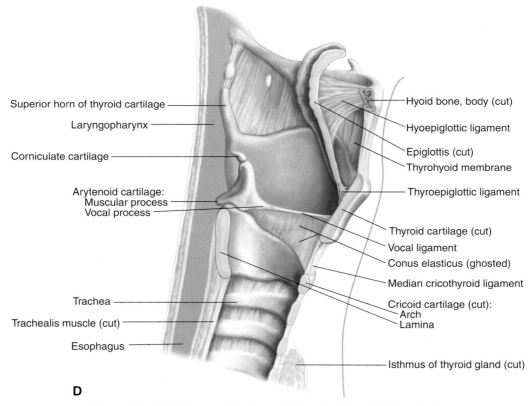

Superior horn of thyroid cartilage

Laryngopharynx

Corniculate cartilage

Arytenoid cartilage:
Muscular process
Vocal process

Trachea

Trachealis muscle (cut)

Esophagus

Hyoid bone, body (cut)

Hyoepiglottic ligament

Epiglottis (cut)
Thyrohyoid membrane

Thyroepiglottic ligament

Thyroid cartilage (cut)
Vocal ligament
Conus elasticus (ghosted)
Median cricothyroid ligament
Cricoid cartilage (cut):
Arch
Lamina

Isthmus of thyroid gland (cut)

D

Figure 1.10C,D. Laryngeal Cartilages. **C.** Anterior View. **D.** Sagittal Section.

V. Clinical Considerations

A. Cricoid cartilage

  1. Palpable just below thyroid cartilage at level of C6

  2. Used as guideline to approximate level of the following

    a. Passage of inferior thyroid artery behind common carotid artery

    b. Entrance of vertebral artery into transverse foramen of C6

    c. Entrance of recurrent laryngeal nerve into larynx

    d. Middle cervical sympathetic ganglion

    e. Junction of larynx and trachea

    f. Junction of pharynx and esophagus

    g. Opening of a pharyngoesophageal diverticulum

B. Vestibule of larynx is very sensitive to foreign objects

  1. When these come in contact with its epithelium, violent coughing begins in order to expel them

  2. Involves first a marked abduction of the vocal cords, by posterior cricoarytenoid muscles, to enlarge airway as much as possible and allow a "gasp for breath"

  3. Next, larynx is closed, primarily via vestibular folds and, therefore, thyroepiglottic muscle

  4. When this closure is suddenly released following increase in pressure in thorax, air erupts as cough

C. Foreign bodies in laryngopharynx

  1. Food passes through laryngopharynx in swallowing, with some entering piriform recess

  2. Foreign bodies (fishbone, chicken bone, etc.) can lodge in recess and can pierce mucous membrane and injure neurovascular structures there

  3. Most young children can swallow a variety of objects, which pass to stomach and through alimentary canal without any problem; in some cases, foreign objects stop at inferior end of laryngopharynx (its narrowest part); they can be visualized by a pharyngoscope or by X-ray or CT scans

  4. **Heimlich maneuver**

    a. Foreign object may aspirate through laryngeal inlet into laryngeal vestibule and become trapped above vestibular folds; laryngeal muscles go into spasm, tensing vocal folds; rima glottidis closes and shuts off air entering trachea; may even be complete laryngeal obstruction and leave individual choking and without speech; death may occur in 5 minutes from lack of oxygen if obstruction is not removed

    b. Sudden compression of abdomen (Heminlich maneuver) by subdiaphragmatic abdominal thrusts using closed fist with base of palm facing inward placed between umbilicus and xiphoid process of sternum, causes diaphragm to elevate and compress lungs, which still contain air, sending air from trachea into larynx, dislodging object from larynx

D. **Laryngoscopy**

  1. Visualization of laryngeal structures accomplished directly, by deflecting tongue and epiglottis with laryngoscope blade or indirectly, using mirror positioned in posterior pharynx, while pulling tongue forward

  2. Care must be taken to avoid touching the oropharynx, which would trigger gag reflex and make visualization very difficult

(Continued)

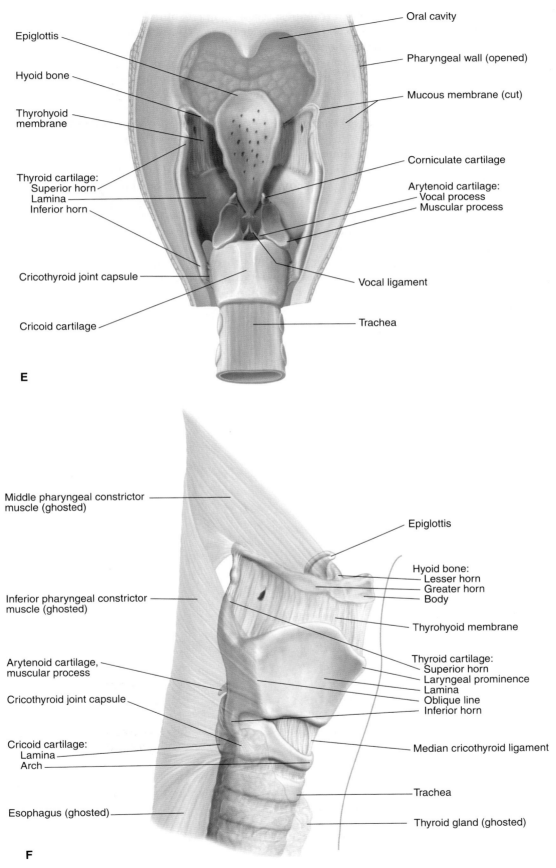

E

Epiglottis

Hyoid bone

Thyrohyoid membrane

Thyroid cartilage:
Superior horn
Lamina
Inferior horn

Cricothyroid joint capsule

Cricoid cartilage

Oral cavity

Pharyngeal wall (opened)

Mucous membrane (cut)

Corniculate cartilage

Arytenoid cartilage:
Vocal process
Muscular process

Vocal ligament

Trachea

F

Middle pharyngeal constrictor muscle (ghosted)

Inferior pharyngeal constrictor muscle (ghosted)

Arytenoid cartilage, muscular process

Cricothyroid joint capsule

Cricoid cartilage:
Lamina
Arch

Esophagus (ghosted)

Epiglottis

Hyoid bone:
Lesser horn
Greater horn
Body

Thyrohyoid membrane

Thyroid cartilage:
Superior horn
Laryngeal prominence
Lamina
Oblique line
Inferior horn

Median cricothyroid ligament

Trachea

Thyroid gland (ghosted)

Figure 1.10E,F. Laryngeal Cartilages. **E.** Posterior View. **F.** Lateral View.

E. **Laryngeal fractures:** resulting in crushing injury to skeletal elements of larynx may interfere with laryngeal patency and ability to breathe

F. **Laryngectomy (larynx removal)**

1. Performed in cases of serious malignancy; presence of palpable lymph nodes anterior to upper tracheal rings signals possibility of laryngeal cancer; symptoms include hoarseness, frequently associated with otalgia (earache), dysphagia, and severe constant coughing

2. After laryngectomy, patient may produce some intelligible sound by learning to govern escape of swallowed air from stomach and esophagus

G. Sexual dimorphism of larynx

1. At puberty, in males, length of vocal cord almost doubles and supporting cartilages become stronger and thicker; men generally have both longer and heavier vocal folds than women, thus deeper voices

2. Changes also seen in females, but to lesser degree

3. With aging, laryngeal cartilages tend to calcify, which may affect speech patterns and breathing

H. **Cricothyrotomy:** incisions through median cricothyroid ligament just below skin can be easily made; due to large cricoid lamina, there is less danger in penetrating laryngeal pharynx and creating laryngopharyngeal fistula

Larynx: Muscles and Neurovasculature

I. Muscles (Fig. 1.11A,B)

Muscle	Origin	Insertion	Action
Cricothyroid	Arch of cricoid cartilage	Inferior horn and lower border of thyroid cartilage	Pulls thyroid cartilage and cricoid arch together anteriorly, tensing vocal cords
Posterior cricoarytenoid	Cricoid lamina	Muscular process of arytenoid	Abducts vocal cords
Lateral cricoarytenoid	Arch of cricoid cartilage	Muscular process of arytenoid cartilage	Adducts vocal cords, closing glottis
Arytenoid, transverse	Posterior border of arytenoid cartilage	Posterior border of opposite arytenoid cartilage	Adducts arytenoid cartilages, closing glottis
Arytenoid, oblique	Posterior border of arytenoid cartilage near base	Apex of arytenoid cartilage of opposite side	Adducts arytenoid cartilages, closing glottis
Thyroarytenoid	Inner surface of thyroid laminae near laryngeal prominence	Lateral borders of arytenoid cartilage	Pulls arytenoid cartilage anteriorly, relaxing vocal cord
Vocalis	Portion of thyroarytenoid attaching onto vocal ligament	Vocal ligament	Selectively relaxes segment of vocal cord, providing fine control of pitch
Thyroepiglottic	Superior extension of thyroarytenoid	Lateral border of epiglottis	Helps to pull lateral edge of epiglottis down

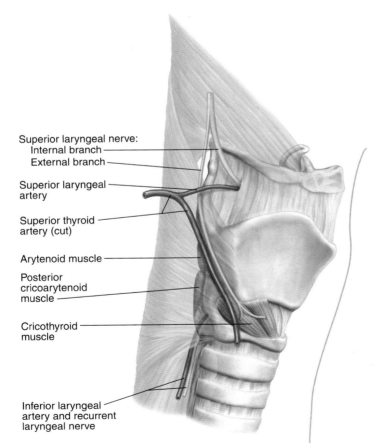

A

Figure 1.11A. Laryngeal Muscles and Neurovascular Supply. **A.** Lateral View.

II. Special Features of Laryngeal Muscles (Fig. 1.11C,D)

A. All derived from 4th and 6th branchial arches, thus innervated by CN X; cricothyroid innervated by external branch of superior laryngeal nerve; all others innervated by inferior laryngeal nerve, the continuation of recurrent laryngeal nerve into larynx

B. Only 1 laryngeal muscle (cricothyroid) found externally, all others located within larynx

1. **Cricothyroid muscle**
   a. Origin: on external surface of larynx, arising from lateral surface of arch of cricoid cartilage
   b. Passes posteriorly and superiorly to insert on inferior horn and inferior border of thyroid lamina
   c. Action: pulls thyroid cartilage anteriorly and inferiorly in rocking action, thus stretching and increasing tension on vocal cords
   d. Innervation: external branch of superior laryngeal nerve (from vagus CN X)

2. **Posterior cricoarytenoid muscle**
   a. Arises from posterior surface of lamina of cricoid cartilage
   b. Passes superiorly and laterally to attach to muscular process of arytenoid cartilage
   c. Action: pull is in posteromedial direction, and when muscular process is pulled in this direction, vocal process moves in opposite direction (laterally), and vocal cords are abducted due to rotation of arytenoid cartilage; widens intercartilaginous and intermembranous (space between 2 vocal cords) of rima glottidis

3. **Lateral cricoarytenoid muscle**
   a. Origin: superior border of lateral part of arch of cricoid cartilage
   b. Insertion: passes superiorly and posteriorly to be inserted onto muscular process of arytenoid cartilage
   c. Action: rotates or pulls muscular process anteriorly and laterally and vocal process moves medially, adducting vocal cords

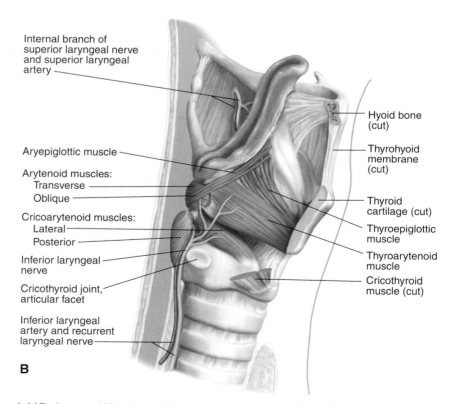

B

Figure 1.11B. Laryngeal Muscles and Neurovascular Supply. Right Thyroid Lamina Removed, Lateral View.

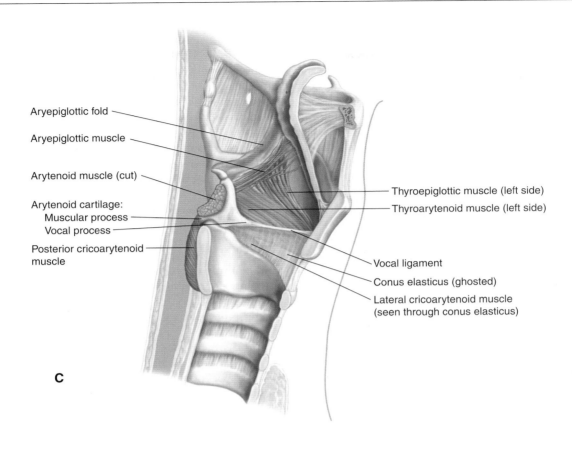

Aryepiglottic fold

Aryepiglottic muscle

Arytenoid muscle (cut)

Arytenoid cartilage:
Muscular process
Vocal process

Posterior cricoarytenoid muscle

Thyroepiglottic muscle (left side)
Thyroarytenoid muscle (left side)

Vocal ligament
Conus elasticus (ghosted)
Lateral cricoarytenoid muscle (seen through conus elasticus)

C

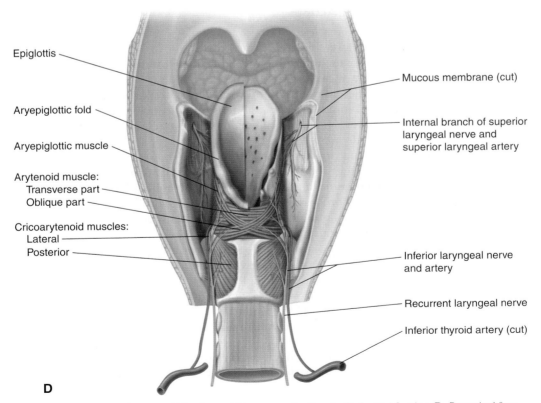

Epiglottis

Aryepiglottic fold

Aryepiglottic muscle

Arytenoid muscle:
Transverse part
Oblique part

Cricoarytenoid muscles:
Lateral
Posterior

Mucous membrane (cut)

Internal branch of superior laryngeal nerve and superior laryngeal artery

Inferior laryngeal nerve and artery

Recurrent laryngeal nerve

Inferior thyroid artery (cut)

D

Figure 1.11C,D. Laryngeal Muscles and Neurovascular Supply. **C.** Sagittal Section. **D.** Posterior View.

4. **Arytenoideus muscle**
   a. Oblique and transverse fibers
   b. Oblique arytenoid
      i. Origin: lies superficial to transverse arytenoid and extends from base near muscular process of arytenoid cartilage
      ii. Insertion: apex of opposite arytenoid cartilage on opposite side; superior extension, called *aryepiglottic muscle*, continues into aryepiglottic folds and reaches epiglottic cartilage
      iii. Action: adduct arytenoid cartilages, pulling them closer together and forming sphincter of laryngeal aditus by tightening aryepiglottic folds, to help prevent foreign bodies from entering vestibule; important in process of swallowing
   c. Transverse arytenoid muscle
      i. Origin: posterior surface of arytenoid cartilage
      ii. Insertion: posterior surface of opposite arytenoid
      iii. Action: adducts arytenoid cartilages
5. **Thyroarytenoid muscle**
   a. Origin: inner surface of thyroid lamina near laryngeal prominence
   b. Insertion: passes posteriorly to insert on arytenoid cartilage on its anterior and lateral surfaces
   c. Action: pulls arytenoid cartilage anteriorly, thereby decreasing tension on vocal cords
   d. 2 specialized portions, vocalis and thyroepiglottic muscles
   e. **Vocalis muscle**: inner fibers of thyroarytenoid that attach onto vocal ligament and selectively relax precise segments of vocal ligament to fine-tune pitch
   f. **Thyroepiglottic muscle**: extends from upper portion of thyroarytenoid into aryepiglottic folds where they blend with aryepiglottics and insert, in part, into quadrangular membrane and into epiglottic cartilage; part of sphincteric mechanism of laryngeal inlet and vestibule

III. Summary of Muscle Actions

A. 2 types of laryngeal muscles described
   1. Tensor muscles: stretch or relax vocal cords
   2. Positioning muscles: determine width of rima glottidis by way of arytenoid cartilages
B. Altering tension on vocal cords
   1. Cricothyroid: increases tension on vocal cords, preparing for phonation
   2. Thyroarytenoid muscles decrease tension of vocal cords; vocalis muscle, due to attachment to vocal ligament, allows for selective relaxation of part of vocal cord rather than entire cord
C. Opening and closing rima glottidis
   1. Arytenoid cartilages rotate and glide on cricoid lamina
   2. Lateral cricoarytenoid muscles close glottis by pulling laterally on muscular processes and moving vocal processes medially, adducting vocal cords
   3. Transverse and oblique arytenoid muscles help lateral arytenoids in this action by bringing arytenoid cartilages closer to each other in gliding motion
   4. Posterior cricoarytenoid muscles open glottis by pulling muscular process posteriorly and medially, rotating vocal process laterally, abducting vocal cords
D. Closing larynx during swallowing
   1. Epiglottis does not fall down over opening of larynx like a "trapdoor," due in part to attachment of hyoepiglottic ligament
   2. Upward motion of thyroid cartilage under epiglottis primarily responsible for closing inlet
   3. Elevation of thyroid cartilage accomplished by thyrohyoid, salpingopharyngeus, palatopharyngeus, and stylopharyngeus

4. Laryngeal inlet is further protected by action of thyroepiglottic and aryepiglottic muscles in pulling epiglottis inferiorly

5. Because breath is held during swallowing, rima glottidis is closed by action of transverse and oblique arytenoid muscles and lateral cricoarytenoid muscles

6. Note: a large part of epiglottis may be removed without interfering unduly with process of swallowing

E. Larynx in respiration

1. In quiet respiration and in whispering: vocal cords are slightly abducted and somewhat curved, and arytenoid cartilages are also apart, allowing for fair-sized slit at rima glottidis

2. During medium respiration: intermembranous and intercartilaginous parts are opened slightly due to traction of posterior cricoarytenoid muscles, and entire rima forms acute-angled triangle

3. In forced respiration: rima glottidis is widened as much as possible, which means arytenoid cartilages are pulled laterally and vocal processes rotated laterally by posterior cricoarytenoid muscles (abducting the vocal cords); intermembranous and intercartilaginous parts of rima glottidis are opened to form rhombus shape due to extreme traction of posterior cricoarytenoid muscles

F. Larynx in voice production

1. Initially, rima glottidis is closed, which represents phonation position, and the vocal folds are simultaneously stretched; they are caused to vibrate by expiratory blast of air current, which produces sound waves

2. During phonation, except for lowest tones, vocal cords become straight and move together to meet near midline; this is created by action of several muscles simultaneously

   a. Cricothyroids stretch and tighten the cords and folds because they tilt thyroid and cricoid cartilages upon each other anteriorly

   b. Lateral cricoarytenoids adduct vocal cords by swinging vocal processes together

   c. Vocalis portion of thyroarytenoid muscle apparently acts differentially on vocal fold so that selected portion of cord vibrates

3. Volume: determined by strength of air current

4. Pitch: determined by frequency of vibrations; controlled by length, tension, and thickness of vocal folds, which are coarsely adjusted by cricothyroid muscles and muscles attached to muscular process of arytenoids and then fine-tuned by vocalis muscles; anterior ends of cords vibrate for highest tones, and as progressively lower tones are produced, longer and longer anterior segments of folds vibrate

5. Resonators: beginning at glottis are cavities of ventricle, vestibule, pharynx, mouth, and nose including paranasal sinuses; air column vibrating in these passages determines timbre or quality of tone; air passages altered by movements of soft palate, tongue, lips, and pharynx and supraglottic portion of larynx; larynx as a whole also raised or lowered (raised for high tones, lowered for low tones) so that pharynx, part of resonating chamber above larynx, is altered in length for different tones

G. Larynx in coughing: closed rima glottidis opened by explosive expiration of air

IV. Nerves of Larynx

A. Sensory innervation to mucous membranes and motor supply to intrinsic muscles

B. Sensory nerve supply

1. Cell bodies of nerve fibers that supply sensory fibers to mucous membrane of larynx in inferior (nodose) ganglion of vagus CN X

2. Supraglottic portion (above vocal cords): supplied by internal branch of superior laryngeal nerve (from vagus CN X)

3. Infraglottic portion: supplied by recurrent laryngeal nerves

C. Motor nerve supply
   1. Cell bodies in nucleus ambiguus of brainstem; carried by branches of vagus (CN X)
   2. **External branch of superior laryngeal nerve** (from vagus CN X): innervates cricothyroid muscle
   3. **Recurrent laryngeal nerve** (from vagus CN X): supplies all other laryngeal muscles via its inferior laryngeal nerve (continuation within larynx)

V. Vessels of Larynx

A. **Superior laryngeal artery**
   1. From superior thyroid artery
   2. Accompanies internal branch of superior laryngeal nerve through thyrohyoid membrane
B. **Inferior laryngeal artery**
   1. From inferior thyroid artery
   2. Ascends on back of larynx, under inferior pharyngeal constrictor
   3. Accompanied by recurrent laryngeal nerve
C. Veins: follow same pattern as arteries

VI. Lymphatic Drainage of Larynx

A. Supraglottic portion: lymphatics pierce thyrohyoid membrane and empty into infrahyoid nodes and upper deep cervical nodes
B. Infraglottic portion: follow blood vessels to reach nodes anterior and lateral to larynx and trachea; namely, prelaryngeal, pretracheal, and paratracheal nodes
C. Vocal folds
   1. Some suggest very sparsely formed, fine lymphatic capillary network exists here, which may connect to lymphatic tracts of supraglottic region and with lower regional lymphatic vessels and that there are also connections with opposite side for vessels existing near median plane
   2. Others believe vocal cords have no lymphatic vessels
   3. Either way, edematous, swollen folds take time to return to normal, and tumors in this area can be long confined before metastasizing

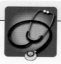

VII. Clinical Considerations

A. **Valsalva maneuver**
   1. Contraction of thoracic and abdominal wall muscles, accompanied by forced closure of glottis, results in marked increase in intrapleural intra-abdominal pressure
   2. Used for urination, defecation childbirth, and lifting heavy objects
   3. Glottic closure necessary because otherwise, pressure in chest and abdomen would be dissipated as air escapes through trachea
B. **Thyroidectomy**: may result in injury to recurrent laryngeal nerves because each nerve is closely related to posterior aspect of gland just before they enter larynx; external branch of superior laryngeal nerve is in jeopardy when superior thyroid vessels are ligated
C. Superior laryngeal nerve damage
   1. Internal branch of superior laryngeal nerve: at great risk when surgery on common carotid artery is performed for atherosclerosis
   2. External branch of superior laryngeal nerve: if damaged, cricothyroid muscle cannot tense vocal cord, causing hoarseness and easy tiring of voice
D. Recurrent laryngeal nerve damage
   1. Because recurrent laryngeal nerve innervates all muscles concerned with movement of vocal cords except for cricothyroid, paralysis of this nerve produces paralysis of vocal cord on 1 side
   2. Paralyzed cord is at first bowed outward and cannot be abducted or adducted and normal vocal cord cannot meet it, causing poor voice

3. Over time, paralyzed cord may gradually move toward the midline, with consequent improvement of voice even to seeming normalcy
4. Paralysis of left recurrent laryngeal nerve may occur as result of mediastinal lesion because nerve turns upward around arch of aorta, or either nerve may be interrupted in neck
5. **Bilateral vocal cord paralysis**
    a. Voice is nearly lost because cords cannot be moved together
    b. Over time, bilaterally paralyzed cords gradually become less bowed and tend to move toward each other through pull of unparalyzed cricothyroid muscles
    c. Voice improves as adduction increases, but cords cannot be abducted and airway simultaneously narrowed
    d. If narrowing becomes too severe, surgery to remove arytenoid cartilage is possible
E. Glottic edema: fluid accumulation in mucosal connective tissue of laryngeal inlet and vestibule can lead to suffocation
F. Incomplete moistening of vocal folds can lead to hoarseness

Pharynx: Parts and Relations

I. General Features (Fig. 1.12A,B)

A. 13–15 cm long fibromuscular tube

B. Lined by mucous membrane

C. Extends from base of skull superiorly to esophagus inferiorly

D. Has posterior and lateral (narrow) walls, but no anterior wall because it is directly continuous anteriorly with nasal cavity, oral cavity, and larynx

E. Serves for passage of both air and food; air passage always open except during swallowing process

F. Located in midline anterior to vertebral column and prevertebral musculature

G. 3 parts
   1. Nasal part (nasopharynx or epipharynx)
   2. Oral part (oropharynx)
   3. Laryngeal part (laryngopharynx or hypopharynx)

II. Parts of Pharynx (Fig. 1.12C)

A. **Nasopharynx**
   1. Mucosa of roof is attached to base of occipital bone, at apex of petrous part of temporal bone and at sphenoid bone
   2. **Choanae**: openings between nasal cavities and nasopharynx
   3. Opening of **auditory tube** (pharyngotympanic or Eustachian tube)
      a. Unites tympanic cavity with pharynx
      b. Opening surrounded at posterior and superior circumference by elevation, **torus tubarius**, which is formed by free end of tubal cartilage
      c. Posterior lip continued down into **salpingopharyngeal fold**, containing **salpingopharyngeus muscle**, which arises from free end of tubal cartilage and passes in fold to lateral wall of pharynx
      d. Lower part of tubal opening bordered by **torus levatorius** produced by levator veli palatini muscle
   4. **Pharyngeal recess** (**fossa of Rosenmuller**): posterior to torus tubarius
   5. **Pharyngeal tonsils** (**adenoids**)
      a. Lymphatic tissue located on roof and upper posterior wall of nasopharynx
      b. Upper part of discontinuous lymphatic tonsillar ring (with palatine and lingual tonsils) called **Waldeyer's ring** of lymphoid tissue, which surrounds entrance to pharynx (palatine and lingual tonsils are features of oral cavity, discussed in Chapter 2)
   6. **Pharyngeal isthmus**
      a. Boundary between naso- and oropharynx
      b. Anteriorly, margins of soft palate; and posteriorly, posterior wall of pharynx

B. **Oropharynx**
   1. Boundaries
      a. Superiorly: level of soft palate; continuous above with nasopharynx
      b. Anteriorly: continuous with oral cavity at palatopharyngeal folds or arches, which mark posterior edge of tonsillar pillars (also called *isthmus of fauces*)
      c. Inferiorly: level of hyoid bone (although superior tip of epiglottis is sometimes used); continuous with laryngopharynx
   2. **Palatopharyngeus muscle**
      a. Arises from palatal aponeurosis and pterygoid hamulus and passes down in palatopharyngeal fold (arch) on inner surface of superior pharyngeal constrictor
      b. Inserts on posterior edge of thyroid cartilage; other fibers pass into posterior pharyngeal wall
      c. Action: forms sling with its opposite muscle, which lifts larynx and posterior pharyngeal wall; strongest elevator of larynx

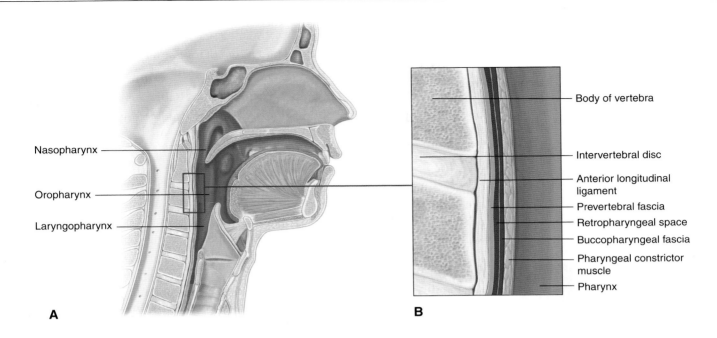

Nasopharynx

Oropharynx

Laryngopharynx

A

Body of vertebra

Intervertebral disc

Anterior longitudinal ligament

Prevertebral fascia

Retropharyngeal space

Buccopharyngeal fascia

Pharyngeal constrictor muscle

Pharynx

B

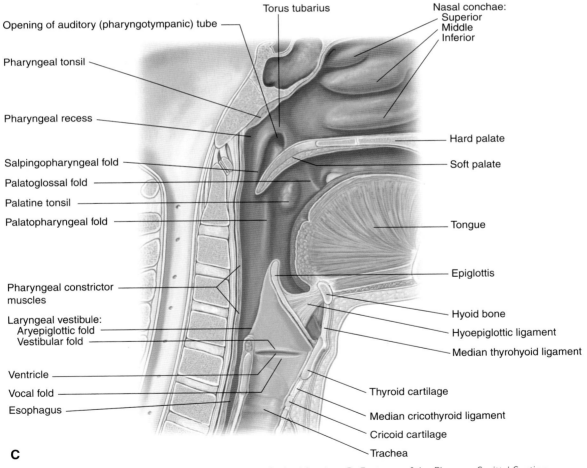

Torus tubarius

Nasal conchae:
Superior
Middle
Inferior

Opening of auditory (pharyngotympanic) tube

Pharyngeal tonsil

Pharyngeal recess

Hard palate

Salpingopharyngeal fold

Soft palate

Palatoglossal fold

Palatine tonsil

Palatopharyngeal fold

Tongue

Epiglottis

Pharyngeal constrictor muscles

Hyoid bone

Laryngeal vestibule:
Aryepiglottic fold
Vestibular fold

Hyoepiglottic ligament

Median thyrohyoid ligament

Ventricle

Vocal fold

Esophagus

Thyroid cartilage

Median cricothyroid ligament

Cricoid cartilage

Trachea

C

Figure 1.12A–C. A,B. Parts of the Pharynx, Sagittal Section. **C.** Features of the Pharynx, Sagittal Section.

3. **Median** and **lateral glossoepiglottic folds**: mucosal folds passing from epiglottis to root of tongue

4. **Epiglottic valleculae**: depressions located between root of tongue and epiglottis, framed by glossoepiglottic folds

C. **Laryngopharynx**

1. Boundaries
   a. Superiorly: level of hyoid bone (or epiglottis, according to some sources)
   b. Anteriorly: laryngeal inlet (aditus) and posterior wall of larynx
   c. Inferiorly: continuous with esophagus at lower border of cricoid cartilage

2. Piriform recesses
   a. Fossae posterolateral to laryngeal inlet of larynx
   b. Lies against thyrohyoid membrane and inner surface of superolateral portion of thyroid lamina
   c. Anterior wall of piriform recess has mucosal fold, fold of laryngeal nerve, for internal branch of superior laryngeal nerve and superior laryngeal artery

III. Clinical Considerations

A. **Adenoiditis**: inflammation of pharyngeal tonsil, with potential obstruction of airflow and consequent noisy breathing, often leading to mouth breathing; severe obstruction of airway or recurrent infection may require surgical intervention; inflamed pharyngeal tonsil may additionally obstruct auditory tube, leading to recurrent middle ear infections (otitis media)

B. **Retropharyngeal abscess**: inflammation of posterior pharyngeal wall can increase distance between air column in pharynx and anterior edge of vertebral column (seen in lateral neck X-ray); likely source for infected area or abscess in patient with fever, pain on swallowing and respiratory distress without any other possible source of problem

C. **Posterior rhinoscopy**: choanae and posterior part of nasal cavities seen through mouth and nasopharynx with laryngoscope

D. **Pharyngeal cysts**: during development, when lateral wall of neck does not close and cervical sinus or space beneath skin surface persists, branchial or pharyngeal cyst (which has the potential of becoming inflamed and filling with fluid) may occur; if also open externally, called **lateral cervical fistula**

E. **Pharyngeal fistula**: quite rare and due to 2nd pharyngeal pouch and cleft remaining confluent with each other during development and thus staying open at both ends, producing fistula; external opening in lateral part of neck and internal opening in region of palatine tonsillar bed

Pharynx: Muscles and Neurovasculature

I. Muscles of Pharynx and Soft Palate (Fig. 1.13A,B)

Muscle	Origin	Insertion	Action	Nerve
Stylopharyngeus	Styloid process of temporal bone	Posterior and superior border of thyroid cartilage and pharyngeal wall	Elevates pharynx and larynx during swallowing and speaking	Glossopharyngeal nerve (CN IX)
Palatopharyngeus	Posterior margin of bony palate, palatine aponeurosis	Posterior border of thyroid cartilage; posterior wall of pharynx	Elevates pharynx and larynx during swallowing and speaking	Vagus nerve (CN X) via pharyngeal plexus
Salpingopharyngeus	Inferior surface of anteromedial end of auditory tube cartilage	Superior border of thyroid cartilage and pharyngeal wall; blends with palatopharyngeus	Elevates pharynx and larynx during swallowing and speaking	Vagus nerve (CN X) via pharyngeal plexus
Superior pharyngeal constrictor	Medial pterygoid plate, pterygoid hamulus, pterygomandibular raphe, mylohyoid line of mandible	Pharyngeal tubercle on basilar part of occipital bone and midline pharyngeal raphe	Constricts pharyngeal cavity	Vagus nerve (CN X) via pharyngeal plexus
Middle pharyngeal constrictor	Greater and lesser horns of hyoid bone, inferior part of stylohyoid ligament	Midline pharyngeal raphe	Constricts pharyngeal cavity	Vagus nerve (CN X) via pharyngeal plexus
Inferior pharyngeal constrictor	Oblique line of thyroid cartilage, lateral surface of cricoid cartilage	Midline pharyngeal raphe; cricopharyngeal part encircles pharyngoesophageal junction	Constricts pharyngeal cavity	Vagus nerve (CN X) via pharyngeal plexus and external branch of superior laryngeal nerve
Levator veli palatini	Apex of petrous part of temporal bone and medial surface of auditory tube cartilage	Muscles and fascia of soft palate; palatine aponeurosis	Elevates soft palate	Vagus nerve (CN X) via pharyngeal plexus
Tensor veli palatini	Scaphoid fossa, lateral wall of auditory tube cartilage	Palatine aponeurosis	Opens auditory tube; tenses soft palate	Mandibular division of trigeminal nerve (CN V3)
Musculus uvulae	Posterior nasal spine	Mucosa of uvula	Shortens uvula	Vagus nerve (CN X) via pharyngeal plexus
Palatoglossus	Palatine aponeurosis	Side of tongue, entering from above	Elevates and retracts tongue	Vagus nerve (CN X) via pharyngeal plexus
Palatopharyngeus	Posterior margin of bony palate and palatine aponeurosis	Posterior wall of pharynx and posterior margin of thyroid cartilage	Elevates larynx	Vagus nerve (CN X) via pharyngeal plexus

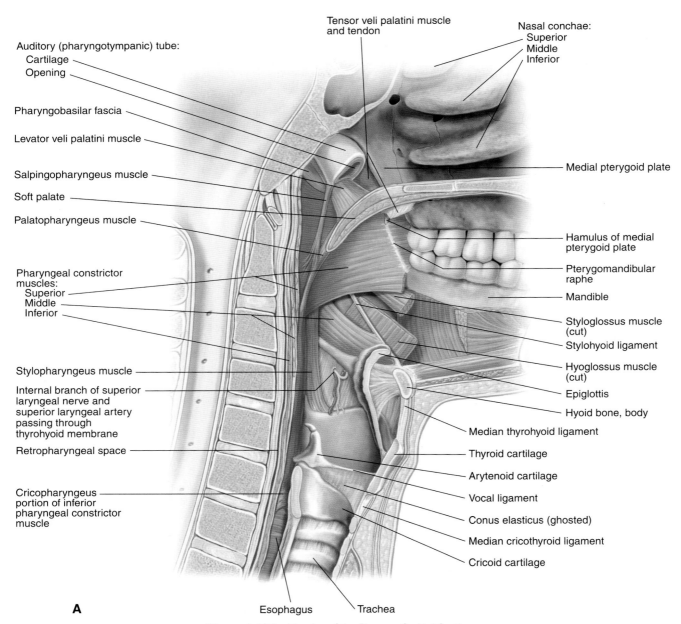

Figure 1.13A. Muscles of the Pharynx, Sagittal Section.

II. Special Features (Fig. 1.13C,D)

A. Pharyngeal wall: 4 layers, from inside to outside

  1. Mucous membrane layer

    a. Composed of pseudostratified, columnar epithelium, some areas being ciliated, others not

    b. Mixed glands lie in mucosal lamina propria lining pharyngeal roof and around laryngeal inlet, whereas many mucosal glands are found in rest of pharyngeal mucosa

  2. Submucosal layer (**pharyngobasilar fascia**)

    a. Continues superiorly above upper border of superior constrictor, underlies all pharyngeal muscles

    b. Penetrated there by auditory tube opening into nasopharynx

  3. Muscle layer

    a. 3 pharyngeal constrictors (superior, middle, inferior), which overlap like nested flowerpots

    b. 3 longitudinal muscles (stylopharyngeus, palatopharyngeus, salpingopharyngeus), which primarily elevate larynx during swallowing

    c. **Cricopharyngeus muscle**

      i. Lowest part of inferior pharyngeal constrictor

      ii. Serves as sphincter between pharynx and esophagus to prevent regurgitation

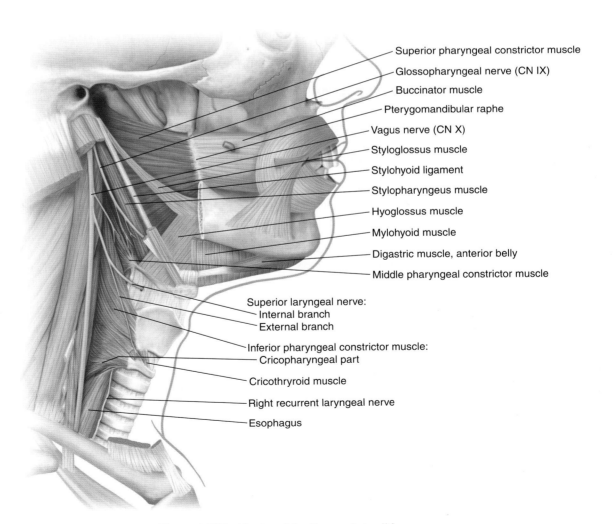

B

Figure 1.13B. Muscles of the Pharynx, Lateral View.

4. Deep fascial layer (buccopharyngeal fascia)
   a. Covers pharyngeal muscles posteriorly
   b. Anterior boundary of retropharyngeal space

B. Recesses
   1. **Pharyngeal recess**: posterolateral to torus tubarius
   2. **Epiglottic valleculae**: depressions between root of tongue and epiglottis
   3. **Piriform recesses**: posterolateral to laryngeal inlet

C. Soft palate
   1. Moveable fibromuscular posterior projection from hard palate
   2. Made up of skeletal muscles (tensor veli palatini, levator veli palatini, musculus uvulae) covered by mucous membrane; contains many mucous (palatine) glands in submucosa
   3. **Uvula**: median projection from posterior free end
   4. During swallowing, uvula presses against arched posterior wall of pharynx and closes off food pathway from nasopharynx
   5. Supplied by **lesser palatine vessels** (from 3rd part of maxillary) and ascending palatine artery (from facial artery)
   6. Nerves: sensory fibers via lesser palatine nerves (from maxillary nerve, CN V_2); sympathetic fibers from superior cervical ganglion; parasympathetics from pterygopalatine ganglion (from CN VII) for supply of glands, smooth muscle, and blood vessels
   7. Muscles
      a. All innervated by CN X, except tensor veli palatini (mandibular division, CN V_3)
      b. **Levator veli palatini**: main action to lift soft palate
      c. **Tensor veli palatini**: opens auditory tube; tenses soft palate
      d. **Musculus uvulae**: helps close off nasopharynx during swallowing
      e. **Palatoglossus muscle**: closes off opening of oral pharynx by pulling tongue up and tensing palate
      f. **Palatopharyngeus muscle**: either lifts larynx during swallowing or tenses soft palate

III. Neurovasculature of Pharynx

A. Arteries
   1. Ascending pharyngeal artery from external carotid artery
   2. Ascending palatine and tonsillar branches of facial artery
   3. Descending palatine and pharyngeal branches of maxillary artery
   4. Inferior thyroid artery

B. Veins
   1. Form **pharyngeal plexus** on either surface of muscle layer (Note: pharyngeal plexus of nerves also exists)
   2. These plexuses drain to pterygoid plexus and into internal jugular vein; make connections with meningeal veins

C. Lymph vessels: drain from pharynx and pharyngeal tonsil into retropharyngeal and upper deep lateral cervical nodes

D. Nerves
   1. Glossopharyngeal nerve (CN IX): innervates stylopharyngeus muscle (derived from 3rd branchial arch)
   2. Vagus nerve (CN X): pharyngeal branch innervates all other muscles of pharynx; external branch of superior laryngeal nerve (from CN X) helps innervate inferior pharyngeal constrictor muscle
   3. **Pharyngeal plexus**: branches of glossopharyngeal nerve, vagus nerve, maxillary division of trigeminal nerve, and sympathetic fibers form plexus, which provides sensory, motor, and autonomic innervation to pharynx
   4. Sensory supply
      a. Mucous membrane receives most sensory supply from glossopharyngeal nerve
      b. Nasopharynx receives pharyngeal branches of maxillary division of CN V
      c. Laryngopharynx receives pharyngeal branches from internal branch of superior laryngeal nerve and recurrent laryngeal nerve

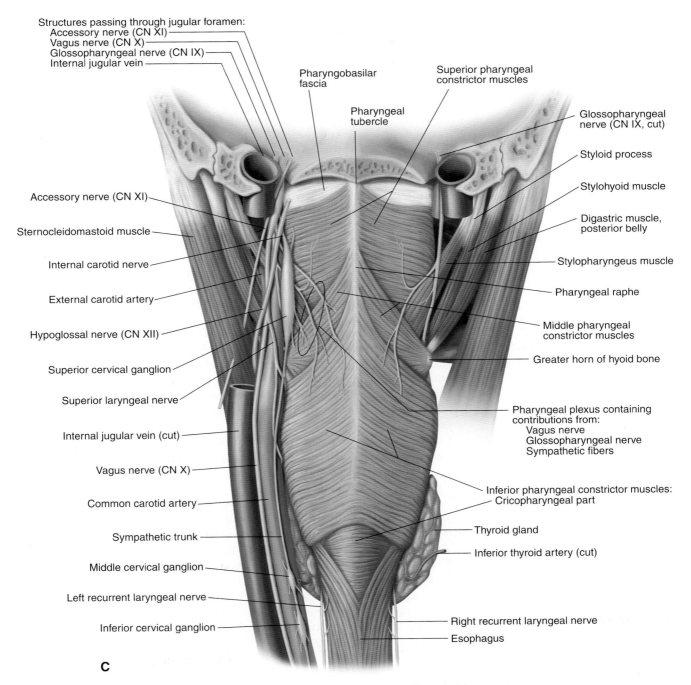

Structures passing through jugular foramen:
Accessory nerve (CN XI)
Vagus nerve (CN X)
Glossopharyngeal nerve (CN IX)
Internal jugular vein

Pharyngobasilar fascia

Superior pharyngeal constrictor muscles

Pharyngeal tubercle

Glossopharyngeal nerve (CN IX, cut)

Styloid process

Stylohyoid muscle

Digastric muscle, posterior belly

Accessory nerve (CN XI)

Sternocleidomastoid muscle

Internal carotid nerve

External carotid artery

Hypoglossal nerve (CN XII)

Superior cervical ganglion

Superior laryngeal nerve

Internal jugular vein (cut)

Vagus nerve (CN X)

Common carotid artery

Sympathetic trunk

Middle cervical ganglion

Left recurrent laryngeal nerve

Inferior cervical ganglion

Stylopharyngeus muscle

Pharyngeal raphe

Middle pharyngeal constrictor muscles

Greater horn of hyoid bone

Pharyngeal plexus containing contributions from:
Vagus nerve
Glossopharyngeal nerve
Sympathetic fibers

Inferior pharyngeal constrictor muscles:
Cricopharyngeal part

Thyroid gland

Inferior thyroid artery (cut)

Right recurrent laryngeal nerve

Esophagus

C

Figure 1.13C. Muscles of the Pharynx, Posterior View.

IV. Clinical Considerations

A. Swallowing (deglutition)

1. Generally, reflex cessation of breathing also takes place for duration of act of swallowing

2. Complex act beginning with chewing and softening of food bolus by muscles of mastication and moistening with saliva

3. Tongue then compresses bolus against palate and forces it posteriorly by contraction of intrinsic muscles of tongue, which stiffen the tongue using palatoglossus muscle to elevate tongue against hard palate, and styloglossus muscle to retract tongue and move bolus of food backward along surface of palate

4. Soft palate made rigid by contraction of levator and tensor veli palatini muscles, which seals off nasopharynx from oropharynx when soft palate pressed against posterior wall of pharynx; posterior pharyngeal wall bulges forward at this level due to circumscribed contraction of superior pharyngeal constrictor muscles

5. Stylopharyngeus, salpingopharyngeus, and palatopharyngeus muscles contract and draw pharynx and larynx superiorly, while stylohyoid and digastric muscles elevate hyoid bone and by extension, the larynx; laryngeal inlet closed by elevation of larynx with assistance of thyrohyoid muscles (inlet brought closer to epiglottis); larynx is compressed upward against epiglottis and laryngeal opening is blocked, permitting food bolus to slide posteriorly and inferiorly, passing over posterior aspect of closed larynx and into laryngopharynx

6. Most food glides through piriform recesses, but some also passes above epiglottis

7. Sequential contraction of pharyngeal constrictors forces food bolus inferiorly into esophagus; cricopharyngeal part of inferior constrictor (cricoesophageal sphincter) relaxes as swallowing is started and descending contraction of esophagus passes bolus into stomach (Note: swallowing reflex maintained when sleeping and ensured by several cranial nerves; afferents and efferents of reflex are coordinated by swallowing center in medulla oblongata)

8. In paralysis of soft palate (i.e., in diphtheria, an acute infection due to *Corynebacterium diphtheriae* and its toxin, affecting membranes of nose, throat, and larynx), food particles can make their way into nasal cavities; also occurs in cleft palate

9. "Swallowing the wrong way": can occur by voluntary disturbance of mechanism (i.e., attempting to eat while swallowing)

B. **Pharyngitis** (sore throat): inflammation of pharynx

C. Other conditions

1. **Pharyngismus** (pharyngeal muscle spasms)
2. **Pharyngodynia** (pain in the pharynx)
3. **Pharyngostenosis** (narrowing of the pharynx)
4. **Pharyngoplegia** (paralysis of the pharynx)
5. **Pharyngomycosis** (infection of the pharynx)

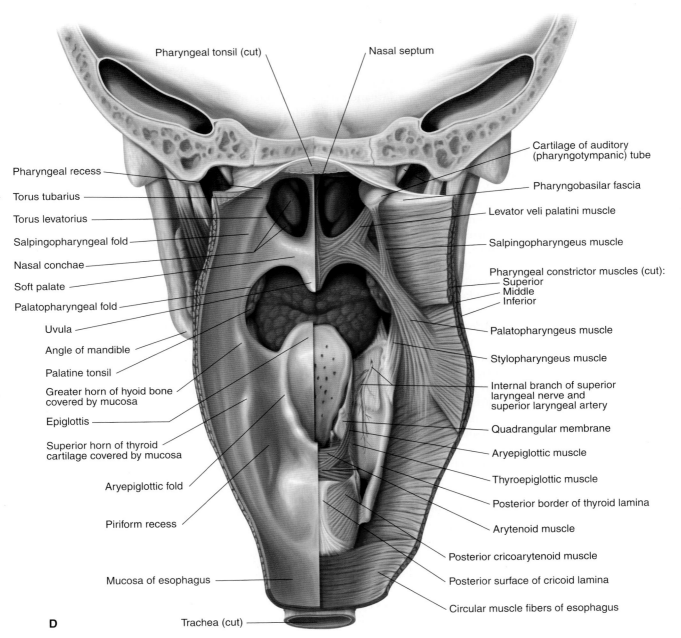

Pharyngeal tonsil (cut)

Nasal septum

Cartilage of auditory (pharyngotympanic) tube

Pharyngeal recess

Torus tubarius

Torus levatorius

Salpingopharyngeal fold

Nasal conchae

Soft palate

Palatopharyngeal fold

Uvula

Angle of mandible

Palatine tonsil

Greater horn of hyoid bone covered by mucosa

Epiglottis

Superior horn of thyroid cartilage covered by mucosa

Aryepiglottic fold

Piriform recess

Mucosa of esophagus

Trachea (cut)

Pharyngobasilar fascia

Levator veli palatini muscle

Salpingopharyngeus muscle

Pharyngeal constrictor muscles (cut):
Superior
Middle
Inferior

Palatopharyngeus muscle

Stylopharyngeus muscle

Internal branch of superior laryngeal nerve and superior laryngeal artery

Quadrangular membrane

Aryepiglottic muscle

Thyroepiglottic muscle

Posterior border of thyroid lamina

Arytenoid muscle

Posterior cricoarytenoid muscle

Posterior surface of cricoid lamina

Circular muscle fibers of esophagus

D

Figure 1.13D. Muscles of the Pharynx, Opened, Posterior View.

Lymphatics of Head and Neck

I. Lymphatic Drainage of Head (Fig. 1.14)

A. Scalp: 3 primary drainage areas
  1. Frontal: ending in preauricular and parotid nodes
  2. Temporal and parietal: ending in parotid and retroauricular nodes
  3. Occipital: ending in occipital and deep cervical nodes
B. External ear: drain into pre- and retroauricular nodes and superficial and deep cervical nodes
C. Face
  1. Eyelids and conjunctiva: to submandibular and parotid nodes
  2. Cheek: to parotid and submandibular nodes
  3. Side of nose, upper lip, and lateral lower lip: to submandibular nodes
  4. Medial lower lip: into submental nodes
  5. Temporal and infratemporal fossae: into deep facial and deep cervical nodes

II. Lymph Nodes of Head

A. **Occipital**
  1. Back of head close to edge of trapezius
  2. Afferents from scalp at back of head
  3. Efferents to superior deep cervical nodes
B. **Retroauricular**
  1. At insertion of SCM on mastoid
  2. Afferents from posterior temporal and parietal regions
  3. Efferents to superior deep cervical nodes
C. **Preauricular**
  1. In front of tragus of ear
  2. Afferents from pinna and temporal region
  3. Efferents to superior deep cervical nodes
D. **Parotid**
  1. 2 sets, either embedded in gland or just below it
  2. Afferents from root of nose, eyelids, anterior temporal region, and external auditory meatus
  3. Efferents to superior deep cervical nodes
E. **Facial**: 3 sets
  1. Infraorbital, buccal, and mandibular
  2. Afferents from eyelids, conjunctiva, skin of nose, nasal mucosa, and cheek
  3. Efferents to submandibular nodes

III. Lymph Nodes of Neck

A. **Submandibular**
  1. Under body of mandible
  2. Afferents from cheek, nose, upper lip, lower lip, and facial and submental nodes
  3. Efferents to superior deep cervical nodes
B. **Submental**
  1. Between anterior bellies of digastric
  2. Afferents from central lower lip and floor of mouth
  3. Efferents to submandibular and deep cervical nodes

C. **Superficial cervical**
   1. Along external jugular vein
   2. Afferents from ear and parotid region
   3. Efferents to superior deep cervical nodes
D. **Deep cervical**
   1. Along carotid sheath; separated by crossing of inferior belly of omohyoid muscle into superior and inferior deep cervical nodes
   2. Superior
      a. Beneath SCM muscle, along accessory nerve and internal jugular vein
      b. Afferents from back of head and neck, tongue, larynx, thyroid, palate, nose, esophagus, and all nodes except inferior deep cervical
      c. Efferents to inferior deep cervical nodes and jugular lymph trunk
      d. **Jugulodigastric node**: located behind posterior belly of digastric muscle; receives lymph from oropharynx and palatine tonsils; may enlarge with infection of throat or tonsils
      e. **Jugulo-omohyoid node**: located superior to inferior belly of omohyoid, which separates superior and inferior deep cervical nodes; receives submental lymph drainage; may enlarge with infection of lips or anterior oral cavity
   3. Inferior
      a. Also called **supraclavicular nodes**; extend lateral to border of SCM, close to subclavian vein
      b. Afferents from superior deep cervical nodes, superficial pectoral region, and part of arm
      c. Efferents join efferents of superior deep cervical nodes to form jugular lymph trunk

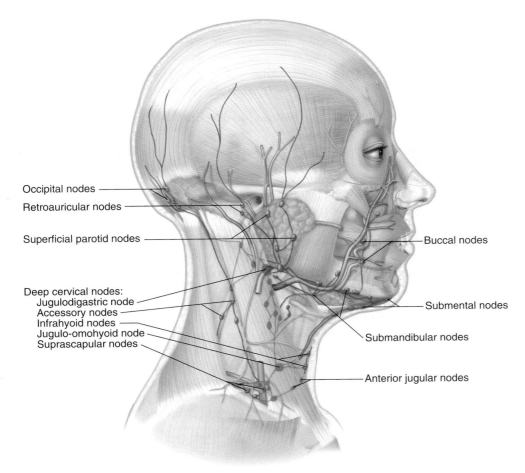

Occipital nodes
Retroauricular nodes
Superficial parotid nodes
Deep cervical nodes:
Jugulodigastric node
Accessory nodes
Infrahyoid nodes
Jugulo-omohyoid node
Suprascapular nodes

Buccal nodes
Submental nodes
Submandibular nodes
Anterior jugular nodes

Figure 1.14. Lymphatics of the Head and Neck, Lateral View.

IV. Jugular Lymph Trunk

A. Formed by union of deep cervical lymph vessels

B. Termination

  1. On right, usually unites with subclavian and bronchomediastinal lymph trunks to form right lymphatic duct, which empties into junction of internal jugular and subclavian veins

  2. On left, empties into thoracic duct

V. Thoracic and Right Lymphatic Ducts

A. Thoracic duct

  1. Arises deep to right crus of diaphragm

  2. Ascends through posterior mediastinum between azygos vein and descending thoracic aorta

  3. Deviates to left side of esophagus at level of sternal angle to continue ascent into root of neck

  4. Anterior to 7th cervical vertebra, arches anterolaterally over left subclavian artery to reach posterior aspect of union of left internal jugular vein and subclavian vein to drain

  5. Usually receives jugular, subclavian, and bronchomediastinal lymph trunk near termination

B. Right lymphatic duct

  1. Formed by union of jugular, subclavian, and bronchomediastinal lymph trunks

  2. Very short, terminates into union of right internal jugular and subclavian veins

VI. Clinical Considerations

A. Enlarged supraclavicular nodes on left side often seen with intra-abdominal cancers of stomach and colon; tumors of gonads may also be involved

B. Most scalp and forehead lymph drains to superficial (collar chain) ring of nodes found at junction of head and neck; some drain directly into deep cervical nodes

C. Clinically, 6 lymph node regions are described and numbered

  1. Submental (zone 1)

  2. Upper jugular (zone 2)

  3. Middle jugular (zone 3)

  4. Lower jugular (zone 4)

  5. Posterior triangle group (zone 5)

  6. Anterior compartment group (zone 6)

D. May also be described clinically as **2 horizontal chains**, divided into **superior** and **inferior group**, and a **vertical chain** consisting of **posterior cervical nodes**, **intermediate (jugular) nodes**, and **anterior (visceral) nodes**

  1. **Superior horizontal chain**: 5 groups of nodes encircling base of head; includes submental, submandibular, preauricular (parotid); postauricular (mastoid); and occipital nodes

  2. **Inferior horizontal chain**: supraclavicular nodes, which lie in subclavian triangle and receive afferents from upper limb, thoracic wall, and superior nodal groups of vertical chain; efferents enter either jugular or subclavian trunks; these nodes have also been called **scalene nodes** because many lie anterior to anterior scalene muscle and are important in diagnosis of thoracic diseases insofar as bronchomediastinal trunk may drain into these nodes before entering thoracic or right lymphatic duct

3. **Vertical chain**: consists of 3 longitudinal groups of nodes in cervical region
   a. **Posterior cervical nodes**: located in relation to external jugular vein and CN XI in posterior triangle
      i. Superficial: usually 1 or 2 nodes along external jugular vein as it crosses SCM muscle
      ii. Deep: associated with CN XI where nerve enters posterior triangle at posterior border of SCM muscle
   b. **Intermediate (jugular) nodes**: extend along internal jugular vein
      i. **Juguloparotid (subparotid)**: near angle of mandible
      ii. **Jugulodigastric (subdigastric)**: at junction of common facial with internal jugular vein
      iii. **Jugulocarotid (bifurcation)**: at bifurcation of common carotid artery
      iv. **Jugulo-omohyoid**: where omohyoid crosses internal jugular vein
   c. **Anterior (visceral)**: related to pharynx, esophagus, larynx, trachea, and adjacent viscera
      i. **Parapharyngeal**: nodes along lateral pharyngeal wall and in retropharyngeal space; afferents from deep in face and upper digestive tract
      ii. **Paralaryngeal:** from larynx and thyroid gland
      iii. **Paratracheal:** from thyroid gland, trachea, and esophagus
      iv. **Prelaryngeal** (Delphian node): on cricothyroid ligament; from thyroid and larynx
      v. **Pretracheal:** continuous with mediastinal group of nodes as is paratracheal

Head

Surface Anatomy of the Head

I. Palpable Features of Head (Fig. 2.1A–C)

A. **Frontal bone**
  1. Mostly palpable, except for orbital part
  2. Surface features
      a. **Frontal tuberosities**: prominences on forehead laterally, especially noticeable in infants
      b. **Superciliary arches**: variable ridges arching above supraorbital margins
      c. **Glabella**: midline union of superciliary arches; usually slightly depressed
      d. **Supraorbital margin**: may have palpable supraorbital notch
      e. **Pterion**: not easily palpable due to overlying temporalis muscle; lies at union of frontal and greater wing of sphenoid bone approximately 1 cm posterior to lateral orbital margin

B. **Zygomatic bone** ("cheekbone")
  1. Palpable on its anterolateral surface
  2. Surface features
      a. Unites with frontal bone to form lateral orbital margin
      b. Unites with temporal bone to form zygomatic arch

C. **Nasal bones** and cartilages
  1. Bones making bridge of nose palpable on anterior surfaces
  2. **Nasion**: midline depression where nasal bones meet frontal bone
  3. Anterior nasal cartilages are palpable

D. **Maxilla**
  1. Anterior surface palpable
  2. Surface features
      a. Forms infraorbital margin
      b. Helps to form nares or nostrils

E. **Mandible**
  1. Palpable along most of its anterolateral surface, except coronoid process
  2. Surface features
      a. **Mental protuberance**: chin, variably prominent
      b. Inferior border easily felt from chin to mandibular angle
      c. **Mandibular ramus** difficult to palpate due to overlying masseter muscle and parotid gland

F. **Temporal bone**
  1. Lateral portions are palpable
  2. Surface features
      a. **Zygomatic arch**: union with zygomatic bone
      b. **External acoustic meatus**: just posteroinferior to root of zygomatic arch
      c. **Mastoid process**: posteroinferior to external acoustic meatus
      d. **Squamous portion**: overlying temporalis muscle makes palpation difficult (except for posterior portion)

G. **Parietal bone**
  1. Palpable through scalp and upper temporalis muscle fibers
  2. Surface features
      a. **Bregma**: union of parietal and frontal bones; site of anterior fontanelle in newborns
      b. **Vertex**: highest point on top of skull, usually several cm posterior to bregma along midline sagittal suture

H. **Occipital bone**
  1. Only its highest portion palpable posterolaterally
  2. Surface features
      a. **External occipital protuberance** (**inion**): midline posterior projection
      b. **Superior nuchal lines**: extend laterally from inion toward mastoid process

II. Surface Topography of Vessels

A. Arteries

1. **Facial**: on line from premasseteric notch on inferior border of mandible (~3 cm from angle) to medial corner of eye; line passes 1 cm lateral to angle of mouth
2. **Superficial temporal**: runs upward just in front of ear, crossing posterior root of zygomatic arch
3. **Middle meningeal** and its anterior branch: by line beginning at midpoint of zygomatic arch, curving slightly forward, then back through pterion, then upward and backward toward vertex

B. Veins

1. **Internal jugular**: follows same line as internal carotid artery
2. **Superior sagittal sinus**: from nasion to external occipital protuberance, running in midsagittal plane
3. **Transverse sinus**: on line from external occipital protuberance laterally, approximating superior nuchal line, to point just posterosuperior to external auditory meatus

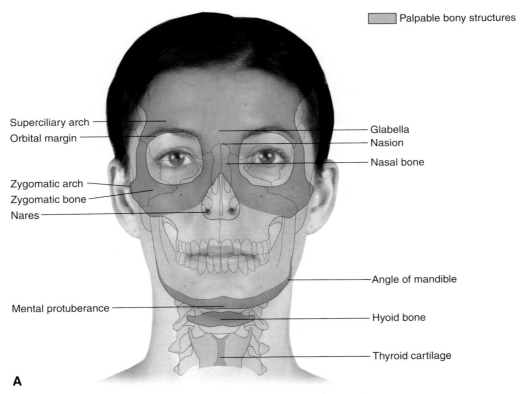

Figure 2.1A. Palpable Features of the Head.

III. Surface Topography of Viscera and Sinuses

A. Brain

1. **Lateral fissure**: begins at pterion with posterior ramus extending upward and backward to parietal eminence
2. **Central sulcus**: along line extending from point halfway between nasion and external occipital protuberance downward and forward to point 2 cm behind pterion
3. Base of cerebrum: lies 1 fingerbreadth above **Reid's line** (i.e., line drawn between lower border of orbit and center of external acoustic meatus)

B. Paranasal sinuses

1. Vary greatly in size, shape, and position
2. Frontal sinus: deep to superciliary arch
3. Maxillary sinus: occupies body of maxilla (i.e., area between orbit, nasal cavity, and upper teeth)

IV. Clinical Considerations

A. Forensic anthropology: sexual dimorphism of skull (rugosity of surface features, prominence of superciliary arches, glabella, etc.) used in forensic identification

B. Growth of face and jaw depends largely on teeth development and closely correlated with emergence of deciduous teeth and their replacement by permanent teeth; thus, jaw has growth spurt after completion of brain growth, after approximately year 6 and particularly at puberty

C. Insignificant asymmetries regularly seen in head and skull; in approximately 60% of cases, right 1/2 of face has slightly greater mass than left, probably due to random variations in growth

D. Natural asymmetry of any face must be distinguished from abnormal asymmetry resulting from paralysis, growth disturbances, inflammation, or tumors

E. Limit of facial hairiness (beard) and beginning of baldness in frontal region (frontal alopecia) can be symptoms of overproduction of male sex hormones in females (i.e., adrenal cortical tumors)

F. Obliteration of nasolabial fold can indicate inflammatory process in region of upper or lower jaw or sign of facial paralysis

G. "Bluish" discoloration of face (strong facial pallor) indicates oxygen deficiency of arterial blood, signaling possible circulatory collapse or strong sympathetic tone (reaction to fright)

H. Aging skin loses elasticity (resiliency); thus ridges and wrinkle lines (Langer's lines) appear in skin perpendicular to direction of facial muscle fibers; incisions along these lines tend to heal without scarring

I. Facial lacerations: tend to "gap" (part widely) because face has no distinct deep fascia and subcutaneous tissue between cutaneous attachment of facial muscles is loose

    a. Looseness of subcutaneous tissue allows fluid and blood to accumulate in loose connective tissue after facial bruising

    b. Facial inflammation results in much swelling

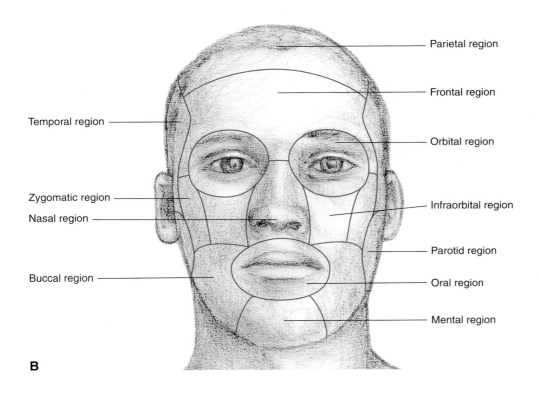

B

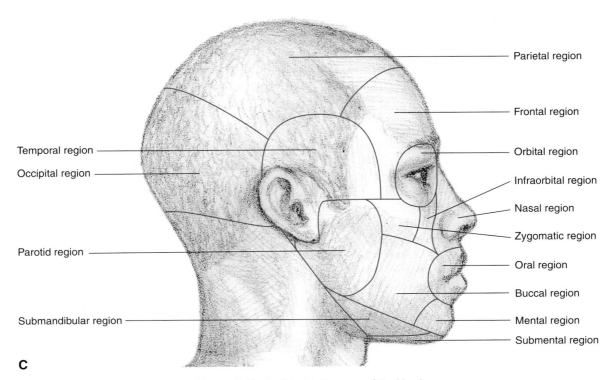

C

Figure 2.1B,C. Palpable Features of the Head.

Superficial Veins and Cutaneous Nerves of the Head

I. Superficial Veins of Head (Fig. 2.2A)

A. Supraorbital vein
 1. Drains scalp and forehead; communicates with superficial temporal vein laterally
 2. Sends branch through supraorbital notch to join superior ophthalmic vein and continues to join frontal vein, forming angular vein

B. Supratrochlear vein
 1. Drains forehead near midline
 2. Descends to medial angle of eye, where it joins supraorbital vein to form angular vein

C. Angular vein
 1. Runs down side of nose to level of lower orbit, where it becomes facial vein
 2. Receives tributaries from sides of nose and communicates, through nasofrontal vein at medial angle of orbit, with superior ophthalmic vein

D. Facial vein
 1. Continuation of angular vein
 2. Runs beneath facial muscles, crosses mandibular margin at premasseteric notch, passes under platysma muscle posteroinferiorly to join anterior division of retromandibular vein, forming common facial vein, which drains into internal jugular vein
 3. Communicates through deep facial vein with pterygoid plexus
 4. Receives tributaries from eyelids, lips, cheeks, and masseter muscles
 5. In submandibular region, receives submental, submandibular, and palatine tributaries

E. Superficial temporal vein
 1. Drains side of head and scalp
 2. Communicates with supraorbital vein
 3. Crosses zygomatic arch to enter parotid gland where it joins maxillary vein to form retromandibular vein
 4. Tributaries from parotid gland, external ear, side of face

F. Retromandibular vein
 1. Not a superficial vein; lies within parotid gland
 2. Formed by union of superficial temporal and maxillary veins
 3. Descends in parotid gland, lateral to external carotid artery, crossed posterolaterally by facial nerve
 4. Ends as anterior and posterior divisions
    a. Anterior division: joins facial vein to form common facial vein
    b. Posterior division: joined by posterior auricular vein to form external jugular vein

G. Posterior auricular vein
 1. Drains side of head behind ear
 2. Descends behind auricle and joins posterior division of retromandibular vein to form external jugular vein, which descends obliquely across sternocleidomastoid (SCM) muscle to drain into subclavian vein

H. Occipital vein
 1. Drains back of head to deep cervical and vertebral veins

I. Anterior jugular vein
 1. Drains submandibular region as small submental veins
 2. Descends vertically in anterior cervical triangle to bend laterally above manubrium, pass deep to SCM origin, and enter external jugular vein

II. Cutaneous Nerves of Head (Fig. 2.2B,C)

A. Spinal nerve branches
 1. **Greater occipital nerve**
    a. Supplies scalp posteriorly to vertex and laterally to behind ear
    b. Cutaneous branch of posterior ramus of C2 spinal nerve

2. **Lesser occipital nerve**
   a. Supplies skin behind ear
   b. Cutaneous branch of anterior ramus of C2 spinal nerve from cervical plexus
3. **Great auricular nerve**
   a. Supplies skin of external ear
   b. From anterior cutaneous branches of C2 and C3 from cervical plexus
B. **Trigeminal nerve branches** (cranial nerve [CN] V)
   1. Supplies skin of face, from vertex to lower border of mandible and just anterior to external ear laterally
   2. 3 divisions

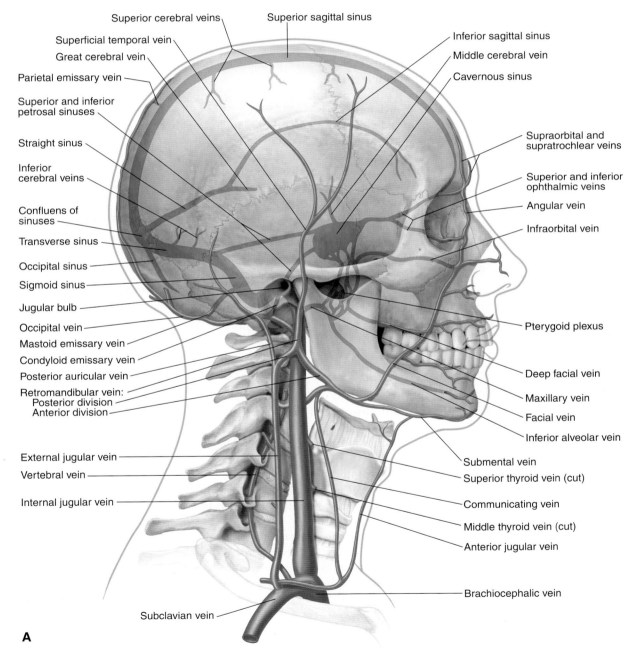

Figure 2.2A. Superficial Veins of the Head.

a. **Ophthalmic division** (**CN V₁**)

   i. Supplies skin of forehead, upper eyelid, and bridge of nose to tip

   ii. Cutaneous branches

      a) **Supraorbital**: from frontal branch; supplies forehead after passing around supraorbital margin in supraorbital notch or foramen

      b) **Supratrochlear**: from frontal branch; supplies forehead near midline and upper eyelid medially

      c) **Infratrochlear**: from nasociliary branch; supplies lacrimal caruncle and sac

      d) **Lacrimal**: supplies upper eyelid laterally

      e) **External nasal**: from anterior ethmoidal branch of nasociliary branch; supplies skin of nose

b. **Maxillary division** (**CN V₂**)

   i. Supplies skin of midface from lower eyelid to upper lip and laterally over cheekbone and lateral orbital margin

   ii. Cutaneous branches

      a) **Infraorbital**: supplies skin of midface from lower eyelid to upper lip and gingiva

      b) **Zygomaticofacial**: from zygomatic branch; supplies skin over cheekbone

      c) **Zygomaticotemporal**: from zygomatic branch; supplies skin over and behind lateral orbital margin

c. **Mandibular division** (**CN V₃**)

   i. Supplies skin overlying mandible, including lower lip, extending superiorly anterosuperior to external ear

   ii. Cutaneous branches

      a) **Mental**: from inferior alveolar; supplies chin, lower lip, and gingiva

      b) **Buccal**: supplies skin of cheek and skin overlying masseter and mucosa of oral vestibule

      c) **Auriculotemporal**: supplies skin anterosuperior to external ear

III. Clinical Considerations

A. Thrombosing inflammations of veins of face: caused by skin infections of upper lip or nose (danger triangle of face), can enter cavernous sinus of skull via connections between angular and superior ophthalmic veins and can produce potentially fatal sinus thrombosis

B. Veins of 1 side of face anastomose with each other and with veins of contralateral side

C. Neuralgias

   1. Paroxysmal pain extending along course of 1 or more nerves; characterized by severe throbbing or stabbing pain in nerve pathway

   2. Common cause of diffuse sensation of facial pain (facial neuralgia)

   3. Occipital neuralgia: pain in distribution of greater occipital nerve may be source of migraine headache pain; may be treated with greater occipital nerve block

   4. Other areas of localized pain may include earache (otalgia) or toothache (odontalgia)

D. Nerve blocks

   1. Infraorbital: local anesthesia of midface

      a. For treating wounds of upper lip and cheek or repairing maxillary incisor teeth

      b. Care must be taken because infraorbital vessels also leave infraorbital foramen with nerve and orbit is just above

   2. Mental and incisive nerve block: anesthetizes skin and mucous membranes of lower lip and chin; used prior to suturing of severe lip lacerations

   3. Buccal nerve block: in mucous membrane over retromolar area, just behind mandibular molar; anesthetizes skin and mucous membrane of cheek and used to repair cheek wounds

   4. Trigeminal ganglion block: made through foramen ovale and has been used to treat trigeminal neuralgia by injecting only sensory division of CN V

E. Headache and facial pain: most common and frequent complaint, but tend generally to be benign and are commonly associated with tension, fatigue, depression, or mild fever

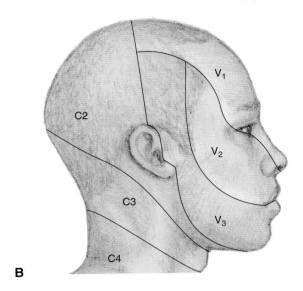

B

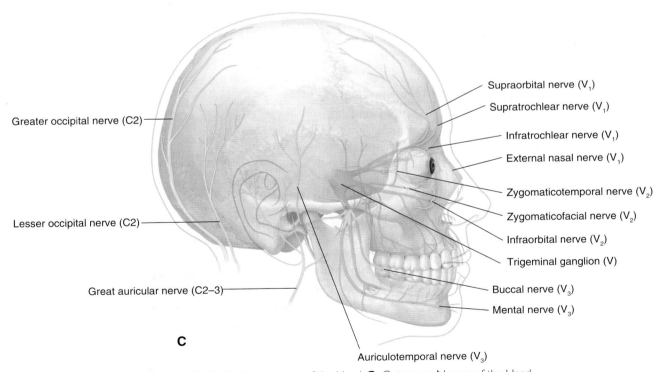

Greater occipital nerve (C2)

Lesser occipital nerve (C2)

Great auricular nerve (C2–3)

Supraorbital nerve (V₁)

Supratrochlear nerve (V₁)

Infratrochlear nerve (V₁)

External nasal nerve (V₁)

Zygomaticotemporal nerve (V₂)

Zygomaticofacial nerve (V₂)

Infraorbital nerve (V₂)

Trigeminal ganglion (V)

Buccal nerve (V₃)

Mental nerve (V₃)

C

Auriculotemporal nerve (V₃)

Figure 2.2B,C. B. Dermatomes of the Head. **C.** Cutaneous Nerves of the Head.

Skull: General Considerations

I. Skull (Cranium) as a Whole

A. Consists of 22 bones, 21 of which are firmly bound together; mandible is moveable and articulates with remainder of skull through paired synovial joints

B. Subdivisions

  1. Neurocranium

    a. Derived from occipital somites and somitomeres

    b. Contains and protects brain

    c. Encloses inner and middle ear

    d. Includes calvaria or skullcap and cranial base

    e. Component bones (8)

      i. Occipital

      ii. Sphenoid

      iii. Frontal

      iv. Ethmoid

      v. Parietals (paired)

      vi. Temporals (paired)

  2. Viscerocranium

    a. Derived from neural crest

    b. Skeleton of face

    c. Component bones (14)

      i. Maxillae (paired)

      ii. Palatines (paired)

      iii. Zygomatic bones (paired)

      iv. Vomer

      v. Inferior nasal conchae (paired)

      vi. Lacrimals (paired)

      vii. Nasals (paired)

    d. Mandible

II. Subdivisions of Neurocranium

A. Calvaria (cranial vault or skullcap)

  1. Forms roof of cranial cavity, which houses brain

  2. Flat bones of skull or flat portions of bones

    a. Squamous part of frontal bone (uppermost portion forming forehead)

    b. Parietal bones

    c. Greater wings of sphenoid bones

    d. Squamous portions of temporal bones (uppermost portion)

    e. Squamous part of occipital bone (uppermost portion)

  3. Except for area of frontal sinus and near sutures, consists of 3 layers

    a. Outer table: relatively thin layer of compact bone

    b. Inner table relatively thin layer of compact bone; may be pitted by arachnoid granulations

    c. Diploe: relatively dense cancellous bone; contains diploic veins, which anastomose with emissary veins and dural venous sinuses

B. Cranial base

  1. Forms solid base for articulation with vertebral column and facial skeleton

  2. Irregular bones which complete enclosed brain case

    a. Orbital part of frontal bone

    b. Ethmoid bone

    c. Sphenoid bone (except greater wings)

    d. Petrous portions of temporal bones

    e. Basal part of occipital bone

  3. Cradles brain and brainstem in 3 cranial fossae: anterior, middle, and posterior

  4. Contains many foramina for passage of nerves and vessels

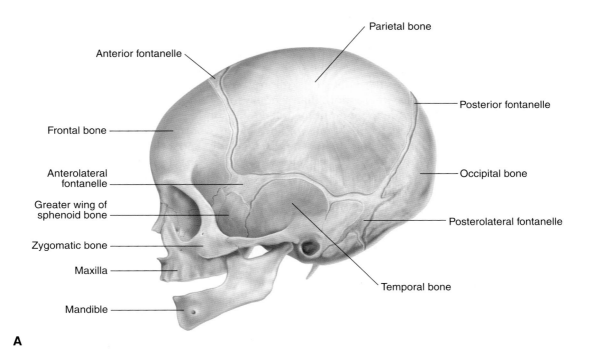

Figure 2.3A,B. Fetal Skull.

III. Skull Ossification (Fig. 2.3A,B)

A. **Neurocranium**

   1. **Membranous part** (**desmocranium**)

     a. Flat bones of cranial vault

     b. Develop from mesenchyme and undergo membranous ossification (bony spicules form from primary ossification centers toward periphery)

     c. Enlarge by apposition (new layers) on outer surface and by osteoclastic resorption from inside

     d. At birth, flat bones of skull are separated by narrow seams of connective tissue, **sutures**; where more than 2 bones meet, sutures are wide and are called **fontanelles**

     e. 6 fontanelles: membrane-filled "soft spot" spaces between incompletely developed (ossified) cranial bones of fetus and newborn at junctions of sutures; allow skull to deform during delivery and later ossify and become rigid, taking approximately 14–24 months; membrane covered by pericranium externally and dura mater internally; permit continued brain growth in an expansible compartment and help mold skull during birth

        i. **Anterior or frontal**: large, rhomboid-shaped, bounded by frontal and parietal bones at intersection of coronal and sagittal sutures (bregma); closes by 2nd year (~18 months)

        ii. **Posterior or occipital**: small, triangle-shaped; bounded by parietal and occipital bones at junction of sagittal and lambdoid sutures (lambda); closes by 2 months after birth

        iii. **Anterolateral or sphenoidal** (bilateral): located at intersection of parietal, temporal, frontal and sphenoid bones; marked in adult by H-shaped area of bony union called **pterion**; closes at 3 months

        iv. **Posterolateral or mastoid** (bilateral): at intersection of temporal, parietal, and occipital bones (asterion); closes at 1 year

   2. **Cartilaginous part** (**chondrocranium**): forms bones at base of skull; consists initially of several separate cartilages; ossify by **endochondral ossification** and fuse to form cranial base

B. **Viscerocranium**: consists of bones of face and formed by cartilages of 1st 2 pharyngeal arches

   1. 1st pharyngeal arch: gives rise to maxillary and mandibular processes

     a. **Maxillary process**: gives rise to maxilla, zygomatic bone, and part of temporal bone

     b. **Mandibular process:** mesenchyme around **Meckel's cartilage** condenses and ossifies by membranous ossification to form mandible, sphenomandibular ligament, and malleus and incus of middle ear

   2. 2nd pharyngeal arch cartilage

     a. **Reichert's cartilage**

     b. Undergoes endochondral ossification to form stapes of middle ear, styloid process, stylohyoid ligament and lesser horn of hyoid bone

C. Ossification centers and growth

   1. 1st ossification center in chondrocranium is seen in endochondral part of occipital bone in 30-mm embryos; enlargement of bones occurs by formation of appositional bone, which is not preformed in cartilage

   2. By end of 3rd month of pregnancy, ossification centers seen in all cartilage models; most skull bones form from 2 or more ossification centers, which fuse with each other

   3. Cartilage and membrane bones unite to form skull

   4. Remodeling (changes in proportions and surface curvatures) is essential part of skull growth

   5. Ossification with membranous bone (seen in 15-mm embryos) begins in mandible and shortly after in maxilla; all membranous bone is present in 37-mm embryo

IV. Clinical Considerations

A. Skull fontanelles

1. Pliability of skull at birth allows for it to mold itself to proportions of mother's pelvis and allow for successful passage of head during birth; when size of baby's head and dimensions of mother's pelvis are not compatible with successful vaginal delivery, cesarean section (delivery through abdominal and uterine incision) is commonly elected

2. Newborn head can be asymmetrical and somewhat misshapen; cranial skeleton assumes regular shape in a few days as molding disappears

3. While fontanelles are open, brain is very vulnerable; care is needed to protect these regions, especially anteriorly, because this fontanelle does not close until middle of 2nd year

B. Cranioschisis

1. Large skull defects (seen at birth) combined with gross brain abnormalities or complete absence of cerebrum (i.e., **anencephaly**)

2. May be small defects in skull through which tissue and/or meninges herniate (**encephalocele** or **cranial meningocele**)

3. Children with severe skull and brain defects are generally not viable, but those with relatively small defects in skull are commonly seen

C. Skull shape abnormalities

1. Sutures begin to obliterate (**synostosis**) at approximately middle age (age 30–40 years); synostosis begins internally and is seen externally 10 years later; begins at bregma and continues sequentially in sagittal, coronal, and lambdoid sutures; **craniostenosis**: premature closure of sutures may lead to deformities; seen in 1/2,000 births; resulting skull shape depends on which sutures close prematurely; appears to be genetic abnormality, more common in males than females, and commonly associated with other skeletal abnormalities

   a. **Scaphocephaly**: premature closure of sagittal suture, resulting in narrow, long, wedge-shaped skull

   b. **Plagiocephaly**: premature closure of lambdoid or coronal sutures on 1 side only, resulting in asymmetric skull

   c. **Oxycephaly** (acrocephaly or turricephaly): premature closure of coronal suture, resulting in high, tower-like skull; more common in females

   d. **Microcephaly**: decrease in cranial volume or abnormal smallness of head (brain fails to grow); bird-headed malformation resulting in formation of greatly flattened calvarium with receding forehead and premature suture closings; child is usually severely mentally retarded

   e. **Crouzon's syndrome**: gross appearance like oxycephaly, but malformation of cranial vault accompanied by malformation of face, teeth, and ears and other parts of body

2. **Hydrocephalus** ("water on the brain"): congenital or acquired enlargement of cranial volume in early childhood caused by obstruction of drainage of brain ventricular system and results in dilatation of cerebral ventricles, causing balloon-like distension of skull, forehead prominence, brain tissue atrophy, mental deterioration, convulsions, and death in childhood; sutures remain open

(Continued)

D. Metopic suture: normal midline suture in squamous portion of frontal bone that usually fuses before birth; found in 8% newborns, usually fuses by age 2 years; present in approximately 5% of adults

E. Head injuries (in general): major cause of death (10%) and disability, occurring mostly in young people between ages of 15–24 years and tend to a large extent (50%) to involve automobile and motor cycle accidents; largely result of falls or blows to head; complications include infection, hemorrhage, and brain and cranial nerve injury with 1/2 of traumatic deaths involving brain

F. Skull fractures

  1. Simple fractures seldom need treatment because there is no displacement downward of any skull parts that might threaten brain; when fractured segment is displaced (depressed), risk of hemorrhagic brain injury and/or infection is much greater; brain itself may be injured from pressure of depressed skull fragment

  2. Fracture lines follow paths of least resistance: through vault between reinforcing pillars; through base within fossae, not at junctions of fossae; and along suture lines; all lines of fracture directed toward base will converge on body of sphenoid bone

  3. Most common cause of death from skull fracture is brain laceration; other causes include subdural hematoma, cerebral concussion, extradural hemorrhage, and meningitis

  4. Classification

   a. Linear: resembling line, most frequent type and occuring at point of contact

   b. Contrecoup: fracture of skull on opposite side of impact area

   c. Closed or simple: fracture with intact overlying scalp and/or mucous membrane

   d. Open or compound: with laceration of overlying scalp and/or mucous membrane

   e. Comminuted: fracture with bone fragmentation

   f. Depressed: fracture with inward displacement of part of calvaria

   g. Expressed: fracture with outward displacement of part of cranium

   h. Diastatic: separation of cranial bones at suture, with marked separation of bone fragments

  5. Fracture at pterion: bone at side of calvaria is thin and may fracture, resulting in intracranial bleeding and hematoma due to tearing of branches of middle meningeal artery lying in bony grooves of inner table of bone; hematoma may exert pressure on underlying cerebral cortex and if untreated, can cause death in a few hours

  6. Skull X-rays: may be used to evaluate patients for possible skull fractures; care must be taken, particularly in children, not to confuse normal suture lines with actual fractures

G. **Stereotaxic surgery**: skull landmarks used as points of reference for stereotaxic triangulation when determining 3-dimensional coordinates of various structures within brain; allows removal of tissue samples for diagnostic purposes or lesions may be placed in brain in order to destroy small brain areas

Skull: Anterior View

I. General Features of Anterior View of Skull (Fig. 2.4)

A. Also known as **Norma frontalis**

B. Consists of anterior part of calvaria (forehead) and most of facial skeleton

II. Bones of Anterior View of Skull

A. Frontal
1. **Frontal tuber** or **eminence**
2. **Superciliary arches**: variable browridges above orbits
   a. More prominent in males
   b. Meet at glabella, a small variable midline depression
3. Supraorbital margin: marked by **supraorbital notch** or foramen for supraorbital neurovascular bundle
4. **Zygomatic process**: meets frontal process of zygomatic bone at frontozygomatic suture
5. Nasal part: meets nasal bones at frontonasal suture

B. Nasal: paired; unite at internasal suture to form base of bridge of nose

C. Maxilla
1. **Frontal process**
   a. Forms most of medial margin of orbit
   b. Meets frontal bone at frontomaxillary suture
   c. Forms most of nasal aperture, completed above by nasal bones
   d. **Anterior nasal spine**: midline protuberance below nasal aperture
2. Forms medial portion of inferior orbital margin
3. **Infraorbital foramen**: transmits infraorbital neurovascular bundle
4. **Alveolar process**: forms sockets for upper teeth; marked by depression called *canine fossa* above canine root

D. Zygomatic (malar or cheek bone)
1. Frontal process meets frontal bone at frontozygomatic suture; forms lower portion of lateral orbital margin
2. Forms lateral portion of inferior orbital margin; unites with maxilla at zygomatico-maxillary suture
3. **Zygomaticofacial foramen**: transmits zygomaticofacial neurovascular bundle
4. Temporal process meets temporal bone to form zygomatic arch

E. Mandible
1. Body
   a. Convex anteriorly; fused at symphysis menti during 1st year
   b. External surface: **mental protuberance** with mental tubercles on either side; **mental foramen** below 2nd premolar tooth; oblique line extends from mental tubercle up to anterior border of ramus
   c. Superior border: alveolar process forming sockets for lower teeth

F. Ramus (paired)
1. Form **angles** with body (~150°)
2. **Condyloid process**, with rounded head for articulation
3. **Neck**: constricted portion below condyle; pterygoid fovea medially
4. **Coronoid process**: thin, separated from condyloid process by wide mandibular notch

III. Sutures on Anterior View of Skull

A. **Frontonasal**: frontal and 2 nasal bones; nasion is midpoint of suture
B. **Zygomaticomaxillary**: zygomatic and maxillary bones forming inferior orbital margin
C. **Frontozygomatic**: zygomatic and frontal bones forming lateral orbital margin
D. **Intermaxillary**: between maxillary bones
E. **Metopic**: between frontal bones (usually not present in adult skull)

IV. Clinical Considerations

A. Fractures of mandible: commonly involves 2 fractures, which tend to occur on opposite sides (e.g., severe blow to jaw may fracture neck and body of mandible in region of opposite canine teeth)
   1. Open type: bone fragments break skin or mucous membrane of mouth
   2. Closed type: vertical breaks between ramus and body of mandible; ramus fragment pulled upward by temporalis and masseter muscles and medially by medial pterygoid muscle; body fragment pulled downward by gravity and geniohyoid muscle and backward by digastric and mylohyoid muscles
   3. Displacement of bone fragments at fracture lines may result in malocclusion
   4. Coronoid process fracture: rare and usually single sided
   5. Neck fracture: commonly transverse and associated with temporomandibular joint (TMJ) dislocation on same side
   6. Angle of mandible fracture: commonly oblique and tends to involve alveolar bony socket of 3rd molar tooth
   7. Body fracture: usually passes through socket of canine tooth
B. Fractures of maxilla
   1. Le Fort I fracture: various horizontal fractures passing superior to alveolar process, crossing bony nasal septum and, at times, even pterygoid plates
   2. Le Fort II fracture: passes from posterolateral part of maxillary sinuses superomedially through infraorbital foramina, lacrimal or ethmoid bones, to bridge of nose (tends to separate middle of face, including hard palate and alveolar processes, from remainder of cranium)
   3. Le Fort III fracture: horizontal fracture through superior orbital fissures and ethmoid and nasal bones and runs laterally through greater wings of sphenoid and frontozygomatic sutures; maxillae and zygomatic bones separate from rest of skull, if zygomatic arches also fractured
C. Tooth loss
   1. Alveolar bone resorbed after loss of individual teeth
   2. With loss of most or all teeth, shape of face changes, mental foramina come to lie closer to upper border of mandible, and their nerves may be compressed there, leading to injury and pain

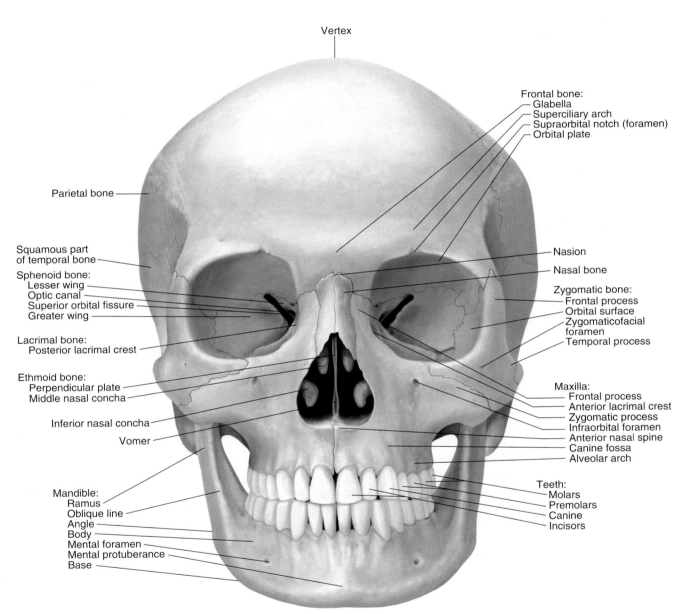

Vertex

Frontal bone:
— Glabella
— Superciliary arch
— Supraorbital notch (foramen)
— Orbital plate

Parietal bone

Nasion

Nasal bone

Squamous part
of temporal bone

Zygomatic bone:
— Frontal process
— Orbital surface
— Zygomaticofacial
  foramen
— Temporal process

Sphenoid bone:
  Lesser wing
  Optic canal
  Superior orbital fissure
  Greater wing

Lacrimal bone:
  Posterior lacrimal crest

Maxilla:
— Frontal process
— Anterior lacrimal crest
— Zygomatic process
— Infraorbital foramen
— Anterior nasal spine
— Canine fossa
— Alveolar arch

Ethmoid bone:
  Perpendicular plate
  Middle nasal concha

Inferior nasal concha

Vomer

Teeth:
— Molars
— Premolars
— Canine
— Incisors

Mandible:
  Ramus
  Oblique line
  Angle
  Body
  Mental foramen
  Mental protuberance
  Base

Figure 2.4. Skull, Anterior View.

Skull: Lateral View

I. General Features of Lateral View of Skull (Fig. 2.5A)

A. Also known as **Norma lateralis**

B. Consists of calvaria superiorly and facial skeleton anteroinferiorly

II. Bones of Lateral View of Skull

A. Frontal (squamous part)

  1. Anterior and anterolateral part of cranium

  2. Superciliary arch: above superior orbital margin

  3. Zygomatic process: attaches to zygomatic bone

  4. Temporal line: for temporalis muscle attachment

B. Zygomatic (cheekbone): zygomaticofacial and zygomaticotemporal foramina

C. Maxilla: anterior nasal spine and alveolar border; frontal process

D. Mandible

  1. Condyle and neck

  2. Coronoid process: for temporalis insertion

  3. Ramus: descends anteroinferiorly

  4. Angle: where ramus meets body; may project laterally slightly

  5. Body: alveolar process for teeth; mental protuberance and foramen

E. Sphenoid

  1. Greater wing

    a. Meets with zygomatic anteriorly, frontal and parietal superiorly, temporal posteriorly

    b. Pterion: point where sphenoparietal and sphenosquamous sutures meet; bone is thin and covered by temporalis muscle

    c. Infratemporal crest: ridge where greater wing turns medially to form part of cranial base

  2. Lateral pterygoid plate

    a. Descends from sphenoid body behind maxilla

    b. Pterygomaxillary fissure: gap between maxilla and lateral pterygoid plate; leads into cleft called **pterygopalatine fossa**

F. Parietal

  1. Part of roof and sides of cranium

  2. Superior and inferior temporal lines: for temporalis muscle and fascia

  3. Parietal foramen (inconsistent): for parietal emissary vein

G. Temporal

  1. Squamous: flat, forming lower part of calvaria

  2. Mastoid: large portion behind ear; mastoid process and foramen are evident

  3. Tympanic: surrounding external auditory meatus; part of wall of tympanic cavity

  4. Styloid process: gives attachment to ligaments and muscles

  5. Zygomatic process of temporal: unites with zygomatic bone to form zygomatic arch

H. Occipital (squamous portion)

  1. External occipital protuberance: midline

  2. Superior nuchal line: for trapezius and SCM muscles

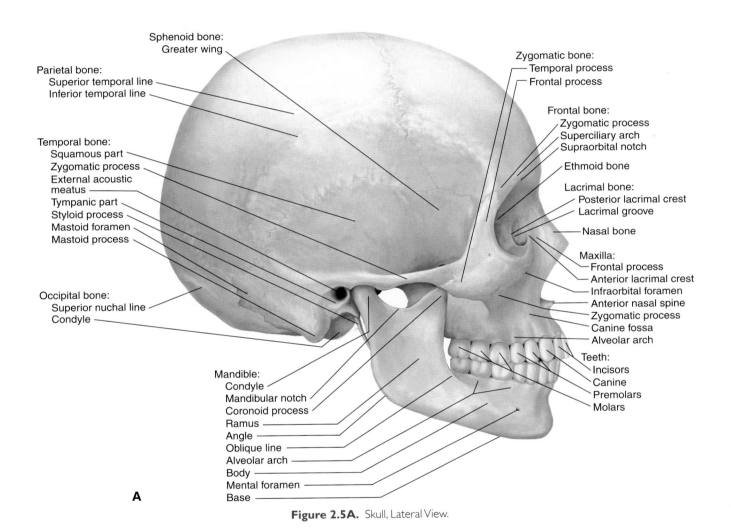

Sphenoid bone:
Greater wing

Parietal bone:
Superior temporal line
Inferior temporal line

Temporal bone:
Squamous part
Zygomatic process
External acoustic
meatus
Tympanic part
Styloid process
Mastoid foramen
Mastoid process

Occipital bone:
Superior nuchal line
Condyle

Zygomatic bone:
Temporal process
Frontal process

Frontal bone:
Zygomatic process
Superciliary arch
Supraorbital notch

Ethmoid bone

Lacrimal bone:
Posterior lacrimal crest
Lacrimal groove

Nasal bone

Maxilla:
Frontal process
Anterior lacrimal crest
Infraorbital foramen
Anterior nasal spine
Zygomatic process
Canine fossa
Alveolar arch

Teeth:
Incisors
Canine
Premolars
Molars

Mandible:
Condyle
Mandibular notch
Coronoid process
Ramus
Angle
Oblique line
Alveolar arch
Body
Mental foramen
Base

A

Figure 2.5A. Skull, Lateral View.

III. Sutures on Lateral View of Skull (Fig. 2.5B)

A. **Coronal**: frontal and parietal bones

B. **Frontozygomatic**: zygomatic and frontal bones

C. **Sphenofrontal**: greater wing of sphenoid and frontal bone

D. **Sphenoparietal**: greater wing of sphenoid and parietal bone; pterion is posterior end of suture

E. **Sphenosquamosal**: great wing of sphenoid and squamous temporal bones

F. **Temporozygomatic**: processes of zygomatic and temporal bones

G. **Squamosal**: squamous temporal and parietal bone

H. **Parietomastoid**: parietal and mastoid temporal bone

I. **Lambdoidal**: parietal and occipital bones

J. **Occipitomastoid**: occipital and mastoid of temporal bone; **asterion** is point at which lambdoidal and occipitomastoid sutures meet

IV. Special Features (Fig. 2.5C)

A. **Temporal fossa**: deep to zygomatic process of temporal bone
1. Bounded above and behind by temporal lines, in front by frontal and zygomatic bones, laterally by zygomatic arch, and below by infratemporal crest
2. Floor is formed by parts of 4 bones (frontal, parietal, temporal, and greater wing of sphenoid) that form pterion
3. Roof of fossa made up of temporalis muscle (and its overlying fascia), which arises from floor

B. **Infratemporal fossa**: deep to ramus of mandible; bounded in front by maxilla, behind by styloid process, above by greater wing of sphenoid, and medially by lateral pterygoid plate

C. **Pterygopalatine fossa**
1. Small, pyramidal space below apex of orbit and medial to infratemporal fossa
2. Bounded above by body of sphenoid, in front by maxilla, behind by pterygoid process and greater wing of sphenoid, and medially by palatine bone
3. 5 foramina open into fossa: foramen rotundum, pterygoid canal, pharyngeal canal, sphenopalatine foramen, and greater and lesser palatine canals; anteriorly, fossa communicates with orbit via inferior orbital fissure and laterally with infratemporal fossa via pterygomaxillary fissure
4. Contains terminal branches of maxillary artery, maxillary nerve and its branches, and pterygopalatine ganglion

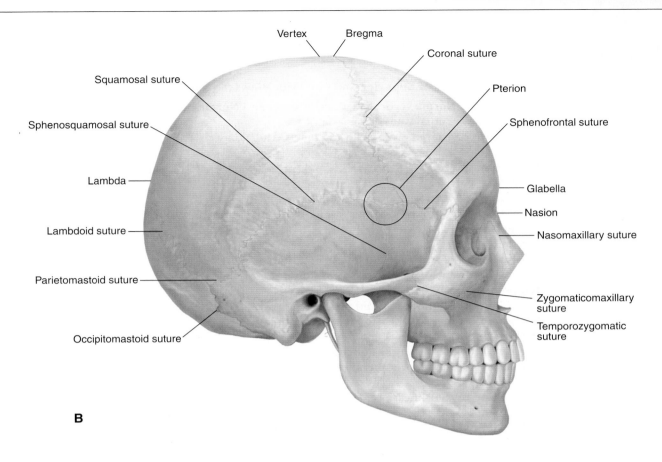

Vertex Bregma Coronal suture Pterion Sphenofrontal suture

Squamosal suture

Sphenosquamosal suture

Glabella

Nasion

Lambda

Nasomaxillary suture

Lambdoid suture

Parietomastoid suture

Zygomaticomaxillary suture

Temporozygomatic suture

Occipitomastoid suture

B

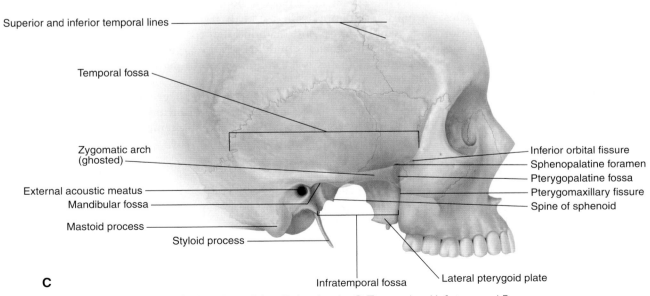

Superior and inferior temporal lines

Temporal fossa

Zygomatic arch (ghosted)

Inferior orbital fissure

Sphenopalatine foramen

Pterygopalatine fossa

External acoustic meatus

Pterygomaxillary fissure

Mandibular fossa

Spine of sphenoid

Mastoid process

Styloid process

Infratemporal fossa

Lateral pterygoid plate

C

Figure 2.5B,C. Skull, Lateral View. **B.** Landmarks. **C.** Temporal and Infratemporal Fossae.

Skull: Superior, Posterior, and Sagittal Views

I. General Features of Superior and Posterior Views (Fig. 2.6A)

A. Also known as **Norma verticalis** (superior view) and **Norma occipitalis** (posterior view)

B. Superior view: cranial vault or calvaria

C. Posterior view: occiput, where calvaria meets cranial base

II. Bones (Fig. 2.6B)

A. Frontal
1. Usually smooth and convex in adult
2. In infancy, 2 frontal bones are joined at frontal (**metopic**) suture; sometimes seen in adults

B. Parietal
1. Forms most of superior and lateral cranium
2. **Parietal foramen** (for emissary vein) and tuberosity

C. Temporal
1. Mastoid portion with mastoid process
2. **Mastoid foramen**: for mastoid emissary vein

D. Occipital
1. Forms lower posterior part of cranium
2. **External occipital protuberance**: in midline, with external occipital crest running inferiorly
3. **Superior nuchal lines**: arch laterally from external occipital protuberance; planum occipital lies above
4. **Inferior nuchal lines**: run laterally from midpoint of median crest; planum nuchale lies between nuchal lines

III. Sutures of Superior and Posterior Views of Skull

A. Coronal: between frontal and 2 parietal bones; **bregma** is that point of union of coronal and sagittal sutures

B. Sagittal: between parietal bones on either side; **vertex** is highest point on skull

C. Lambdoidal: between occipital and 2 parietal bones

D. Fontanelles: portions of skull not ossified at birth, usually 6 in number
1. Anterior (bregmatic): largest and diamond-shaped, located at junctions of coronal, sagittal, and frontal sutures; closes middle of 2nd year; location of bregma
2. Posterior: triangular in shape, is located at union of sagittal and lambdoidal sutures; closes 2 months after birth
3. Sphenoidal: 1 on each side; small gap between parietal, greater wing of sphenoid, and squamous temporal bones; closes 1 to 2 months after birth
4. Mastoid: 1 on each side; small gap between parietal, temporal, and occipital bones; closes 1 to 2 months after birth

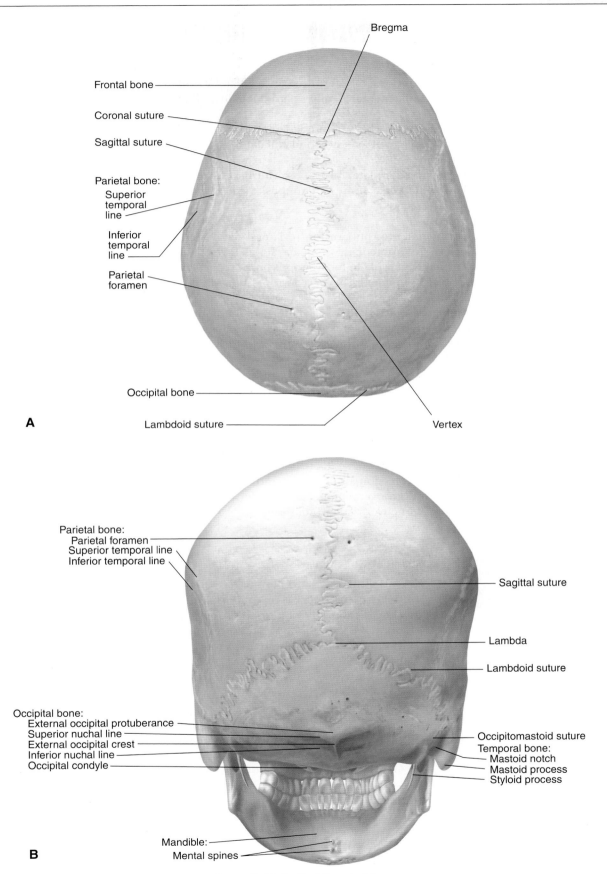

Figure 2.6A,B. Skull, Superior View.

IV. Features of Median Sagittal View (Fig. 2.6C)

A. Nasal bone: forms bridge of nose; anterior to maxilla

B. Maxilla

1. Forms anterior and inferior portion of lateral wall of nasal cavity
2. **Intermaxillary suture**: unites paired maxillae in midline, forming anterior 2/3 of hard palate

C. Inferior nasal concha: surrounded anteriorly by maxillary bone

D. Lacrimal bone: visible between maxilla anteriorly and ethmoid posteriorly

E. Palatine bone

1. **Perpendicular plate:** forms posterior part of lateral wall of nasal cavity
2. **Horizontal plate:** unites with opposite side at interpalatine suture to form posterior 1/3 of hard palate

F. Ethmoid

1. Forms much of midportion of lateral nasal wall; **superior** and **middle nasal conchae** project inferomedially from lateral wall
2. **Perpendicular plate:** forms upper portion of bony nasal septum
3. **Cribriform plate:** forms narrow roof of nasal cavity

G. Sphenoid bone

1. **Sphenoid sinus:** hollow space filling body, immediately below hypophyseal fossa
2. **Medial pterygoid plate:** forms posterior edge of lateral nasal wall, bounding choana

H. Vomer: completes bony nasal septum inferiorly

I. Mandible **(Fig. 2.6D)**

1. **Mental spines** (genial tubercles): projections near symphysis menti
2. **Digastric fossa**: for anterior belly of digastric
3. **Sublingual fossa**: for sublingual glands
4. **Mylohyoid line**: extends posterior from fossa
5. **Submandibular fossa**: for submandibular gland, below mylohyoid line
6. **Mandibular foramen**: for inferior alveolar neurovascular bundle; leads into mandibular canal
7. **Lingula**: projection anterior to mandibular foramen
8. **Mylohyoid groove**: extends anteroinferiorly on medial surface of ramus; location of mylohyoid neurovascular bundle

V. Clinical Considerations

A. Calvaria fracture: hard blow to thin area tends to produce depressed fracture where bone fragment is pushed inward, compressing and/or injuring brain

1. Linear calvarial fracture: most frequent type and usually occurs at impact point, but commonly radiates away from impact site in 1 or more directions
2. Comminuted fracture: bone is broken into several pieces

B. Craniotomy

1. Allows for surgical access to cranial cavity, where section of neurocranium called a "bone flap" is elevated or removed
2. Surgically produced bone flaps are put back in place and wired to other parts of calvaria or held in place temporarily by metal plates
3. Best results occur when bone is reflected with overlying muscle and skin so that blood supply is preserved
4. Craniectomy: bone flap not replaced, but metal or plastic plate permanently replaces original bone

C. With aging, cranial bones normally become progressively thinner and lighter and diploe gradually fills with gray gelatinous material as bone loses its marrow, blood cells, and fat

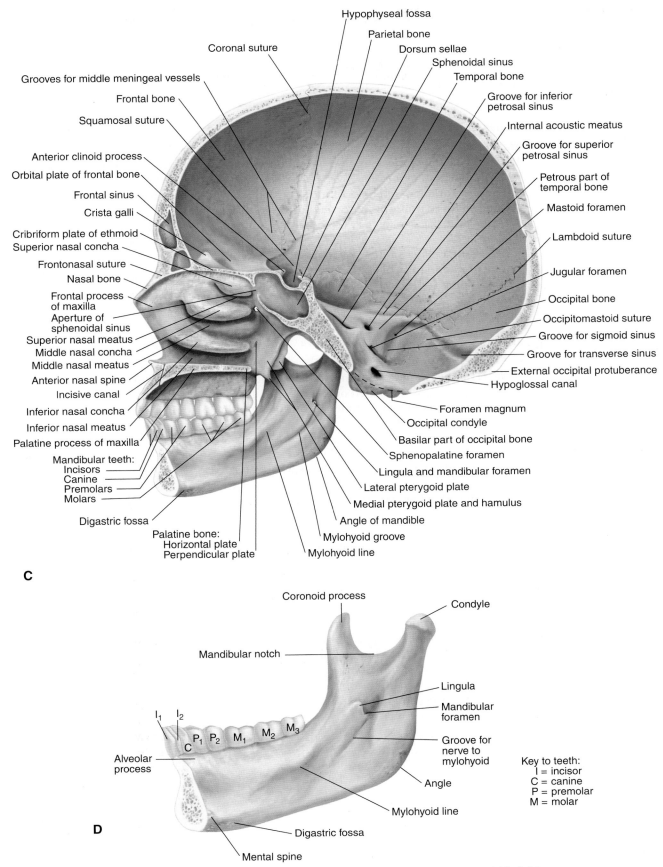

Hypophyseal fossa
Parietal bone
Coronal suture
Dorsum sellae
Sphenoidal sinus
Temporal bone
Grooves for middle meningeal vessels
Groove for inferior petrosal sinus
Frontal bone
Internal acoustic meatus
Squamosal suture
Groove for superior petrosal sinus
Anterior clinoid process
Petrous part of temporal bone
Orbital plate of frontal bone
Frontal sinus
Mastoid foramen
Crista galli
Lambdoid suture
Cribriform plate of ethmoid
Superior nasal concha
Jugular foramen
Frontonasal suture
Nasal bone
Occipital bone
Frontal process of maxilla
Occipitomastoid suture
Aperture of sphenoidal sinus
Groove for sigmoid sinus
Superior nasal meatus
Groove for transverse sinus
Middle nasal concha
External occipital protuberance
Middle nasal meatus
Hypoglossal canal
Anterior nasal spine
Incisive canal
Foramen magnum
Inferior nasal concha
Occipital condyle
Inferior nasal meatus
Basilar part of occipital bone
Palatine process of maxilla
Sphenopalatine foramen
Mandibular teeth:
Incisors
Lingula and mandibular foramen
Canine
Lateral pterygoid plate
Premolars
Medial pterygoid plate and hamulus
Molars
Angle of mandible
Digastric fossa
Mylohyoid groove
Palatine bone:
Horizontal plate
Perpendicular plate
Mylohyoid line

C

Coronoid process
Condyle

Mandibular notch

Lingula
Mandibular foramen

I_1 I_2
P_1 P_2 M_1 M_2 M_3
C

Groove for nerve to mylohyoid

Alveolar process

Angle

Key to teeth:
I = incisor
C = canine
P = premolar
M = molar

Mylohyoid line

D

Digastric fossa

Mental spine

Figure 2.6C,D. C. Skull, Sectioned, Midsagittal View. **D.** Mandible, Sectioned, Medial View.

Skull: Basal View

I. General Features of Basal View (Fig. 2.7)

A. Also known as **Norma basalis**

B. Lower portion of facial skeleton anteriorly, cranial base posteriorly

II. Bones of Basal View

A. Maxilla

  1. Paired **palatine processes** meet at midline to form anterior 2/3 of hard palate, bounded by dental arch of maxilla

  2. **Incisive foramen**: opening of incisive canal behind incisor teeth, usually into shallow incisive fossa; transmits nasopalatine neurovascular bundle

  3. Alveolar process: maxillary teeth sockets

B. Palatine

  1. Horizontal plates unite to form posterior 1/3 of hard palate

  2. **Greater and lesser palatine foramina** (for palatine nerves and arteries) and **posterior nasal spine**

C. Vomer

  1. Lower portion of bony nasal septum

  2. Separates choanae or posterior nasal apertures

D. Sphenoid

  1. **Medial pterygoid plate**

    a. **Hamulus**: at lower extremity; forms pulley for tendon of tensor veli palatini muscle

    b. **Scaphoid fossa**: located on lateral side of base

  2. **Lateral pterygoid plate**: origin of both pterygoid muscles

  3. **Greater wing of sphenoid**

    a. Foramina

      i. **Ovale**: transmits mandibular nerve (CN V_3) and lesser petrosal nerve

      ii. **Rotundum**: transmits maxillary nerve (CN V_2)

      iii. **Spinosum**: transmits middle meningeal artery

    b. **Spine of sphenoid**: attachment of sphenomandibular ligament

    c. Sulcus for auditory tube

E. Temporal

  1. Mandibular fossa: for mandibular condyle; articular tubercle is anterior

  2. **Jugular fossa**: forms anterior margin of jugular foramen

  3. **Foramen lacerum**: between tip of petrous portion and sphenoid body; filled with cartilage and crossed superiorly by internal carotid artery

  4. **Carotid canal**: for internal carotid artery and plexus

  5. **Inferior tympanic canaliculus**: on crest of bone between carotid canal and jugular foramen; transmits tympanic branch of glossopharyngeal nerve (CN IX)

  6. Styloid process: attachment of stylohyoid ligament and 3 muscles, stylohyoid, styloglossus, and stylopharyngeus

  7. Stylomastoid foramen: transmits facial nerve (CN VII)

  8. Mastoid process and notch and occipital groove

  9. Tympanomastoid fissure

F. Occipital

  1. Basilar part

    a. Anterior to foramen magnum

    b. Pharyngeal tubercle: attachment of pharyngeal raphe

  2. Lateral part

    a. Occipital condyles

    b. Condylar fossa and canal: emissary vein

    c. Hypoglossal canal: transmits hypoglossal nerve (CN XII)

    d. Jugular process: forms posterior margin of jugular foramen

    e. Foramen magnum

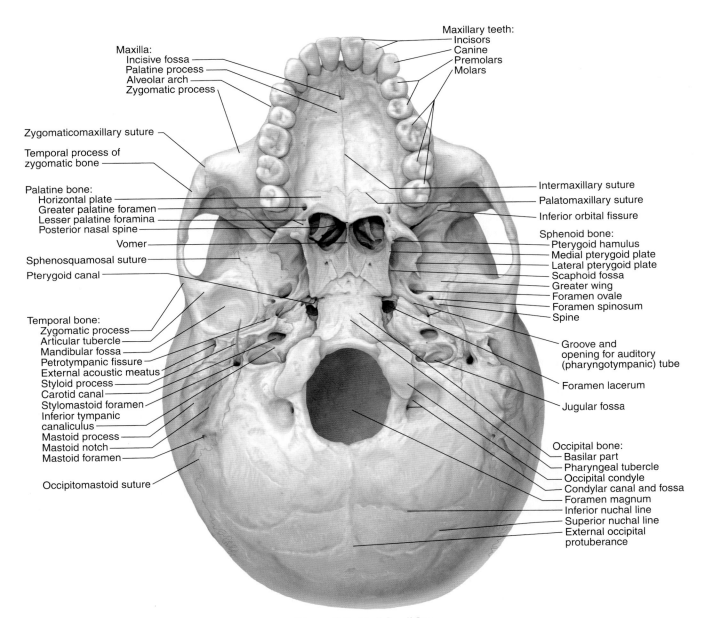

Maxillary teeth:
Incisors
Canine
Premolars
Molars

Maxilla:
Incisive fossa
Palatine process
Alveolar arch
Zygomatic process

Zygomaticomaxillary suture

Temporal process of
zygomatic bone

Palatine bone:
Horizontal plate
Greater palatine foramen
Lesser palatine foramina
Posterior nasal spine

Vomer

Sphenosquamosal suture

Pterygoid canal

Temporal bone:
Zygomatic process
Articular tubercle
Mandibular fossa
Petrotympanic fissure
External acoustic meatus
Styloid process
Carotid canal
Stylomastoid foramen
Inferior tympanic
canaliculus
Mastoid process
Mastoid notch
Mastoid foramen

Occipitomastoid suture

Intermaxillary suture
Palatomaxillary suture
Inferior orbital fissure

Sphenoid bone:
Pterygoid hamulus
Medial pterygoid plate
Lateral pterygoid plate
Scaphoid fossa
Greater wing
Foramen ovale
Foramen spinosum
Spine

Groove and
opening for auditory
(pharyngotympanic) tube

Foramen lacerum

Jugular fossa

Occipital bone:
Basilar part
Pharyngeal tubercle
Occipital condyle
Condylar canal and fossa
Foramen magnum
Inferior nuchal line
Superior nuchal line
External occipital
protuberance

Figure 2.7. Skull, Basal View.

3. Squamous part
   a. External occipital protuberance and external occipital crest
   b. Superior and inferior nuchal lines with planum nuchale between

II. Foramina of Basal View

Foramen/Opening	Bone	Contents
Incisive	Palatine process of maxilla	Nasopalatine nerve, branches of descending palatine vessels
Greater palatine	Palatine	Greater palatine nerve, descending palatine vessels
Lesser palatine	Palatine	Lesser palatine neurovascular bundle
Pterygoid canal	Sphenoid	Nerve of pterygoid canal
Ovale	Sphenoid	Mandibular nerve (CN V$_3$)
Spinosum	Sphenoid	Middle meningeal artery
Petrotympanic fissure	Sphenoid and temporal	Chorda tympani
Lacerum	Sphenoid, temporal and occipital	Occupied by cartilage
Stylomastoid	Temporal	Facial nerve (CN VII)
Carotid canal	Temporal	Internal carotid artery and plexus
Inferior tympanic canaliculus	Temporal	Tympanic branch of glossopharyngeal nerve (CN IX)
Mastoid canaliculus	Temporal	Auricular branch of vagus nerve (CN X)
Jugular	Temporal and occipital	Jugular vein posterolaterally, glossopharyngeal nerve (CN IX), vagus nerve (CN X), and accessory nerve (CN XI) anteromedially
Hypoglossal	Occipital	Hypoglossal nerve (CN XII)
Condyloid	Occipital	Emissary vein

III. Special Features

A. Emissary sphenoidal foramen: at base of lateral plate just medial to foramen ovale (contains emissary vein)

B. Foramen lacerum: between basilar part of occipital bone, petrous part of temporal and sphenoid; filled with cartilage which internal carotid passes across; transmits small vessels, nerves, and lymphatics

IV. Clinical Considerations

A. Basal skull fractures: bleeding from ear is common; **Battle's sign** is discoloration of skin along course of posterior auricular artery

B. Ring fracture of occipital bone around foramen magnum may occur in injuries in which base of skull is jammed against atlas

C. Bony basicranium is variably thick and thin and, thus, not equally strong everywhere; weak points are cribriform plate of ethmoid, roof of orbit, floor of sella turcica, greater wing of sphenoid bordering foramina, region of mandibular fossa and thinner lateral parts of occipital squama

D. Fracture of cranial base: internal carotid artery may be torn, producing arteriovenous fistula within cavernous sinus
   1. Arterial blood rushes into cavernous sinus, enlarging it and forcing retrograde blood flow into its tributaries, especially affecting ophthalmic veins and causing following symptoms
      a. Protruding eyeball (exophthalmos)
      b. Engorged conjunctiva (chemosis)
      c. Eyeball to pulse in symmetry with radial pulse (pulsating exophthalmos)
   2. Because CNs III, IV, V$_1$, and V$_2$, lie within lateral wall of cavernous sinus, and CN VI lies within sinus, these nerves can be affected when sinus is injured

Skull Interior: Cranial Fossae and Foramina

I. Anterior Cranial Fossa (Fig. 2.8A)

A. Boundaries
   1. Anteriorly and laterally: squamous frontal bone
   2. Posteriorly: posterior margin of lesser wings of sphenoid and anterior margin of chiasmatic sulcus
B. Floor: orbital plate of frontal bone, ethmoid bone, body and lesser wings of sphenoid bone
C. Special features
   1. Frontal lobes: lie on orbital plate of frontal bone forming floor of anterior cranial fossa
   2. Cribriform plate of ethmoid: transmits olfactory nerves
   3. Foramen cecum: may transmit emissary vein
   4. Anterior and posterior ethmoidal foramina: transmit anterior and posterior ethmoidal neurovascular bundles
   5. Crista galli: ethmoid bone; anchors falx cerebri anteriorly

II. Middle Cranial Fossa

A. Boundaries
   1. Anteriorly: lesser wings of sphenoid, anterior clinoid processes and anterior margin of chiasmatic groove
   2. Posteriorly: petrous ridge and dorsum sellae
   3. Laterally: squamous temporal, greater wing of sphenoid, and parietal bones
B. Floor: greater wings of sphenoid, squamous and petrous temporal, and sella turcica
C. Special features
   1. Superior orbital fissure
      a. Between lesser and greater wings of sphenoid
      b. Transmits oculomotor (CN III), trochlear (CN IV), ophthalmic (CN V_1), and abducent (CN VI) nerves and superior ophthalmic vein
   2. Optic canal: transmits optic nerve (CN II) and ophthalmic artery
   3. Sella turcica: hypophyseal fossa for pituitary
   4. Foramen rotundum: transmits maxillary nerve (CN V_2)
   5. Foramen ovale: transmits mandibular nerve (CN V_3)
   6. Foramen spinosum: transmits middle meningeal artery
   7. Posterior clinoid processes: anterior attachment for tentorium cerebelli
   8. Carotid canal: opens above foramen lacerum; transmits internal carotid artery and plexus
   9. Carotid sulcus (groove): on side of sphenoid body
   10. Foramen lacerum: filled with cartilage; internal carotid artery passes above
   11. Arcuate eminence: made by anterior semicircular canal
   12. Tegmen tympani: forms roof of tympanic cavity
   13. Hiati and grooves for greater and lesser petrosal nerves
   14. Grooves for branches of middle meningeal arteries
   15. Temporal lobe: lies on floor of middle cranial fossa, filling lateral part of fossa

III. Posterior Cranial Fossa

A. Boundaries
   1. Anteriorly: dorsum sellae and petrous ridge
   2. Laterally: parietal bones
   3. Posteriorly: squamous occipital bone
B. Floor: occipital and temporal bones, clivus, formed by union of basioccipital and sphenoid body
C. Special features
   1. Groove for superior petrosal sinus: along petrous ridge
   2. Groove for inferior petrosal sinus: at anteromedial tip of petrous temporal
   3. Internal acoustic (auditory) meatus: transmits facial (CN VII) and vestibulocochlear (CN VIII) nerves and labyrinthine artery

4. Vestibular aqueduct: for vestibular system
5. Jugular foramen: posterolaterally, transmits sigmoid sinus and inferior petrosal sinus, uniting to become jugular vein; anteromedially, transmits glossopharyngeal nerve (CN IX), vagus nerve (CN X), and accessory nerve (CN XI)
6. Foramen magnum: transmits medulla oblongata becoming spinal cord and its meninges, vertebral arteries; accessory nerve (CN XI)
7. Hypoglossal canal: transmits hypoglossal nerve (CN XII)
8. Condylar canal: transmits emissary vein
9. Grooves for transverse and sigmoid sinuses
10. Mastoid foramen: transmits emissary vein
11. Internal occipital crest: anchors falx cerebelli
12. Cerebellum: lies on floor of posterior cranial fossa
13. Pons and medulla oblongata: lie on clivus

IV. Foramina or Other Openings and Their Principal Contents

Foramen/Opening	Fossa	Transmits
Cribriform	Anterior	Olfactory nerve fibers
Anterior ethmoid	Anterior	Anterior ethmoid neurovascular bundle
Posterior ethmoid	Anterior	Posterior ethmoid neurovascular bundle
Foramen cecum	Anterior	Origin of superior sagittal venous sinus
Optic canal	Middle	Optic nerve and ophthalmic artery
Superior orbital fissure	Middle	Oculomotor (CN III), trochlear (CN IV), abducent (CN VI), and ophthalmic (CN V_1) nerves; sympathetic fibers; superior ophthalmic vein
Rotundum	Middle	Maxillary nerve (CN V_2)
Ovale	Middle	Mandibular nerve (CN V_3)
Spinosum	Middle	Middle meningeal artery
Hiatus for greater petrosal nerve	Middle	Greater petrosal nerve
Carotid canal	Middle	Internal carotid artery and plexus
Magnum	Posterior	Spinal cord, accessory nerve (CN XI), vertebral artery, anterior and posterior spinal arteries
Jugular	Posterior	Inferior petrosal and sigmoid sinuses; CNs IX, X, XI
Hypoglossal canal	Posterior	Hypoglossal nerve (CN XII)
Internal acoustic meatus	Posterior	Facial (CN VII) and vestibulocochlear (CN VIII) nerves; labyrinthine artery

V. Inner Aspect of Calvaria (Fig. 2.8B)

A. Bones
  1. Frontal
  2. Parietal
  3. Occipital
  4. Greater wing of sphenoid and squamous temporal bone (lower portion laterally)
B. Sutures
  1. Coronal
  2. Sagittal
  3. Lambdoidal
C. Grooves and markings
  1. Groove for sagittal sinus: follows sagittal suture; becomes more pronounced posteroinferiorly
  2. Granular fovea: small pits within or lateral to groove for sagittal sinus; for arachnoid granulations, which function to return cerebrospinal fluid (CSF) to venous system
  3. Groove for middle meningeal artery branches: more pronounced laterally near pterion

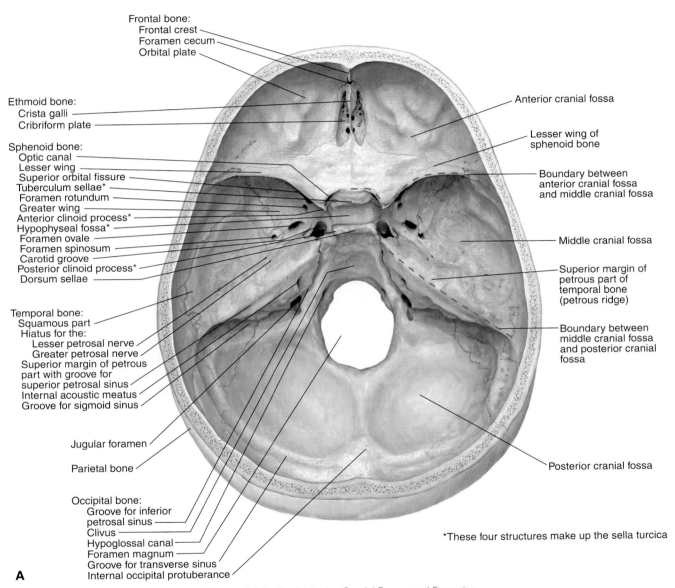

Frontal bone:
Frontal crest
Foramen cecum
Orbital plate

Ethmoid bone:
Crista galli
Cribriform plate

Sphenoid bone:
Optic canal
Lesser wing
Superior orbital fissure
Tuberculum sellae*
Foramen rotundum
Greater wing
Anterior clinoid process*
Hypophyseal fossa*
Foramen ovale
Foramen spinosum
Carotid groove
Posterior clinoid process*
Dorsum sellae

Temporal bone:
Squamous part
Hiatus for the:
Lesser petrosal nerve
Greater petrosal nerve
Superior margin of petrous part with groove for superior petrosal sinus
Internal acoustic meatus
Groove for sigmoid sinus

Jugular foramen

Parietal bone

Occipital bone:
Groove for inferior petrosal sinus
Clivus
Hypoglossal canal
Foramen magnum
Groove for transverse sinus
Internal occipital protuberance

Anterior cranial fossa

Lesser wing of sphenoid bone

Boundary between anterior cranial fossa and middle cranial fossa

Middle cranial fossa

Superior margin of petrous part of temporal bone (petrous ridge)

Boundary between middle cranial fossa and posterior cranial fossa

Posterior cranial fossa

*These four structures make up the sella turcica

A

Figure 2.8A. Skull Interior, Cranial Fossae and Foramina.

VI. Clinical Considerations

A. Fracture lines occur along weak points of basicranium (i.e., in anterior cranial fossa, they commonly course in cribriform plate or toward optic canal; in middle cranial fossa, they can connect nerve exit sites)

B. Transverse fractures in region of sella turcica commonly occur near dorsum sellae because this bone can be of variable strength; in occipital region, fractures may course in lateral parts of squama

C. Bleeding in connective tissue of eyelids, from nose, ear, or throat are common accompanying signs of skull fracture

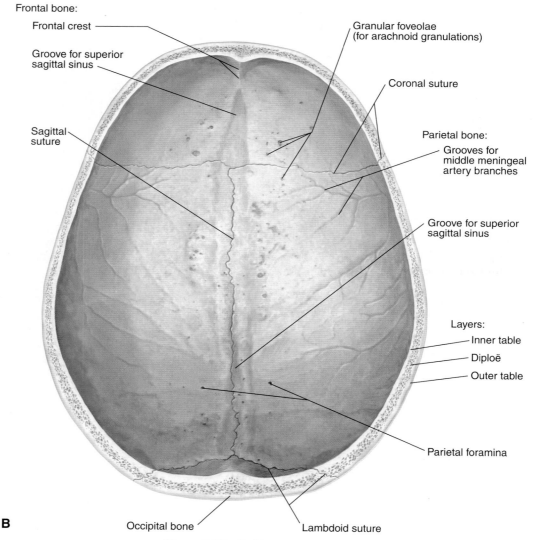

Figure 2.8B. Skull Interior, Cranial Vault.

Scalp and Diploic and Emissary Veins

I. Structure (Fig. 2.9A)

A. Composed of 5 layers that spell S-C-A-L-P

1. Skin (S): thick, with many close-set hair follicles and their associated sebaceous and sweat glands; firmly joined to next deeper layer
2. Subcutaneous connective tissue (C): superficial fascia; thick, strong with fiber bundles woven together and fat interspaced
   a. Contains superficial vessels and nerves in abundance
   b. Hair follicles of skin project into this layer
3. Musculoaponeurotic (A): represents muscles that move scalp and ear, along with aponeurosis and deep fascia
   a. **Epicranius muscle** (occipitofrontalis muscle)
      i. **Galea aponeurotica**: aponeurotic layer connecting frontalis and occipitalis bellies
      ii. **Occipitalis**: arises from superior nuchal line, inserts onto galea aponeurotica
      iii. **Frontalis**: arises from galea aponeurotica and inserts into skin overlying superciliary arches
   b. **Auricular muscles** are also in this layer in temporal region; 3 sets of auricular muscles move ears: anterior, superior, and posterior auricular muscles attach to pinna
4. Loose connective tissue layer (L): subaponeurotic; very loose and scanty; contains a few small vessels; this layer permits easy movement of superficial layers, which act as a unit, over deepest layer
5. Pericranium (P): periosteum of bones of cranial vault

II. Arteries of Scalp (Fig. 2.9B)

A. Occipital: from external carotid artery to back of head
B. Posterior auricular: from external carotid artery to region behind ear and posterior temporal region of scalp
C. Superficial temporal: 1 of terminal branches of external carotid artery to scalp anterosuperior to ear
D. Supraorbital: from ophthalmic artery to skin of forehead and anterior scalp
E. Supratrochlear: from ophthalmic artery to medial part of forehead

III. Superficial Veins (see also Section 2.2)

A. Supraorbital and supratrochlear veins
1. Drain forehead as far as vertex
2. Drain to angular vein in medial corner of eye beside nose
3. Communicate with superficial temporal and superior ophthalmic veins
B. Superficial temporal vein
1. Drains scalp laterally
2. Unites with maxillary vein to form retromandibular vein
C. Occipital vein
1. Drains scalp posteriorly
2. Drains to deep cervical and vertebral veins
D. Emissary veins
1. Defined as veins communicating through skull; in general connect superficial veins with dural venous sinuses
2. Valveless; blood can flow in both directions, although flow is usually away from brain
3. Size and number are variable; usually 6–10 recognized connections
   a. **Parietal emissary veins**: 1 on each side, pass through parietal foramina located beside sagittal suture to connect occipital veins with superior sagittal sinus; may communicate with diploic veins
   b. **Mastoid emissary veins**: pass through mastoid foramina behind mastoid processes to connect occipital and posterior auricular veins with sigmoid sinus

c. **Condyloid emissary veins**: pass through condyloid canals above occipital condyles to connect occipital veins with internal jugular vein
d. **Frontal emissary vein**: seen in children and in some adults; passes through foramen cecum connecting superior sagittal sinus with veins of frontal sinus and nasal cavities
e. Venous plexuses that act as emissary veins
   i. Venous plexus of hypoglossal canal accompanies hypoglossal nerve and connects lower part of occipital sinus with upper end of internal jugular vein (or terminal end of inferior petrosal sinus)
   ii. Venous plexus of foramen ovale accompanies mandibular division of trigeminal nerve and connects cavernous sinus to pterygoid plexus of veins
   iii. Internal carotid venous plexus is found around artery and connects cavernous sinus with internal jugular vein or pharyngeal plexus
f. Ophthalmic veins: although not technically emissary veins, they serve same dangerous function of connecting outside veins with dural sinuses and drain areas likely to become infected

IV. Diploic Veins (Fig. 2.9C)

A. Endothelium-lined channels found between inner and outer tables of calvaria
B. Dilated at intervals, have thin walls, and develop after birth
C. Do not have valves; free communication between diploic veins and dural venous sinuses
D. 4 major diploic veins on each side
   1. **Frontal diploic vein**: drains anterior portion of frontal bone into supraorbital vein and superior sagittal sinus
   2. **Anterior temporal diploic vein**: drains posterior portion of frontal bone and anterior portion of parietal and temporal bones into sphenoparietal sinus and into temporal veins via emissary veins in greater wing of sphenoid
   3. **Posterior temporal diploic veins**: drain posterior portions of parietal and temporal bones into transverse and sigmoid sinuses and mastoid emissary vein
   4. **Occipital diploic veins**: drain occiput into confluence of sinuses, transverse sinuses, occipital veins, and mastoid emissary vein

V. Nerves of Scalp (Fig. 2.9D; see also Section 2.2)

A. Cutaneous nerves
   1. Anteriorly: supraorbital and supratrochlear branches of ophthalmic nerve (CN V_1) follow arteries of same name to supply forehead to vertex
   2. Laterally: auriculotemporal branch of mandibular nerve (CN V_3) follows superficial temporal artery
   3. Posteriorly: greater occipital (C2) accompanies branches of occipital artery
   4. Posterolaterally: lesser occipital from cervical plexus (C2); in general, follows posterior auricular artery
B. Motor nerves of scalp
   1. Posterior auricular branch of facial nerve (CN VII): innervates occipital belly (occipitalis) of epicranius muscle and posterior auricular muscle
   2. Temporal branches of facial nerve (CN VII): innervate frontal belly (frontalis) of epicranius muscle and superior and anterior auricular muscles

VI. Lymphatics of Scalp

A. Tend to follow vascular supply of scalp
B. Drainage patterns
   1. Occipital area: end in nodes in occipital region near attachment of trapezius muscle
   2. Posterior parts of parietal and temporal regions: end in posterior auricular or mastoid nodes
   3. Anterolateral part of scalp drains into parotid or preauricular nodes on parotid gland surface
   4. Forehead: may be to submandibular region, following facial artery

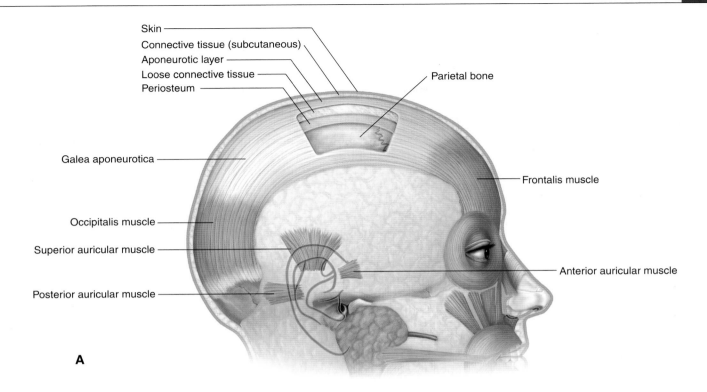

Skin
Connective tissue (subcutaneous)
Aponeurotic layer
Loose connective tissue
Periosteum

Parietal bone

Galea aponeurotica

Frontalis muscle

Occipitalis muscle

Superior auricular muscle

Posterior auricular muscle

Anterior auricular muscle

A

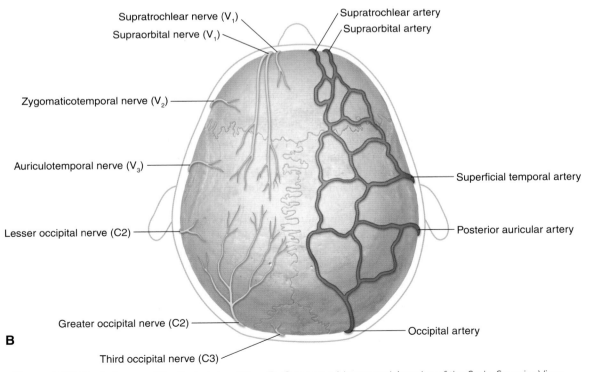

Supratrochlear nerve (V₁)
Supraorbital nerve (V₁)

Supratrochlear artery
Supraorbital artery

Zygomaticotemporal nerve (V₂)

Auriculotemporal nerve (V₃)

Superficial temporal artery

Lesser occipital nerve (C2)

Posterior auricular artery

Greater occipital nerve (C2)

Occipital artery

B

Third occipital nerve (C3)

Figure 2.9A,B. **A.** Layers of the Scalp, Lateral View. **B.** Cutaneous Nerves and Arteries of the Scalp, Superior View.

VII. Hair of Scalp

A. Grow approximately 1 cm per month

B. Lifespan is approximately 2–4 years

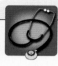

VIII. Clinical Considerations

A. Anesthesia of scalp: should be placed into dense connective tissue layer (C) where neurovasculature of scalp lies

B. "Danger zone" of scalp: infections within loose connective tissue layer (L) can spread into skull via emissary veins and diploic veins and forward onto face itself

   1. Infection here cannot pass into posterior neck because occipital bellies of occipitofrontalis muscle attach to occipital bone and mastoid part of temporal bone

   2. Infection cannot pass laterally beyond zygomatic arches because epicranial aponeurosis is continuous with temporal fasciae that attaches to arches

   3. Infection or fluid can pass anteriorly and enter eyelids and root of nose because frontalis mucles insert into skin and subcutaneous tissue and does not attach to bone

C. Injuries to scalp

   1. Vessels in scalp bleed profusely when cut or injured because they are held open by dense connective tissue (C) and cannot easily collapse to occlude flow; in addition, there are vast anastomoses between vessels

   2. Lacerations of head gape only mildly if galea is not severed completely; subcutaneous bleeding thus does not spread significantly into surrounding tissues; if galea is completely severed, injury gapes widely due to pull of frontal and occipital bellies of occipitofrontalis muscle, and hemorrhage and effusions spread extensively below galea into subaponeurotic space

   3. Hemorrhage between pericranium and parietal bone (**cephalic hematomas**) commonly seen after difficult or traumatic delivery; can lead to pericranial detachment from skull; usually do not extend beyond edges of bones because pericranium merges into connective tissue of bony sutures and anchors it to bone margins

   4. Due to looseness of subaponeurotic layer, large amounts of blood can form enormous hematomas after blows on head

   5. **Periorbital eccymosis** ("black eyes"): can occur from injury to scalp or forehead, causing soft tissue damage around eye and into eyelid

D. **Sebaceous cysts** (**wens**): obstruction of ducts of sebaceous glands associated with hair follicles and retention of secretions

E. Emissary veins may enlarge to carry considerable blood with chronic increase in intracranial pressure

F. Infections outside skull can pass by way of emissary veins into dural venous sinuses; inflammation in walls of emissary veins can lead to thrombophlebitis of dural venous sinuses

G. Diploic veins are additional drainage pathways for blood in case of dural venous drainage stagnation, but may also have importance as pathways for spread of infections from soft parts of head to interior of cranium

H. Partially detached scalp (accident) can be replaced because major scalp arteries enter from sides of head and are protected by dense connective tissue and freely anastomose, allowing for reasonable healing capability, as long as its vessels remain intact

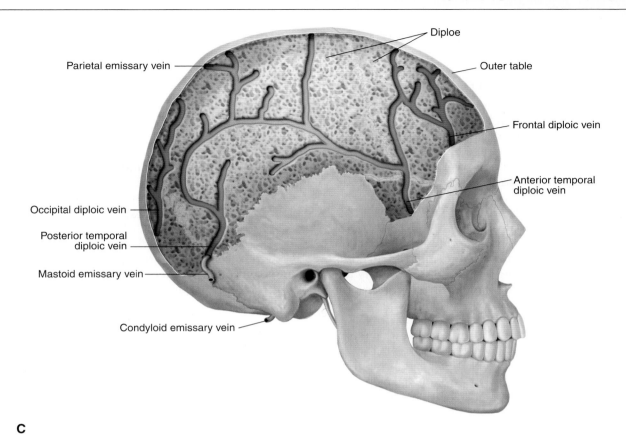

Diploe

Outer table

Parietal emissary vein

Frontal diploic vein

Anterior temporal
diploic vein

Occipital diploic vein

Posterior temporal
diploic vein

Mastoid emissary vein

Condyloid emissary vein

C

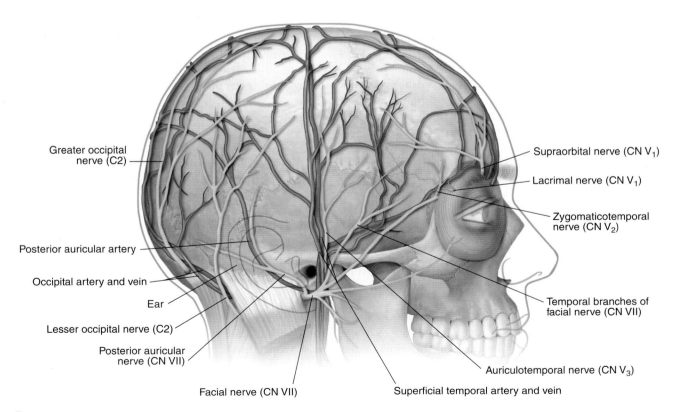

Greater occipital
nerve (C2)

Supraorbital nerve (CN V₁)

Lacrimal nerve (CN V₁)

Zygomaticotemporal
nerve (CN V₂)

Posterior auricular artery

Occipital artery and vein

Ear

Temporal branches of
facial nerve (CN VII)

Lesser occipital nerve (C2)

Posterior auricular
nerve (CN VII)

Auriculotemporal nerve (CN V₃)

Facial nerve (CN VII)

Superficial temporal artery and vein

D

Figure 2.9C,D. C. Diploic and Emissary Veins, Lateral View. **D.** Neurovasculature of the Scalp, Lateral View.

Muscles of Facial Expression

I. General Features (Fig. 2.10A)

A. Cutaneous muscles lie in superficial fascia and may arise from either fascia or bone and insert into skin

B. Also called *mimetic muscles*

C. Innervated by branches of facial nerve (CN VII)

D. Grouped according to location or principal action, although many individual muscles are indistinctly separated from those closely adjoining

II. Groupings of Facial Muscles with Principal Actions (Fig. 2.10B)

A. Scalp and ear
1. For major muscles, see Section 2.9
2. **Corrugator supercilii**: deep to eyebrows; arises from nasal part of frontal bone (from medial end of superciliary arch) and inserts into skin of eyebrows; draws skin toward midline in direction of root of nose and produces perpendicular folds on forehead, forming wrinkling typical of a scowl

B. Eye
1. **Orbicularis oculi**: surrounds palpebral fissure approximating shape of circle
   a. 3 parts
      i. Orbital part: arises from nasal part of frontal bone, at frontal process of maxilla, and at medial palpebral ligament; for closing eyes tightly to protect against glare of light (squinting) and dust
      ii. Palpebral part: thin portion within upper and lower eyelids; for closing eyelids lightly to keep cornea from drying (responsible for blinking)
      iii. Lacrimal part: deep, medial portion continuous with palpebral part and commonly considered part of it; attaches to lacrimal sac and pulls it laterally when eyelids are closed, creating siphon effect or "lacrimal pump" that sucks tears into lacrimal canaliculi and sac
   b. When all parts contract, eyes are firmly closed and adjacent skin is wrinkled; these wrinkles become permanent by age 30–35 years and are called "crow's feet"
   c. Paralysis results in drooping of lower lid (**ectropion**) and spilling of tears (**epiphora**)

C. Nose
1. **Procerus**: small muscle continuous with occipitofrontalis, passing from forehead over bridge of nose where it inserts; draws medial angle of eyebrow downward and produces wrinkles over bridge of nose
2. **Depressor septi**: runs from maxilla above incisors to mobile part of nasal septum; assists dilator nares in widening aperture during deep inspiration and also depresses nasal septum
3. **Nasalis**: consists of transverse (compressor naris) and alar (dilator naris) portions
   i. Compressor nares: from maxilla above incisor teeth to dorsum of nose; compress anterior nasal openings
   ii. Dilator nares: from maxilla into alar cartilages of nose; widens anterior nasal opening; in children, a marked or increased action of these muscles suggests respiratory distress (pneumonia)

D. Mouth
1. **Levator labii superioris**: descends from maxilla just above infraorbital foramen (below infraorbital margin) to insert into upper lip; raises upper lip
2. **Levator labii superioris alaeque nasi**: from frontal process of maxilla to insert on ala of nose and on lip; raises lip and dilates nares
3. **Zygomaticus major**: from zygomatic bone to insert into orbicularis oris near angle of mouth; draws angle of mouth up and back, as in laughing and smiling
4. **Zygomaticus minor**: occasional muscle slip almost continuous with orbicularis oculi; inserts on angle of mouth; helps form nasolabial groove; helps lift angle of mouth in smiling and deepens nasolabial groove in sorrow

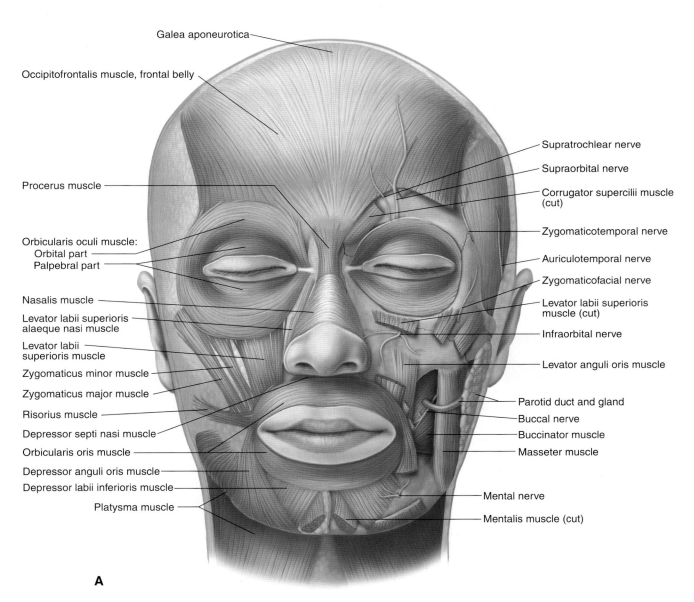

Galea aponeurotica

Occipitofrontalis muscle, frontal belly

Procerus muscle

Orbicularis oculi muscle:
　Orbital part
　Palpebral part

Nasalis muscle

Levator labii superioris
alaeque nasi muscle

Levator labii
superioris muscle

Zygomaticus minor muscle

Zygomaticus major muscle

Risorius muscle

Depressor septi nasi muscle

Orbicularis oris muscle

Depressor anguli oris muscle

Depressor labii inferioris muscle

Platysma muscle

Supratrochlear nerve

Supraorbital nerve

Corrugator supercilii muscle
(cut)

Zygomaticotemporal nerve

Auriculotemporal nerve

Zygomaticofacial nerve

Levator labii superioris
muscle (cut)

Infraorbital nerve

Levator anguli oris muscle

Parotid duct and gland

Buccal nerve

Buccinator muscle

Masseter muscle

Mental nerve

Mentalis muscle (cut)

A

Figure 2.10A. Muscles of Facial Expression, Anterior View.

5. **Levator anguli oris** (caninus): from canine fossa of maxilla below infraorbital foramen to insert on corner of mouth (on deeper plane than zygomaticus and levator labii superioris muscles); with levator labii superioris, alaeque nasi, and zygomaticus minor, it helps express contempt or disdain by raising angle of mouth

6. **Risorius**: extends posterior from corners of mouth as a small, very superficial muscle which pulls corners of mouth laterally, retracting angle of mouth; so-called "laughter" muscles

7. **Depressor anguli oris**: from mandible near attachment of platysma to insert on corners of mouth; pulls down or depresses corner of mouth; expression of disatisfaction or sorrow

8. **Depressor labii inferioris**: deep to depressor anguli oris, arising from mandible just above depressor anguli oris, and inserts into lower lip; depresses lower lip, drawing lip down and back

9. **Mentalis**: named for its location, not its action; small muscle just anterior to mental foramen, arising from mandible and inserting just inferior to incisor teeth; raises and wrinkles skin of chin and pushes up lower lip

10. **Platysma**: thin sheet of muscle in superficial fascia of neck, from pectoral region to mandible; retracts and depresses angle of mouth

11. **Orbicularis oris**: completely surrounds mouth, with no bony attachments; a complex muscle with layers, some parts intrinsic to lips, and others derived from buccinator, levator anguli oris, depressor anguli oris, and zygomaticus major and minor; closes lips, protrudes and purses lips, and presses lips to teeth aiding in articulation and mastication (chewing)

12. **Buccinator**: from pterygomandibular raphe and lateral surfaces of mandible and maxilla to insert into muscles around mouth, with fibers crossing to upper and lower lips; compresses cheek, holds food between teeth in mastication, and is important in blowing when cheeks are distended with air

III. Clinical Considerations

A. Due to deficiency of deep fascia and because superficial fascia between cutaneous attachments of muscles is loose, lacerations of face tend to open wide; suturing of skin of face must be done with great care to avoid scarring

B. Facial inflammation results in much swelling because of looseness of superficial fascia that permits fluid and blood to accumulate in loose connective tissue

C. Facial nerve injury and impairment

1. Produces variable amounts of weakness or paralysis of facial muscles, called **Bell's palsy**; weakness is particularly noticeable around mouth, where it may be evidenced by a sagging corner of mouth and possibly drooling, and becomes very obvious as asymmetry when attempting to smile; upper facial weakness can similarly be brought out by having patient attempt to frown, raise the eyebrows, or close the eyes tightly

2. Paralysis of entire side of face indicates that facial nerve as a whole has been damaged along its course; results in smooth, immobile face; if 1 side is involved, contrast to normal side is obvious: lower eyelid droops, tears trickle, angle of mouth droops, and saliva trickles; eating is difficult and speech is affected

3. Lesions paralyzing orbicularis oculi muscle and denervating lacrimal gland (also supplied by facial nerve CN VII) may result in corneal ulceration and ultimately scarring and impaired vision because patient cannot maintain corneal lubrication

4. Lesion of facial nerve within temporal bone may also cause disturbance of taste (loss of chorda tympani) or hyperacousis (loss of stapedius innervation)

(Continued)

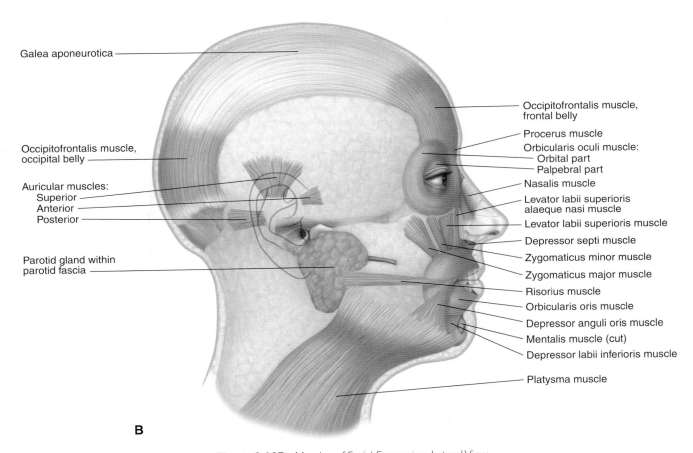

Galea aponeurotica

Occipitofrontalis muscle, frontal belly

Procerus muscle

Orbicularis oculi muscle:
Orbital part
Palpebral part

Occipitofrontalis muscle, occipital belly

Nasalis muscle

Auricular muscles:
Superior
Anterior
Posterior

Levator labii superioris alaeque nasi muscle

Levator labii superioris muscle

Depressor septi muscle

Zygomaticus minor muscle

Zygomaticus major muscle

Parotid gland within parotid fascia

Risorius muscle

Orbicularis oris muscle

Depressor anguli oris muscle

Mentalis muscle (cut)

Depressor labii inferioris muscle

Platysma muscle

B

Figure 2.10B. Muscles of Facial Expression, Lateral View.

5. Supranuclear lesion of CN VII
   a. Leads to sparing of upper muscles of facial expression (above palpebral fissure) and contralateral paralysis of lower muscles of facial expression
   b. Patients are able to close both eyes and wrinkle both brows
   c. No accompanying atrophy of muscles and patients retain facial reflexes (ability to smile reflexly or show other emotional expressions)
6. If buccinator and orbicularis oris muscles are weakened or paralyzed, food tends to accumulate in oral vestibule during chewing, needing a finger to remove it
7. Weakened lip muscles tend to affect speech due to impaired ability to produce labial letters (i.e., B, M, F, and W); patient cannot whistle or blow on a musical instrument
8. Weakness rather than complete paralysis of group of muscles typically results from injury to facial nerve branches because of overlap of their distribution
9. Clinical testing of facial muscles and their nerve supply is done by asking patient to close eye, show teeth (as wide as possible), and whistle (tests ability to purse lips and ability of buccinator to raise pressure in mouth
10. Some potential causes of facial paralysis
   a. Most common nontraumatic cause is inflammation of nerve near stylomastoid foramen due to viral infection, which produces swelling (edema) and compression of nerve in facial canal
   b. Fracture of temporal bone with paralysis noted after injury
   c. Unknown cause (idiopathic), but commonly follows exposure to cold (sleeping near open window with wind blowing on ear area)
   d. Complication of surgery (i.e., in case of parotidectomy) or associated with dental manipulation, vaccination, pregnancy, HIV infection, Lyme disease, and infections in middle ear
   e. Result of injury by stab or gunshot wounds, cuts, or even childbirth injuries
D. In Parkinson's disease or syndrome, emotional changes of facial expression are usually lost, giving face masklike, expressionless appearance

Parotid Gland, Facial Nerve, and Blood Vessels of Face

I. General Features of Parotid Gland

A. Largest of major salivary glands; weight = 14–28 g

B. Compound, branched tubuloalveolar gland; purely serous

C. Traversed by facial nerve and its branches, retromandibular vein, and external carotid artery

II. Location and Relations (Fig. 2.11A)

A. Anterior: lies against posterior border of ramus of mandible, extending anterolaterally onto masseter

  1. Medial projection: extends between pterygoid muscles medial to mandible

  2. Lateral projection: lies on lateral surface of masseter muscle, with small piece, commonly detached, just below zygomatic arch (accessory part or socia parotidis)

B. Posterior: SCM muscle

C. Superior: external acoustic meatus and root of zygomatic arch

D. Medial (deep portion): posterior part extends to styloid process and its muscles, entering infratemporal fossa

E. Relations

  1. Superficially: lobulated, covered by skin, fascia, lymph nodes, and branches of great auricular nerve

  2. Medially: internal carotid artery, internal jugular vein, vagus and glossopharyngeal nerves

  3. Within: facial nerve passing lateral to retromandibular vein and external carotid artery

III. Parotid Fascia

A. Continuous with superficial layer of deep cervical fascia; dense and closely united with gland (parotideomasseteric fascia)

B. Between styloid process and angle of mandible this fascia forms **stylomandibular ligament**, which separates parotid from submandibular gland; anteriorly it fuses with masseteric fascia

IV. Parotid Duct (Stensen's)

A. Approximately 5 cm long, passing anteriorly transversely and then medially

B. From anterior border of gland, crosses masseter muscle 1 fingerbreadth below zygomatic arch, turns medialward to pierce fat pad of cheek and buccinator muscle to open into oral vestibule opposite 2nd upper molar tooth

V. Innervation

A. Parasympathetic

  1. Presynaptic fibers arising in inferior salivatory nucleus pass by way of tympanic branch of glossopharyngeal nerve, through tympanic plexus and into lesser petrosal nerve; synapsing in otic ganglion

  2. Postsynaptic fibers enter auriculotemporal branch of mandibular nerve (CN V_3) to reach gland (secretomotor)

B. Sympathetics

  1. Presynaptic fibers from intermediolateral cell column of upper thoracic spinal cord, through anterior roots and white rami to synapse in superior cervical ganglion

  2. Postsynaptic fibers run in plexus on external carotid artery to reach gland (vasomotor)

VI. Structures Embedded in Gland (Fig. 2.11B,C)

A. **External carotid artery**: enters gland from below, gives posterior auricular branch and its terminal branches, superficial temporal and maxillary; transverse facial artery also arises from superficial temporal in gland

B. **Retromandibular vein**: union of maxillary and superficial temporal veins within gland; lies lateral to external carotid artery; in lower part, it branches into anterior and posterior divisions; anterior division joins facial vein to form **common facial vein** and posterior division unites with posterior auricular vein to form **external jugular vein**

C. Facial nerve

1. Enters posteromedial part of gland after emerging from stylomastoid foramen; gives rise to nerves to stylohyoid and posterior belly of digastric before entering gland and posterior auricular branch, which passes posterosuperiorly to innervate posterior auricular and occipitalis muscles

2. Passes inferolaterally, then anteriorly within gland to cross retromandibular vein laterally

3. 2 divisions; buccal branches of each commonly unite across parotid duct
   a. **Temporofacial division**: passes anterosuperiorly; 3 types of branches
      i. **Temporal branches**: pass superiorly across zygomatic arch to innervate superior and anterior auricular muscles and forehead muscles
      ii. **Zygomatic branch**: passes anterosuperiorly toward corner of eye to innervate orbicularis oculi
      iii. **Buccal branches**: pass transversely above parotid duct to innervate muscles of upper midface
   b. **Cervicofacial division**: passes anteroinferiorly; 3 types of branches
      i. **Buccal branches**: pass transversely below parotid duct to innervate muscles of lower midface
      ii. **Marginal mandibular branch**: passes anteroinferiorly then transversely across facial vessels near lower border of mandible to innervate facial muscles on mandible
      iii. **Cervical branch**: passes inferiorly and slightly anteriorly beneath platysma to innervate this muscle

D. **Auriculotemporal nerve**

1. Arises from mandibular nerve (CN V_3) below foramen ovale, receives postsynaptic fibers from otic ganglion (lying on medial surface of mandibular nerve)

2. Passes transversely posteriorly against TMJ capsule, then bends laterally behind joint to deliver secretomotor fibers into uppermost portion of parotid gland before coursing superiorly to innervate skin anterosuperior to ear

VII. Arteries of the Face

A. Predominantly branches of external carotid artery, although forehead and bridge of nose are supplied by ophthalmic branch of internal carotid artery

B. Branches of ophthalmic artery from internal carotid artery
   1. **Supratrochlear artery**: medially to upper eyelid and forehead
   2. **Supra-orbital artery**: forehead as high as vertex
   3. **Lacrimal artery**: upper eyelid laterally
   4. **Dorsal nasal artery**: bridge of nose

C. Branches of external carotid artery
   1. **Superficial temporal artery**: passes in temporalis fascia between head of mandible and external acoustic meatus and divides into anterior and posterior branches to scalp
   2. **Transverse facial artery**: branch of superficial temporal artery; passes anteriorly parallel to lower margin of zygomatic arch over masseter muscle
   3. **Posterior auricular artery**: behind and above ear and mastoid process
   4. **Occipital artery**: to posterior aspect of head
   5. **Facial artery**: crosses lower border of mandible anterior to masseter insertion; gives off inferior labial branches to lower lip; superior labial branches to upper lip; and anastomoses as angular artery with branch of ophthalmic in medial angle of eye
   6. **Maxillary artery**: supplies deep structures and muscles of face

VIII. Lymphatic Drainage of Superficial Structures of Head

A. Face: to submandibular nodes at submandibular gland; to facial nodes (i.e., buccinator node on buccinator muscle); nasolabial nodes, below nasolabial groove; mandibular node

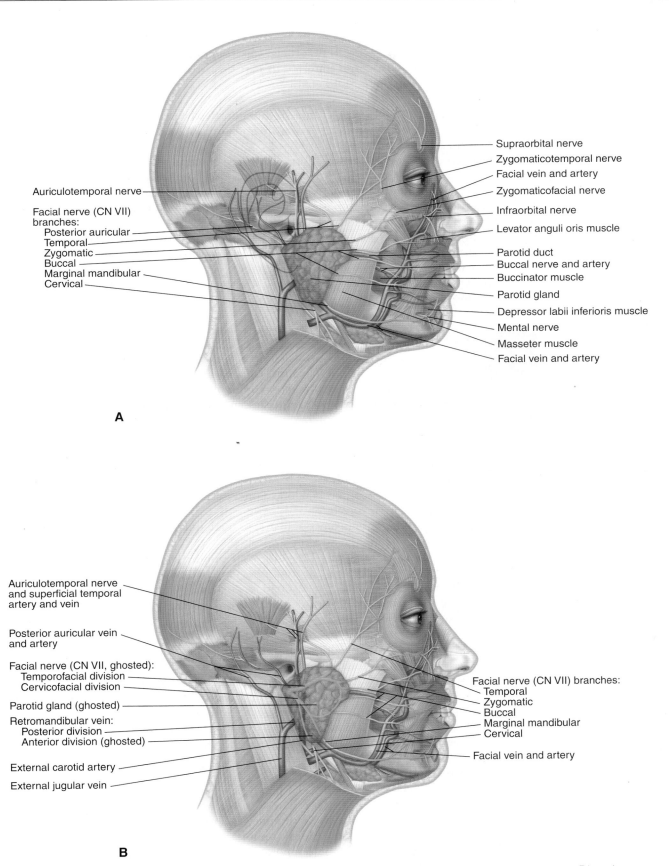

Auriculotemporal nerve

Facial nerve (CN VII) branches:
Posterior auricular
Temporal
Zygomatic
Buccal
Marginal mandibular
Cervical

Supraorbital nerve
Zygomaticotemporal nerve
Facial vein and artery
Zygomaticofacial nerve
Infraorbital nerve
Levator anguli oris muscle
Parotid duct
Buccal nerve and artery
Buccinator muscle
Parotid gland
Depressor labii inferioris muscle
Mental nerve
Masseter muscle
Facial vein and artery

A

Auriculotemporal nerve
and superficial temporal
artery and vein

Posterior auricular vein
and artery

Facial nerve (CN VII, ghosted):
Temporofacial division
Cervicofacial division

Parotid gland (ghosted)

Retromandibular vein:
Posterior division
Anterior division (ghosted)

External carotid artery

External jugular vein

Facial nerve (CN VII) branches:
Temporal
Zygomatic
Buccal
Marginal mandibular
Cervical

Facial vein and artery

B

Figure 2.11A,B. Parotid Gland, Facial Nerve, and Blood Vessels of the Face. **A.** Superficial Dissection. **B.** Deeper Dissection.

(at facial vein on body of mandible); or submental nodes, located below chin, especially from lower lip

B. Angle of jaw and upper neck: to superficial cervical nodes

C. Frontal and temporal regions anterior to ear: to preauricular or superficial and deep parotid nodes, on and in parotid gland

D. Parotid area

   1. Superficial or preauricular group: lie in superficial fascia, receiving channels from upper part of face, temporal area of scalp and anterior part of auricle; drain into chain of nodes along external jugular vein

   2. Deep group: found in gland substance; receive channels from gland itself, part of nasopharynx, and from nose, palate, auditory tube, middle ear, and external acoustic meatus; drains into subparotid node and then to deep cervical nodes

E. Posterior to and above ear: to postauricular (mastoid) nodes on mastoid process

F. Posterior part of head: to occipital nodes

G. Above nodes, serve as primary barriers and subsequently connect, directly or indirectly, with secondary nodes called *upper deep cervical nodes* (along internal jugular vein); latter connect with *lower deep cervical nodes*, which form jugular trunk that drains into venous system at point where internal jugular and subclavian veins unite by joining right lymphatic duct or thoracic duct

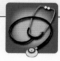

IX. Clinical Considerations

A. Calculus formation: obstruction of parotid duct may be associated with recurrent or chronic parotitis; calculi can form in major ducts of 3 major salivary glands, but occurs most commonly in submandibular duct

B. Salivary fistulas: can occur due to some surgical procedure in area of gland or duct; most close spontaneously; duct ligation in mouth has been performed to control salivary incontinence after radical surgery for malignant tumors of mouth floor

C. Neoplasms: 85%–90% of mixed tumors of salivary glands involve parotid; tumors are generally excised

   1. May involve superficial lobe alone, rarely deep lobe alone; sometimes both lobes are involved

   2. Have high recurrence rate due to inadequate excision with residual tumor in remaining gland after surgery

   3. Approximately 5%–12% of mixed tumors show evidence of malignancy, whereas 30% of all parotid tumors are malignant

D. Frey's syndrome: gustatory sweating; if parotid gland is cut, secretomotor fibers of gland may grow out to innervate sweat glands of face, causing sweating during meals

E. Mumps: most common inflammatory lesion of gland; acute contagious paramyxoviral infection seen mostly in childhood, leading to inflammation of parotid (other salivary glands and other tissues may be involved) causing pain due to swelling within tight cervical fascia covering of gland; swallowing also causes pressure on inflamed gland and subsequent pain; duct may become obstructed and also cause pain

F. Parotid disease commonly causes pain in auricle, external acoustic meatus, temporal areas, and TMJ, because auriculotemporal nerve supplies sensory fibers to parotid gland (and secretomotor fibers) and to skin over temporal fossa and auricle

G. Bell's palsy: unilateral facial paralysis of sudden onset, which involves facial nerve (CN VII)

   1. May be due to facial trauma; lacerations; injury to nerve surgically; inflammation; infections; tumors; cold drafts and other temperature changes, resulting in temporary palsy of areas supplied by CN VII

2. Test for nerve function by asking patient to: raise eyebrows; close eyelids tightly; show teeth; purse lips to whistle; pull down corners of mouth; blow out cheeks; etc.

3. Signs: affected side of face sags; speech is muffled; food and saliva tend to collect between affected cheeks and teeth; marked asymmetry of face when trying to smile; patient cannot whistle; eyelid on affected side cannot be closed and lower lid tends to droop; patient cannot raise eyebrow or wrinkle forehead on affected side; and sound may be exaggerated and seem louder than usual if stapedius muscle innervation is affected

H. Trigeminal neuralgia (tic douloureux): severe, sharp pain in face (paroxysm) precipitated by stimulation of "trigger point" on face by touch, wind, speaking, chewing, etc. and resulting in spasmotic contractions of face

   1. Cause is unknown; may involve any or all of branches of trigeminal nerve (CN V), with maxillary nerve most commonly affected and ophthalmic nerve least commonly affected

   2. Seen most commonly in elderly and middle-aged people; pain may last 15 minutes or more and patient "winces" or has a "tic" (twitch); may lead to depression and suicide if pain is very severe and continuous

(Continued)

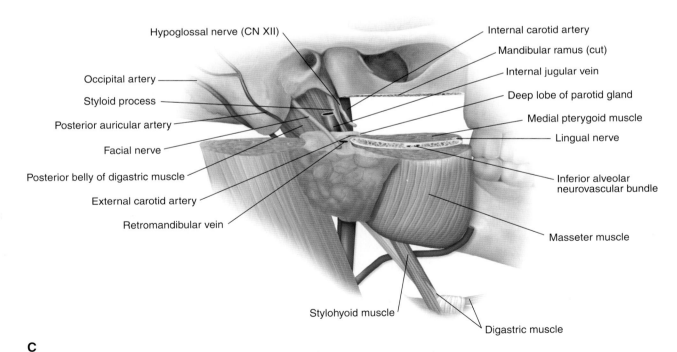

C

Figure 2.11C. Parotid Gland, Facial Nerve, and Blood Vessels of the Face, Deep Dissection.

3. Surgical treatment involves dividing CN V, injecting nerve with alcohol, etc., or balloon compression of nerve root

4. Following surgery, anesthesia usually occurs over 1/2 of face (or affected area), from which patient may recover over time

I. **Horner's syndrome**

1. Interruption of sympathetic supply to head and neck anywhere along its pathway (brainstem, sympathetic trunk, or superior cervical ganglion), leading to denervation of glands and smooth muscles to area supplied

2. Symptoms include: sinking in of eyeball; ptosis (drooping of upper eyelid) due to denervation of smooth muscle component of levator palpebrae superioris muscle; narrowing of palpebral fissure; constriction or miosis of pupil on affected side; lack of sweating (anhidrosis) on affected side; skin of face is warm, dry, and flushed due to interruption of innervation of vascular smooth muscle and sweat glands; nasal congestion also noticeable; heart rate may increase because cardiac branches arise from cervical sympathetic ganglia

J. Arterial pulses of face and scalp: superficial temporal and facial arteries may be used for taking pulse

1. Superficial temporal pulse: where superficial temporal artery crosses zygomatic process just anterior to auricle

2. Facial pulse: with teeth clenched, feel facial artery as it crosses inferior border of mandible just anterior to masseter muscle

K. Facial artery compression

1. Can be occluded by placing pressure against mandible where vessel crosses it

2. Due to numerous branches and anastomoses of facial vessels, compression of 1 side does not stop bleeding from lacerated facial artery or 1 of its branches; thus, in case of bleeding lip, pressure must be applied to both sides of cut; facial wounds tend to bleed freely, and they tend to heal quickly

Temporal, Infratemporal, and Pterygopalatine Fossae

I. General Features of Temporal, Infratemporal, and Pterygopalatine Fossae (Fig. 2.12)

A. Temporal fossa
  1. Space on side of calvaria
  2. Contents: temporalis muscle, deep temporal nerves and vessels, auriculotemporal nerve, superficial temporal vessels
  3. Boundaries
      a. Posterosuperiorly: superior temporal line
      b. Inferiorly: infratemporal crest
      c. Anteriorly: frontal process of zygomatic bone
      d. Laterally: zygomatic arch
      e. Floor: formed by 4 bones: frontal, parietal, temporal, and sphenoid forming pterion

B. Infratemporal fossa
  1. Deep lateral region of face, between ramus of mandible and pharynx beneath base of skull; continuous with temporal fossa above infratemporal crest of sphenoid and zygomatic arch
  2. Boundaries
      a. Anteriorly: posterior surface of maxilla
      b. Posteriorly: styloid and mastoid process
      c. Superiorly: greater wing of sphenoid bone
      d. Medially: lateral pterygoid plate of sphenoid
      e. Laterally: ramus of mandible
      f. Inferiorly: medial pterygoid muscle attaching to mandible near its angle
  3. Foramina
      a. Foramen spinosum: for middle meningeal artery into middle cranial fossa
      b. Foramen ovale: for mandibular nerve (CN V$_3$) and accessory meningeal artery
      c. Pterygomaxillary fissure: medial cleft leading into pterygopalatine fossa; for terminal part of maxillary artery
      d. Inferior orbital fissure: leads anteriorly into orbit; for zygomatic and infraorbital branches of maxillary nerve (CN V$_2$), infraorbital artery, and communication between pterygoid plexus and inferior ophthalmic vein

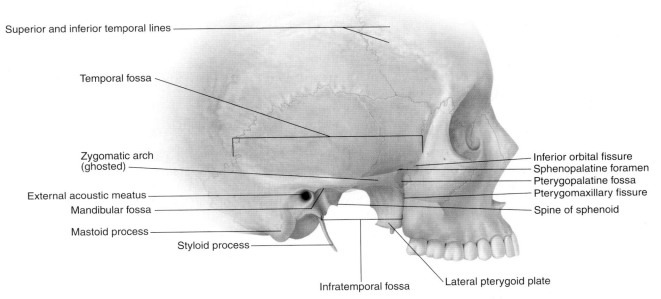

Figure 2.12. Temporal, Infratemporal, and Pterygopalatine Fossae, Lateral View.

4. Contents

    a. Muscles of mastication (masseter and most of temporalis lie outside of infratemporal fossa)

        i. Lower portion of temporalis muscle: passes medial to zygomatic arch to insert on coronoid process and anterior border of ramus of mandible

        ii. Lateral pterygoid muscle: from lateral pterygoid plate and greater wing of sphenoid to neck of mandible and articular disc of TMJ

        iii. Medial pterygoid muscle: from medial surface of lateral pterygoid plate and tuberosity of maxilla to medial surface of ramus and angle of mandible

    b. Mandibular nerve (CN V$_3$) and its branches, chorda tympani, and otic ganglion

    c. Maxillary artery

    d. Pterygoid plexus

    e. Lymphatics

C. Pterygopalatine fossa: narrow cleft located deep in face

  1. Boundaries

    a. Anteriorly: posterior surface of maxilla

    b. Posteriorly: anterior margin of pterygoid process of sphenoid

    c. Medially: perpendicular plate of palatine bone

    d. Superiorly: greater wing of sphenoid

    e. Laterally: communicates with infratemporal fossa through pterygomaxillary fissure (between pterygoid process posteriorly and maxillary bone anteriorly)

  2. Multiple foramina communicate with pterygopalatine fossa

    a. Sphenopalatine foramen: medially into nasal cavity for sphenopalatine artery and nasopalatine nerve

    b. Pharyngeal canal: courses posteriorly and medially into pharynx, for pharyngeal artery

    c. Pterygoid canal: directed posteriorly; ends in superior part of foramen lacerum; transmits nerve of pterygoid canal

    d. Foramen rotundum: transmits maxillary division of CN V anteriorly from middle cranial fossa

    e. Inferior orbital fissure: anterolateral into orbital floor

    f. Greater palatine canal (for greater palatine nerves) and **lesser palatine canals** (for lesser palatine arteries and nerves); pass inferiorly to reach roof of mouth

  3. Contents of pterygopalatine fossa

    a. Pterygopalatine ganglion: parasympathetic, greater petrosal fibers from facial nerve (CN VII) synapse; for lacrimal gland and nasal mucosa

    b. Maxillary nerve and its branches

    c. Maxillary artery and its terminal branches

II. Clinical Considerations

  A. Infratemporal fossa is a deep portion of face with major clinical significance due to its many relations

    1. Parotid gland extends into it

    2. Mandibular nerve branches course through it

    3. Maxillary artery passes through it

  B. Posterior superior alveolar and inferior alveolar nerves to upper and lower teeth are accessible for anesthesia within infratemporal fossa

  C. Electrode pushed against its roof can pick up electroencephalograms from temporal lobe because it abuts anterior part of wing of sphenoid of floor of middle cranial fossa

Infratemporal Fossa: Muscles of Mastication

I. General Features

A. Represent musculature of 1st pharyngeal arch

B. All insert on mandible and are innervated by mandibular nerve (CN V₃)

C. Other muscles are active in mastication but are not considered muscles of mastication (i.e., muscles of cheek, floor of mouth, and tongue)

D. 4 muscles on each side: temporalis, masseter, and medial and lateral pterygoid muscles

II. Special Features (Fig. 2.13A)

A. Temporalis

  1. Origin: from temporal fascia and temporal fossa from temporal lines to infratemporal crest
  2. Insertion: coronoid process and anterior border of ramus of mandible
  3. Action: closes jaw, posteroinferior part retracts jaw
  4. Innervation: anterior and posterior deep temporal branches of mandibular nerve (CN V₃), which curve around infratemporal crest to pass beneath temporalis

B. Masseter

  1. Origin
      a. Superficial part: anterior 2/3 of lower border of zygomatic arch
      b. Deep part: posterior and medial side of zygomatic arch

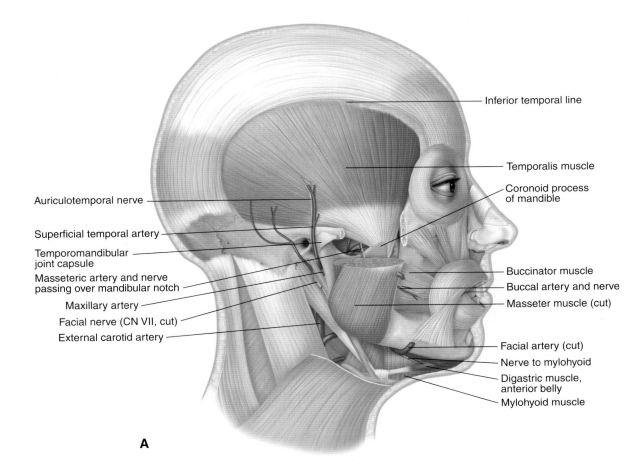

A

Figure 2.13A. Infratemporal Fossa: Muscles of Mastication, Lateral View, Superficial Dissection.

    2. Insertion
      a. Superficial part: angle and lower lateral surface of ramus of mandible
      b. Deep part: upper lateral surface of ramus
    3. Action: closes jaw
    4. Innervation: masseteric nerve from mandibular nerve (CN V_3), which passes over mandibular notch to enter muscle

C. Medial pterygoid (internal pterygoid) **(Fig. 2.13B,C)**
    1. Origin: medial surface of lateral pterygoid plate of sphenoid, pyramidal process of palatine and tuberosity of maxilla
    2. Insertion: lower and posterior part of angle and medial surface of ramus of mandible
    3. Action: closes jaw with bilateral contraction; helps grinding movements with 1-sided contraction (moving jaw side to side)
    4. Innervation: nerve to medial pterygoid from mandibular nerve (CN V_3), which also sends branches to innervate tensor tympani and tensor veli palatini

D. Lateral pterygoid (external pterygoid)
    1. Origin
      a. Superior head: from inferior surface of greater wing of sphenoid
      b. Inferior head: from lateral surface of lateral pterygoid plate
    2. Insertion
      a. Superior head: articular disc of TMJ
      b. Inferior head: pterygoid fovea on neck of mandibular condyle
    3. Action: protrudes mandible, opening mouth by drawing mandible and articular disc forward onto articular tubercle; unilateral contraction moves mandible from side to side, assisting in grinding motion (Note: anterior belly of digastric, geniohyoid, mylohyoid, and platysma help in opening mouth)
    4. Innervation: nerve to lateral pterygoid from mandibular nerve (CN V_3)

III. Mastication: Summary of Muscle Action

A. Opening jaw: lateral pterygoid muscle pulls condyle and articular disc forward onto articular tubercle, whereas stylomandibular and sphenomandibular ligaments restrict forward movement of angle and midpoint of ramus, thereby opening mouth; muscles of floor of mouth and force of gravity assist in opening

B. Closing jaw: temporalis, masseter, and medial pterygoid close mouth

C. Grinding motion: primarily due to alternating unilateral contraction of lateral and medial pterygoid and posterior fibers of temporalis; lateral pterygoid protrudes jaw, whereas posteroinferior fibers of temporalis retract it

D. Lips, tongue, and cheek muscles position food between teeth so that muscles of mastication can produce effective pressure to crush and grind food; muscles of floor of mouth help with movements of tongue

IV. Clinical Considerations

A. Lesions of mandibular division of trigeminal nerve will cause unilateral paralysis of muscles of mastication followed by atrophy; results in a sunken-in appearance along ramus of mandible and above zygomatic arch

B. Masseter, temporalis, and medial pterygoid muscles are powerful jaw closers, accounting for strength of bite; temporalis is strongest individual jaw constrictor; its torque, however, is exceeded by momentum of muscle sling formed by masseter and medial pterygoid muscles

C. Posteroinferior fibers of temporalis are primary retractor of mandible

D. Alternating action of lateral pterygoid muscles can assist in moving jaw from side to side, but important action of these muscles is to act bilaterally and help to open mouth

(Continued)

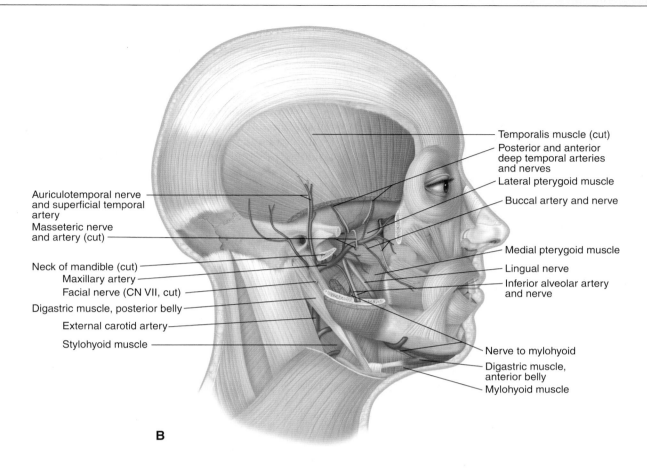

Temporalis muscle (cut)

Posterior and anterior deep temporal arteries and nerves

Lateral pterygoid muscle

Buccal artery and nerve

Medial pterygoid muscle

Lingual nerve

Inferior alveolar artery and nerve

Auriculotemporal nerve and superficial temporal artery

Masseteric nerve and artery (cut)

Neck of mandible (cut)

Maxillary artery

Facial nerve (CN VII, cut)

Digastric muscle, posterior belly

External carotid artery

Stylohyoid muscle

Nerve to mylohyoid

Digastric muscle, anterior belly

Mylohyoid muscle

B

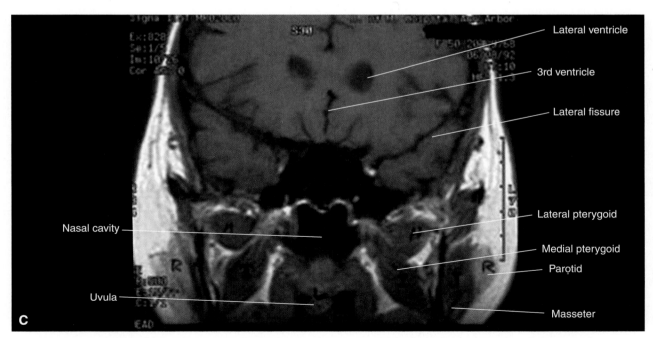

Lateral ventricle

3rd ventricle

Lateral fissure

Lateral pterygoid

Medial pterygoid

Parotid

Masseter

Nasal cavity

Uvula

C

Figure 2.13B,C. B. Infratemporal Fossa: Muscles of Mastication, Lateral View, Deep Dissection. **C.** Muscles of Mastication, Magnetic Resonance Images, Coronal View.

E. Anterior belly of digastric, geniohyoid, and mylohyoid muscles help to open mouth against resistance, if hyoid bone is fixed by contraction of infrahyoid muscles

F. Clinical tests of muscles of mastication: ask patient to clench teeth (to feel masseter and temporalis muscles contract) and to move chin from side to side

G. Jaw dislocation

　1. Muscles that close jaw are far more powerful than those that open it, and jaw may become displaced anterior to articular tubercle

　2. When relocating dislocated jaw by pushing mandible downward and backward over articular tubercle, protect the fingers by wrapping them thoroughly when placing them on mandible to avoid having them caught in sudden snap back of mandible

Infratemporal Fossa: Temporomandibular Joint and Neurovasculature

I. Temporomandibular Joint (Fig. 2.14A–C)

A. Hinge type (ginglymus) synovial joint with 2 synovial cavities separated by oval, biconcave, fibrocartilaginous (may be purely fibrous) intra-articular disc; disc is attached circumferentially to joint capsule and is also attached, in front, to superior head of lateral pterygoid muscle, to ensure forward movement of disc with protrusion of condyle

B. Condyle or head of mandible is cylindrical and extends relatively far medially; mandibular fossa of temporal bone is larger than condyle, allowing for mobility; only anterior part of fossa forms articular surface; posterior part is covered by compact connective tissue and lies outside of joint capsule

C. Anteriorly, articular surface of mandibular fossa is covered by fibrocartilage and continues onto **articular tubercle**; thus, tubercle lies within capsule

D. Capsule of TMJ is lax and relatively flaccid between disc and temporal bone, but stronger both medially and laterally between disc and mandible, actually passing downward over head and neck of mandible; fuses with circumference of disc

E. TMJ is thickened laterally by collateral **temporomandibular ligament** (from zygomatic arch to neck of mandible) and assisted medially by 2 ligamentous tracts (which are not part of capsule); namely, **sphenomandibular** and **stylomandibular ligaments**

  1. Sphenomandibular ligament

    a. From spine of sphenoid to lingula of mandible

    b. Maxillary vessels pass between sphenomandibular ligament and neck of condyle; inferiorly, deep anterior part of parotid gland and inferior alveolar vessels and nerve lie between this ligament and ramus of mandible

  2. Stylomandibular ligament

    a. From styloid process to angle and lower posterior border of mandible

    b. Thickening of parotid fascia

    c. Separates parotid and submandibular salivary glands

F. 3 possible TMJ movements (Note: displacements always take place at both right and left joints simultaneously)

  1. Opening (protrusion)

  2. Closing (retraction)

  3. Grinding (alternating oblique protrusion and retraction)

G. Proprioception (sensory receptors) from TMJ follow auriculotemporal and masseteric branches of mandibular nerve (CN V$_3$)

II. Neurovasculature of Infratemporal Fossa

A. Mandibular nerve (**CN V₃**) **(Fig. 2.14D)**

1. Only division of CN V with both sensory and skeletal motor fibers (CN V₁ and CN V₂ are entirely sensory)
2. Branches from undivided nerve in foramen ovale
   a. **Nerve to medial pterygoid** (also innervates tensor tympani and tensor veli palatini)
   b. Meningeal branch
3. Below foramen ovale, divides into anterior and posterior divisions
   a. Anterior division: primarily to muscles of mastication
      i. 2 **deep temporal branches** to temporalis
      ii. **Masseteric nerve**
      iii. **Nerve to lateral pterygoid**
      iv. **Buccal nerve**
         a) Passes above or through lateral pterygoid and anterior inserting fibers of temporalis to lie on buccinator
         b) Sensory supply to skin of cheek and mucous membrane of oral vestibule (Note: buccal *nerve* is sensory to cheek, inner and outer, whereas buccal *branches* of facial nerve are motor to buccinator muscle and other facial muscles
   b. Posterior division
      i. **Lingual nerve**
         a) Passes anteroinferiorly between medial pterygoid and ramus and under lower border of superior pharyngeal constrictor muscle to leave infratemporal fossa and enter paralingual space
         b) Carries general sensation from anterior 2/3 of tongue and from mucous membrane of front of mouth
         c) **Chorda tympani** from facial nerve joins lingual nerve below cranial base and travels with this nerve to reach tongue for taste; chorda also carries presynaptic parasympathetic fibers to submandibular ganglion, from which postsynaptic fibers pass to submandibular and sublingual glands
      ii. **Inferior alveolar nerve**
         a) Passes inferiorly and slightly anteriorly toward mandibular foramen against sphenomandibular ligament
         b) Gives off **mylohyoid branch** to mylohyoid and anterior belly of digastric muscles; mylohyoid nerve descends in groove on inner surface of ramus then passes anteromedially through submandibular triangle to lie on mylohyoid and enter anterior belly of digastric
         c) Enters mandibular canal to provide sensation for lower teeth and gums; gives off **mental nerve** through mental foramen for skin of chin and lower lip
      iii. **Auriculotemporal nerve**
         a) Passes transversely posteriorly against TMJ, turns superiorly to travel with superficial temporal artery into temporal region
         b) Sensory to TMJ and skin of temporal region of side of head
         c) Carries postsynaptic fibers from otic ganglion to parotid gland; middle meningeal artery usually passes between sensory and secretomotor roots of nerve

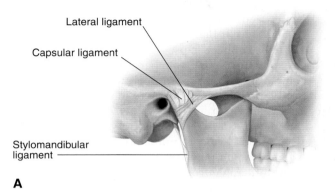

Lateral ligament

Capsular ligament

Stylomandibular
ligament

A

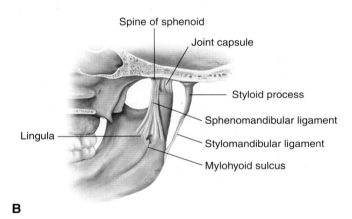

Spine of sphenoid

Joint capsule

Styloid process

Sphenomandibular ligament

Stylomandibular ligament

Mylohyoid sulcus

Lingula

B

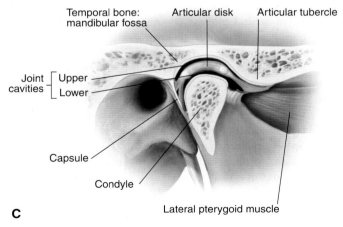

Temporal bone:
mandibular fossa

Articular disk

Articular tubercle

Joint
cavities
Upper
Lower

Capsule

Condyle

Lateral pterygoid muscle

C

Figure 2.14A–C. Temporomandibular Joint. **A.** Lateral View. **B.** Medial View. **C.** Parasagittal Sectional View.

B. Otic ganglion

1. Located on medial surface of mandibular nerve below foramen ovale
2. Parasympathetic ganglion
   a. Presynaptic fibers arise from glossopharyngeal nerve (CN IX)
      i. **Tympanic branch** passes up through inferior tympanic canaliculus to reach promontory of middle ear cavity
      ii. Forms **tympanic plexus** on promontory
      iii. **Lesser petrosal nerve** leaves plexus superiorly, emerges onto floor of middle cranial fossa at hiatus of lesser petrosal, passes through foramen ovale to reach otic ganglion to synapse
   b. Postsynaptic fibers innervate parotid gland
      i. Leave otic ganglion posteriorly to join **auriculotemporal branch of CN V$_3$**
      ii. Leave auriculotemporal nerve to enter parotid gland at its superior portion

C. Maxillary artery (Fig. 2.14E)

1. Largest branch of external carotid artery
   a. External carotid artery terminates within parotid gland by branching into maxillary and superficial temporal arteries
   b. Arises at right angle from bifurcation of external carotid
   c. Passes posterior to neck of mandible, continues anteromedially between sphenomandibular ligament and neck of mandible and temporalis and lateral pterygoid muscles and then either deep or superficial to lateral pterygoid muscle to enter pterygopalatine fossa, where it divides into its terminal branches
2. Supplies muscles of mastication, mucous membranes of oral and nasal cavities, teeth, palate, and a large part of cranial dura and bones of skull
3. Branches in lateral deep facial regions arise in 3 sections, accompanied by branches of mandibular nerve in infratemporal fossa and branches of maxillary nerve in area of pterygopalatine fossa
   a. 1st part (medial to TMJ): branches to TMJ; **deep auricular** to external acoustic meatus; **anterior tympanic branch** to tympanic cavity; **inferior alveolar branch** to mandible and **lower** teeth and gingiva, which terminates as mental artery to supply chin and lower lip; **middle meningeal branch** passes through foramen spinosum to supply dura and skull bones in middle cranial fossa
   b. 2nd part (between muscles of mastication): branches for pterygoids, masseter, temporalis, and buccinator muscles
   c. 3rd part (near or within pterygopalatine fossa):
      i. **Posterior superior alveolar artery**: to maxillary molar teeth and their gingiva and mucosa of maxillary sinus
      ii. **Infra-orbital artery**: through inferior orbital fissure and infraorbital groove, canal, and foramen to midface; in orbit, it supplies inferior rectus and inferior oblique muscles and inferior eyelid (palpebral); mucosa of maxillary sinus and maxillary premolar, canine, and incisor teeth; and gingiva via middle and anterior **superior alveolar arteries**
      iii. **Descending palatine**: to roof of oral cavity via greater palatine canal to supply mucosa of hard palate and gingiva as **greater palatine artery**, soft palate as **lesser palatine artery**, and tonsillar area with **pharyngeal branches**
      iv. **Sphenopalatine artery**: to nasal cavity via sphenopalatine foramen; **lateral posterior nasal** and **posterior septal branches** supply posterior lateral and septal mucosa of nasal cavity

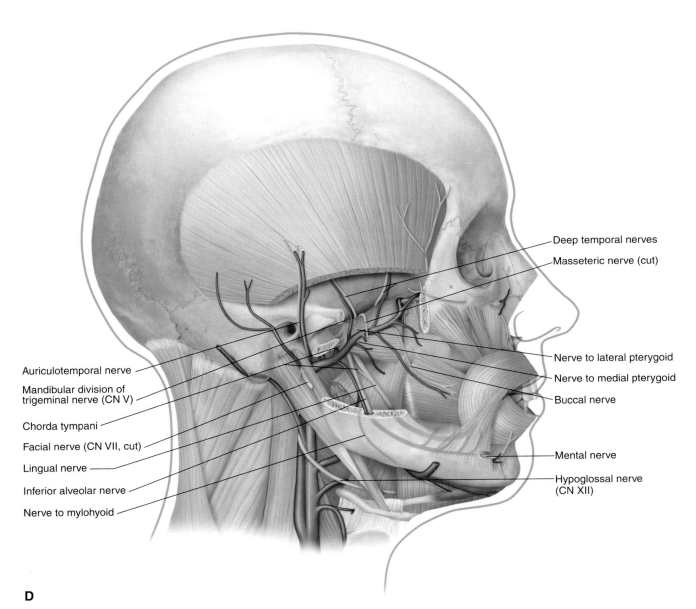

Deep temporal nerves

Masseteric nerve (cut)

Nerve to lateral pterygoid

Nerve to medial pterygoid

Buccal nerve

Mental nerve

Hypoglossal nerve (CN XII)

Auriculotemporal nerve

Mandibular division of trigeminal nerve (CN V)

Chorda tympani

Facial nerve (CN VII, cut)

Lingual nerve

Inferior alveolar nerve

Nerve to mylohyoid

D

Figure 2.14D. Infratemporal Fossa, Nerves, Lateral View.

D. Pterygoid plexus

   1. Extensive venous network in infratemporal fossa between temporalis, medial, and lateral pterygoid muscles

   2. Drains into retromandibular vein via maxillary veins

   3. Receives tributaries from cranial dura mater, muscles of mastication, tympanic cavity, and external ear

   4. Communicates below zygomatic arch with facial vein via deep facial vein

E. Lymphatics: pass to deep cervical lymph nodes along internal jugular vein and to retropharyngeal lymph nodes behind nasopharynx

III. Clinical Considerations

A. Dislocation of TMJ

   1. Always anterior as condyle slides forward too far past articular tubercle and cannot return to mandibular fossa

   2. Must be depressed before it will retract

   3. Bilateral dislocation can occur in absence of external violence (even by yawning)

B. Unilateral injury to V_3 will produce asymmetric protrusion of jaw; can be useful in clinical testing for nerve injury

C. Blows against jaw: may drive mandibular condyle upward and backward, resulting in injury to external auditory meatus and may cause bleeding from ear

D. Pressure produced by muscles that close jaw is normally borne almost entirely by molar teeth and TMJ, which extends in part over articular surfaces; thus, malocclusion or any factor that leads to spastic contraction of muscles (i.e., **trismus**, or **lockjaw**) may cause pain

E. Mandibular nerve block: local anesthesia may be applied to mandibular nerve as it emerges from foramen ovale and enters infratemporal fossa

   1. Extraoral approach: via mandibular notch, anesthetizing auriculotemporal, inferior alveolar, lingual, and buccal nerves; all skin areas innervated by mandibular division of trigeminal are thus anesthetized

   2. Intraoral approach: through buccal mucosa and buccinator muscle just medial to ramus of mandible, near mandibular foramen; anesthetizes inferior alveolar and lingual nerves and their subdivisions; areas involved are body and inferior ramus of mandible, mandibular teeth and gingivae, and mucous membrane of anterior 2/3 of tongue

F. Fractures of mandible: common

   1. TMJ may be disrupted; bone fragment displacements may necessitate wiring of jaw closed to stabilize it during healing

   2. Fractures in children may disrupt arrangement of tooth primordia, which lie deep within mandible

G. Mandibular developmental changes

   1. At birth, mandibular halves are not yet fused at chin

   2. By year 2, fusion at mental symphysis is usually complete

   3. In 1st 2 decades of life, angle between neck and body of mandible is less acute than in later life

   4. In old age, most teeth of mandible may be lost, alveolar bone of tooth sockets is resorbed, body becomes much thinner, and angle between neck and head once again becomes more oblique

H. TMJ arthritis: joint may become inflamed from degenerative arthritis leading to structural problems (i.e., dental occlusion and "joint clicking" (crepitus); latter may be due to delayed movements of anterior disc during elevation and depression of mandible)

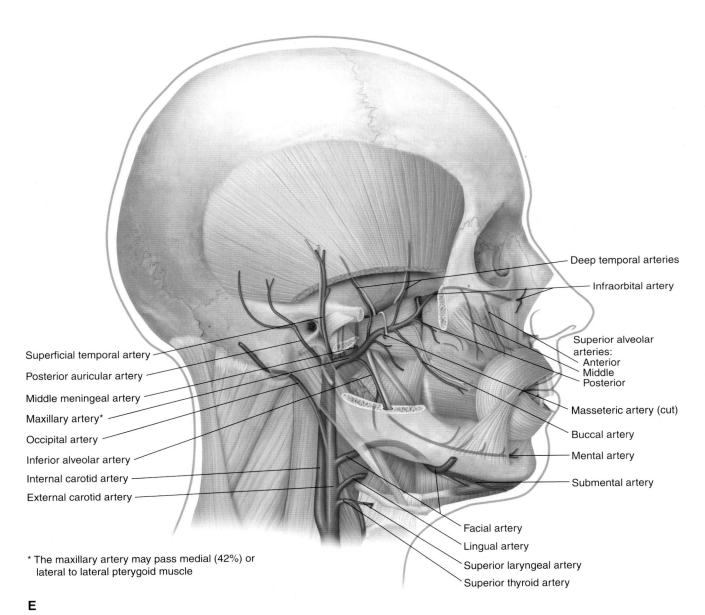

Deep temporal arteries

Infraorbital artery

Superior alveolar
arteries:
Anterior
Middle
Posterior

Masseteric artery (cut)

Buccal artery

Mental artery

Submental artery

Superficial temporal artery

Posterior auricular artery

Middle meningeal artery

Maxillary artery*

Occipital artery

Inferior alveolar artery

Internal carotid artery

External carotid artery

Facial artery

Lingual artery

Superior laryngeal artery

Superior thyroid artery

* The maxillary artery may pass medial (42%) or
lateral to lateral pterygoid muscle

E

Figure 2.14E. Infratemporal Fossa, Arteries, Lateral View.

Submandibular Region

I. Submandibular (Digastric or Submaxillary) Triangle

A. Boundaries (Fig. 2.15A,B)
1. Anterior and posterior bellies of digastric muscle, inferior border of mandible
2. Subdivision of anterior cervical triangle

B. Roof
1. Skin and branches of transverse cervical nerve
2. Platysma and branches of cervical branch of facial nerve; in some people, especially elderly, marginal mandibular branch of facial nerve may swing below lower border of mandible
3. Superficial layer of deep cervical fascia

C. Floor: mylohyoid muscle

D. Contents (Fig. 2.15C,D)
1. Superficial portion of submandibular gland
   a. Invested by superficial layer of deep cervical fascia, which also thickens as stylomandibular ligament attaching to mandibular angle and separating submandibular and parotid salivary glands
   b. Wraps posterior edge of mylohyoid muscle to enter paralingual space, becoming small deep part of submandibular gland
2. Facial vein
   a. Crosses lower border of mandible anterior to masseter insertion
   b. Lies on superficial surface of submandibular gland
   c. Unites with anterior division of retromandibular vein to form common facial vein, which drains to internal jugular vein
3. Facial artery
   a. Arises as 3rd anterior branch of external carotid artery
   b. Lies deep to submandibular gland
   c. Crosses lower border of mandible anterior to masseter insertion to enter face
   d. Supplies submandibular gland, muscles of submandibular region; submental artery supplies submental triangle
4. Nerve to mylohyoid muscle
   a. Arises from inferior alveolar branch of mandibular nerve
   b. Travels in mylohyoid groove on medial surface of ramus
   c. Crosses on inferior surface of mylohyoid muscle to end in anterior belly of digastric muscle
   d. Innervates mylohyoid and anterior belly of digastric muscle
5. Hypoglossal nerve
   a. Emerges from hypoglossal canal, passes through carotid sheath between internal carotid artery and internal jugular vein
   b. Joined by fibers from C1 and C2, runs inferiorly and curving anteriorly just below lower border of posterior belly of digastric muscle within upper portion of carotid triangle
   c. Passes deep to posterior belly of digastric and stylohyoid muscles to enter inferomedial portion of submandibular triangle
   d. Passes from submandibular triangle into paralingual space by passing above posterior edge of mylohyoid muscle
6. Lingual artery
   a. 2nd anterior branch from external carotid artery
   b. Passes deep to posterior belly of digastric and stylohyoid muscles to enter inferomedial part of submandibular triangle
   c. Enters tongue by passing deep to posterior edge of hyoglossus muscle
7. Lymphatics
   a. 3 groups of submandibular nodes: preglandular, prevascular, and retrovascular
   b. Receive afferent channels from submental nodes, oral cavity, and anterior face
   c. Efferent channels drain primarily into deep cervical nodes including jugulodigastric and jugulo-omohyoid nodes

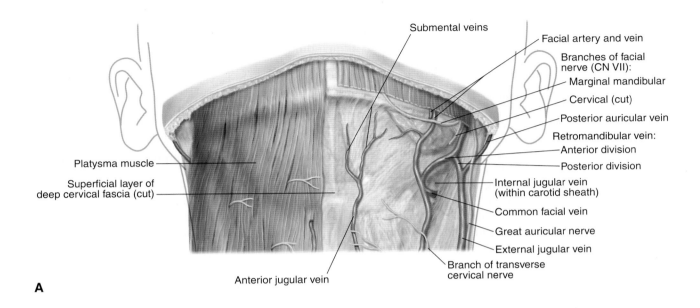

Submental veins

Facial artery and vein

Branches of facial
nerve (CN VII):

Marginal mandibular

Cervical (cut)

Posterior auricular vein

Retromandibular vein:

Anterior division

Posterior division

Platysma muscle

Internal jugular vein
(within carotid sheath)

Superficial layer of
deep cervical fascia (cut)

Common facial vein

Great auricular nerve

External jugular vein

Branch of transverse
cervical nerve

Anterior jugular vein

A

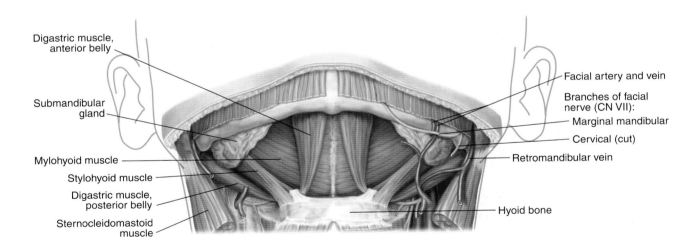

Digastric muscle,
anterior belly

Facial artery and vein

Branches of facial
nerve (CN VII):

Submandibular
gland

Marginal mandibular

Cervical (cut)

Mylohyoid muscle

Retromandibular vein

Stylohyoid muscle

Digastric muscle,
posterior belly

Sternocleidomastoid
muscle

Hyoid bone

B

Figure 2.15A,B. Submandibular Region, Anterior View. **A.** Superficial Dissection. **B.** Deep Dissection.

II. Submental Triangle

A. Boundaries
   1. Midline, hyoid bone, and anterior belly of digastric muscle
   2. Subdivision of anterior cervical triangle
B. Floor: mylohyoid muscle
C. Contents
   1. Submental lymph nodes
      a. Drain skin of chin, lower lip, floor of mouth, and tip of tongue
      b. Efferent channels pass to submandibular nodes or jugulo-omohyoid node of inferior deep cervical chain
   2. Submental veins: small, usually unite with submandibular veins to begin anterior jugular vein

III. Muscles of Submandibular Region (Suprahyoid Muscles)

A. Digastric muscle
   1. Origin
      a. Anterior belly: digastric fossa on lower inner aspect of symphysis of mandible
      b. Posterior belly: mastoid notch of temporal bone
   2. Insertion: body of hyoid bone via fibrous loop around intermediate tendon
   3. Action: elevate hyoid bone, pull mandibular symphysis down to open mouth
   4. Innervation
      a. Anterior belly: nerve to mylohyoid from inferior alveolar branch of mandibular nerve (CN V_3)
      b. Posterior belly: facial nerve (CN VII) as it emerges from stylomastoid foramen
B. Stylohyoid muscle
   1. Origin: styloid process of temporal bone; passes anteroinferiorly on superior surface of posterior belly of diagastric
   2. Insertion: splits to pass to either side of intermediate tendon of digastric to insert on body of hyoid bone lateral to lesser horn
   3. Action: elevate hyoid bone, pull hyoid bone posteriorly
   4. Innervation: facial nerve (CN VII) as it emerges from stylomastoid foramen
C. Mylohyoid muscle
   1. Origin: mylohyoid line on inner surface of body of mandible
   2. Insertion: body of hyoid bone and midline raphe
   3. Action: pulls hyoid bone forward, pulls mandibular symphysis down to open mouth, supports tongue
   4. Innervation: nerve to mylohyoid from inferior alveolar branch of mandibular nerve (CN V_3)
D. Geniohyoid muscle
   1. Origin: mental spine on inner aspect of symphysis of mandible
   2. Insertion: body of hyoid bone
   3. Action: pulls hyoid bone forward, pulls mandibular symphysis down to open mouth, supports tongue
   4. Innervation: C1 via fibers traveling with hypoglossal nerve (CN XII)

IV. Clinical Considerations

A. Superficial part of submandibular gland commonly becomes pendulous with advanced age, giving "jowls" of old age
B. Ludwig's angina: pain and swelling in submandibular region resulting from infections in floor of mouth; a severe form of cellulitis of submandibular space and secondary involvement of sublingual and submental spaces usually due to an infection or penetrating injury to floor of mouth
C. Mumps: painful swelling of submandibular gland may occur, although major target is usually parotid gland
D. Branchial cleft cysts: common in posterior part of submandibular region and are result of remnants of upper 2–3 original pharyngeal clefts, which normally completely disappear
E. Lymph node enlargement in submandibular region
   1. Commonly due to upper respiratory infection
   2. Less commonly seen with malignancy in lateral part of tongue (tip of tongue tumors tend to drain into submental region); usually there is long history of smoking

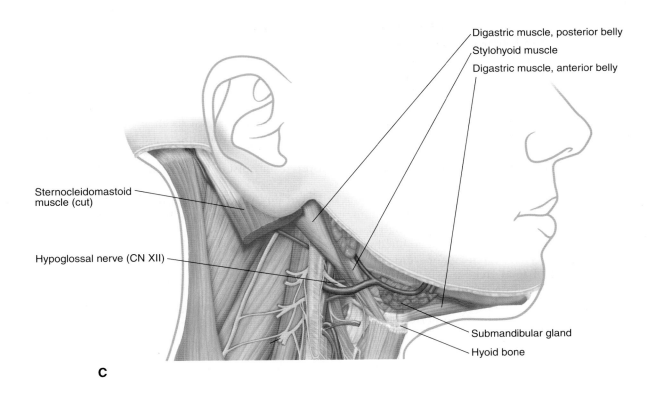

Digastric muscle, posterior belly

Stylohyoid muscle

Digastric muscle, anterior belly

Sternocleidomastoid muscle (cut)

Hypoglossal nerve (CN XII)

Submandibular gland

Hyoid bone

C

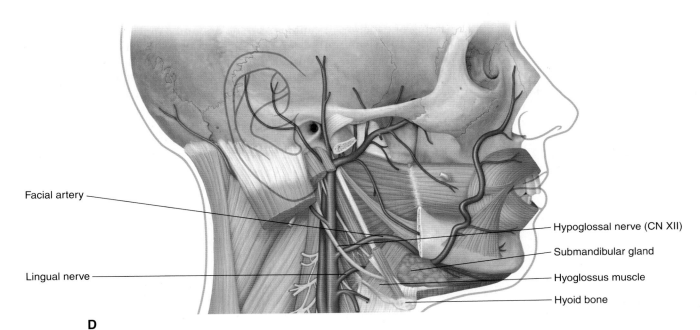

Facial artery

Lingual nerve

Hypoglossal nerve (CN XII)

Submandibular gland

Hyoglossus muscle

Hyoid bone

D

Figure 2.15C,D. Submandibular Region, Lateral View. **C.** Intermediate Dissection. **D.** Deep Dissection.

Oral Cavity and Teeth

I. Oral Cavity (Mouth) (Fig. 2.16A,B)

A. Divided into oral vestibule and oral cavity proper

B. Oral vestibule
1. Narrow space between lips, cheeks, and teeth
2. Communicates with oral cavity proper behind last molar teeth
3. Parotid duct opens into vestibule opposite upper 2nd molar tooth
4. **Labial frenula**: folds of mucous membrane in midline from upper and lower lips to gums

C. Lips
1. Formed by orbicularis oris muscle, covered on outside by facial skin (possesses adult hair) and on inside by oral mucosa
2. Transition zone bears epithelium of red of lips, which is covered by weakly cornified, stratified, squamous epithelium, into which lamina propria of mucosa deeply projects with capillary loops in high papillae
3. Red color of blood visible through epithelium
4. There are no glands and epithelium is moistened when speaking and eating
5. Labial mucosa
   a. Loosely connected with orbicularis oris muscle
   b. In loose mucosal connective tissue are small salivary glands, which commonly develop at puberty and can extend into buccal mucosa

D. Cheek
1. Contains buccinator muscle
2. Externally, buccal fat pad adjoins this muscle in front of anterior border of masseter muscle
3. Buccal mucosa, like labial, possesses small buccal salivary glands

E. Oral cavity proper
1. Extends from lips to palatoglossal folds (isthmus of fauces) and opens posteriorly into oropharynx
2. Roof
   a. Formed by mucous membrane covering hard and soft palate and gingiva of upper teeth, consisting of 2 incisors, 1 canine, 2 premolars, and 3 molars on either side
   b. Soft palate (velum palatinum) extends posteriorly from hard palate; uvula is centrally located extension of soft palate, which projects into pharynx
3. Anteriorly and laterally: teeth separate oral cavity proper from oral vestibule
4. Posteriorly: palatoglossal folds extend from soft palate to sides of tongue and mark posterior boundary of oral cavity and beginning of oropharynx; folds (also called *isthmus of fauces*) contain small palatoglossal muscles
5. Floor: mucous membrane of floor of mouth from tongue to gingiva of lower teeth, which covers paralingual space

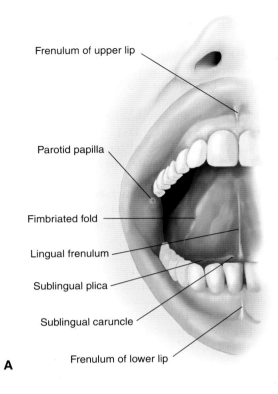

Frenulum of upper lip

Parotid papilla

Fimbriated fold

Lingual frenulum

Sublingual plica

Sublingual caruncle

Frenulum of lower lip

A

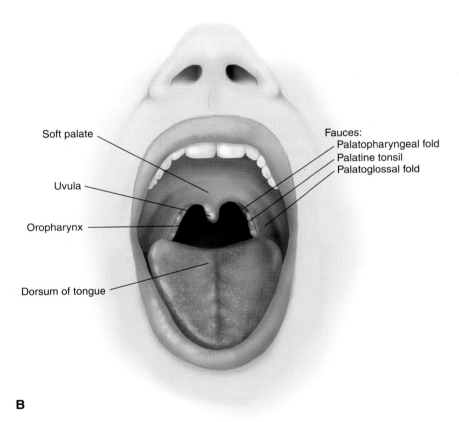

Soft palate

Uvula

Oropharynx

Dorsum of tongue

Fauces:
Palatopharyngeal fold
Palatine tonsil
Palatoglossal fold

B

Figure 2.16A,B. Oral Cavity. **A.** Tongue Elevated. **B.** Tongue Depressed.

II. General Features of Teeth and Gums

A. Located between oral vestibule and oral cavity proper

B. Teeth in both jaws should fit close together with their crowns and have no spaces (**diastemae**) in between, except for small interdental spaces at base of crowns

C. Humans, being mammals, have **heterodont dentition**; namely, teeth vary structurally and are adapted to handle food in different ways

D. Humans are also **diphyodont**; 2 sets of teeth develop in lifetime (deciduous or milk teeth are formed 1st and subsequently are superceded by permanent teeth)

E. **Occlusion**: refers to position that both rows of teeth occupy with respect to each other when jaw is closed (crowns of teeth make contact in occlusal plane)

F. Tooth orientation

   1. Masticatory surface of a tooth is its **occlusal surface**

   2. External surface facing oral vestibule is its **labial** or **buccal surface**

   3. Internal surface, facing oral cavity proper, is its **lingual surface**

III. Classification of Teeth (Fig. 2.16 C–E)

A. **Incisors**: 4 pairs of upper and lower anteriormost teeth; chisel-shaped crown with sharp horizontal edge adapted for cutting and shearing food

B. **Canines**: 2 pairs of cone-shaped teeth (also called *cuspids*)

   1. Located at anterior corners of mouth and are adapted for holding and tearing

   2. Longest tooth protected against tilting stress by long tooth root

C. **Premolars** (**bicuspids**): 4 pairs of upper and lower intermediate-size grinding teeth with 2 cusps behind canines

D. **Molars**: 6 pairs of large, somewhat rounded, irregular surfaces called *cusps* for crushing and grinding food

E. **Deciduous teeth**: 20 total, erupting between age 6–24 months

   1. 1st deciduous teeth are lower central incisors, between age 6–9 months

   2. Deciduous dental formula: 2-1-2 (2 incisors; 1 canine; 2 premolars, bilaterally and in both upper and lower jaws)

   3. 1st deciduous teeth shed at age 6–12 years

F. **Permanent teeth**

   1. Total of 32 teeth (4 × 8)

   2. Permanent dental formula: 2-1-2-3 (2 incisors; 1 canine; 2 premolars, 3 molars bilaterally and in both upper and lower jaws)

G. Age at time of eruption of permanent teeth

1st molar	6–7 years
Central incisors	7–8 years
Lateral incisors	8–9 years
1st premolar	10–11 years
Canine	10–12 years
2nd premolar	11–12 years
2nd molars	12–13 years
3rd molars	13–25 years

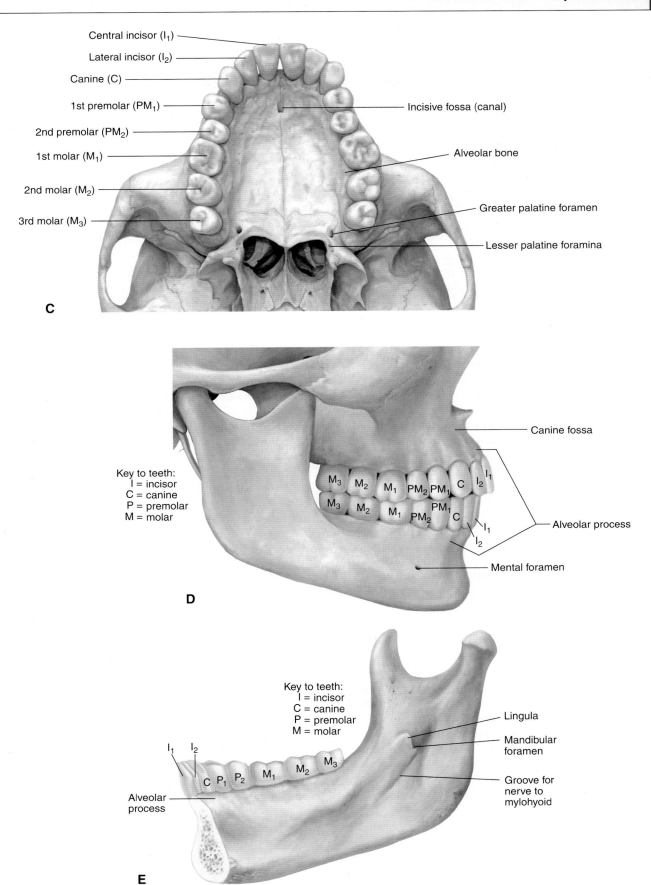

Central incisor (I₁)
Lateral incisor (I₂)
Canine (C)
1st premolar (PM₁)
2nd premolar (PM₂)
1st molar (M₁)
2nd molar (M₂)
3rd molar (M₃)

Incisive fossa (canal)

Alveolar bone

Greater palatine foramen

Lesser palatine foramina

C

Canine fossa

Key to teeth:
I = incisor
C = canine
P = premolar
M = molar

M₃ M₂ M₁ PM₂ PM₁ C I₁ I₂

M₃ M₂ M₁ PM₂ PM₁ C I₁ I₂

Alveolar process

Mental foramen

D

Key to teeth:
I = incisor
C = canine
P = premolar
M = molar

Lingula

Mandibular foramen

Groove for nerve to mylohyoid

I₁ I₂

C P₁ P₂ M₁ M₂ M₃

Alveolar process

E

Figure 2.16C–E. C. Maxillary Teeth, Inferior View. **D.** Maxillary and Mandibular Teeth, Lateral View. **E.** Mandibular Teeth, Medial View.

IV. Tooth Structure (Fig. 2.16F)

A. **Crown**: visible, exposed part; flattened, with hollow area posteriorly in incisor teeth; conical in canines; has 2 tubercles in premolars; and has 3–4 tubercles in molars

B. **Neck** or **cervix**: marginal zone between crown and root, surrounded by gums

C. **Roots**: anchored firmly in bone
   1. Roots fit into sockets called **alveoli**, in alveolar process of mandible and maxillae
   2. Incisors and canines have 1 root, premolars 2 roots, and molars have 2–3 roots

D. **Pulp cavity**: central region of tooth containing **pulp**, composed of connective tissue, blood vessels, and nerves

E. **Root canal**: continuous with pulp cavity through root to opening at base called **apical foramen**, through which vessels and nerves enter pulp cavity

F. **Dentine**: forms basic structure of tooth; similar to bone, but harder; forms nucleus of tooth and contains pulp cavity

G. **Enamel**
   1. Covers dentine to form crown
   2. Crown projects into oral cavity and bears cutting edge, or masticatory surface
   3. Avascular and aneural and consists of enamel prisms, which course from enamel–dentine border to enamel surface and are united by calcified organic cement substance
   4. Hardest substance in body with 96%–97% inorganic substance (90% in form of hydroxyapatite)

H. **Cementum**
   1. Covers dentine of roots
   2. 65% inorganic substances and closely resembles network bone
   3. In cementum, bundles of collagenous fibers are anchored to **periodontal membrane** (connective tissue periosteum) with which it is surrounded; periodontal membrane is covered and protected by gingiva; **periodontium** helps anchor tooth in alveolus; its collagen fibers pass in different directions between alveolar wall and cementum

V. Gums (Gingivae)

A. Mucous membrane over alveolar processes firmly attached to bone and extend into interdental spaces in form of interdental papillae

B. Surround necks of teeth and are firmly attached to alveolar jaw margins

C. Gums consist of fairly dense connective tissue covered by mucous membrane

D. Gingival epithelium, which surrounds neck of tooth is called **border epithelium**

VI. Vessels and Nerves of Teeth, Alveolar Processes, and Gingivae (Fig. 2.16G)

A. Blood supply
   1. Upper teeth
      a. Posterior superior alveolar artery from maxillary artery supplies upper molar teeth
      b. Middle superior alveolar artery from infraorbital branch of maxillary artery supplies upper premolar teeth
      c. Anterior superior alveolar artery from infraorbital branch of maxillary artery supplies upper canine and incisors
   2. Lower teeth: receive blood supply from inferior alveolar branch of maxillary artery

B. Nerves
   1. Upper teeth
      a. Innervated by anterior, middle, and posterior superior alveolar branches of maxillary nerve (CN V_2)
      b. Branches of greater palatine nerve pass to palatal gingiva
      c. Region posterior to incisor teeth, palatal gingiva is innervated by nasopalatine nerve
   2. Lower teeth
      a. Innervated by branches of inferior alveolar nerve from mandibular nerve (CN V_3) which forms **inferior dental plexus** in mandibular canal
      b. Innervates mandibular teeth with inferior dental branches and vestibular gingiva with inferior gingival branches, except for region of 2nd premolar and 1st molar, where buccal gingiva of mandible, like buccal mucosa, is supplied by buccal nerve

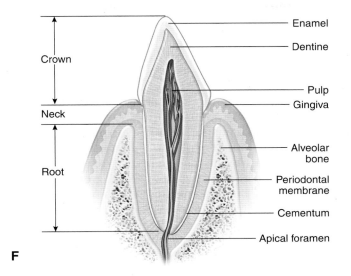

Enamel
Dentine
Crown
Pulp
Gingiva
Neck
Alveolar bone
Root
Periodontal membrane
Cementum
Apical foramen

F

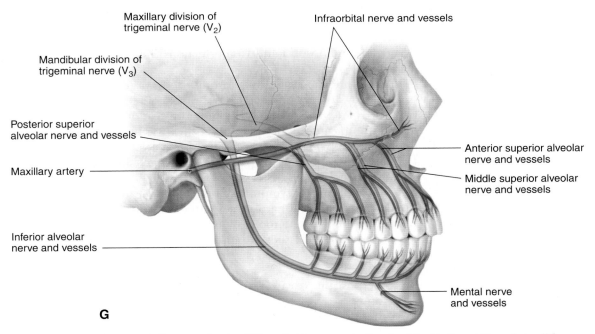

Maxillary division of trigeminal nerve (V₂)

Infraorbital nerve and vessels

Mandibular division of trigeminal nerve (V₃)

Posterior superior alveolar nerve and vessels

Anterior superior alveolar nerve and vessels

Maxillary artery

Middle superior alveolar nerve and vessels

Inferior alveolar nerve and vessels

Mental nerve and vessels

G

Figure 2.16F,G. **F.** Tooth Structure, Sectional View. **G.** Neurovascular Supply of the Teeth and Gums, Lateral View.

C. Lymphatic drainage
   1. Lower teeth, alveoli, and gingiva: lymph passes anteriorly to submental and submandibular nodes
   2. Upper teeth, alveoli, and gingiva: drain more posteriorly across cheek into submandibular, superficial cervical, and parotid nodes
   3. Oral gingiva: lymph passes into deep cervical lymph nodes

VII. Clinical Considerations

A. Oral cavity is common site of **malignancies** as a result of exposure to external environment (e.g., smoking)

B. **Gingivitis**: inflammation of tissue surrounding tooth where it emerges from within bone; untreated, it can lead to deeper inflammation (**periodontitis**), which can destroy attachment of teeth to bone

C. Firm attachment of gingiva to alveolar process does not permit spread of inflammatory fluid accumulations; in looser mucosal connective tissue of lips and cheek, accumulations of blood or fluid can spread easily and lead to much swelling

D. **Eugnathia**: normal condition where 2 rows of teeth contact each other in normal bite

E. **Dysgnathia**: abnormality of faulty position of teeth seen in an anomaly of jaw as result of abnormal development in masticatory system and affects teeth, maxilla, mandible, TMJ, muscles of mastication and facial expression, and tongue

F. **Prognathism** (**mandible protrusion**): usually inherited and characterized by abnormal prominence of chin and reciprocal supraocclusion (overbite) of front teeth

G. **Complete overbite**: inherited; upper front teeth completely cover lower

H. **Occlusion abnormalities** can cause disturbances in swallowing, nasal respiration, and speech formation

I. Severe illness or malnutrition during childhood may affect development of permanent teeth with faults (imperfections) in enamel predisposing to later decay

J. Pulp cavity infections and those around roots of teeth are very painful; if not treated, may develop into abscesses with loss of teeth

K. Exposure of dentine to oral cavity either by wear or faults in enamel or around neck of tooth can produce painful sensitivity to heat and cold

L. Referred pain from teeth: common
   1. Patients complaining of pain over maxillary sinus may have infection of tooth on upper jaw
   2. Pain in ear may be symptom of infected lower tooth

M. Dental caries: decay of hard tissues of tooth results in cavity formation
   1. Invasion of pulp of tooth by carious lesion (cavity) results in infection and irritation of tissues in pulp cavity, which causes inflammatory process (pulpitis)
   2. Toothache
      a. Because pulp cavity is rigid, swollen pulpal tissue causes pain by pressure on nerve
      b. If untreated, small vessels in root canal may die from pressure of swollen tissue, and infected material may pass through apical tissues; an infective process develops and spreads to alveolar bone producing an abscess (periapical disease) and tooth may be lost
      c. Treatment must remove decayed tissue, adds prosthetic dental material ("filling"), and restores tooth

N. Dental implants: after extraction of tooth or fracture of tooth at neck, prosthetic crown can be placed on abutment (metal peg) implanted into alveolar bone

O. Supernumerary teeth

1. May be single, multiple, unilateral or bilateral, erupted or unerupted and in 1 or both maxillary and mandibular alveolar bones

2. May occur in deciduous or permanent dentitions, but most commonly occur in latter

3. Occur in addition to normal number of teeth, but resemble size, shape or placement of normal teeth

4. Most common supernumerary tooth is mestodens, which is malformed peg-like tooth seen between maxillary central incisor teeth

5. Multiple supernumerary teeth rare in people with no other associated diseases or syndromes (i.e., cleft lip or palate or cranial malformations)

6. Can cause problems with eruption and alignment of normal dentition and are usually extracted

Tongue and Paralingual Space

I. General Features of the Tongue

A. Chief organ for taste; important in speech, mastication, and deglutition
B. Muscular organ, covered with mucous membrane, and lying on floor of mouth
C. Root: attached posterior part, through which muscles reach it deep to mucous membrane
D. Dorsum: upper surface
E. Body: major part of tongue, extending from root to tip
F. Ventral surface: inferior or sublingual surface
G. Pharyngeal part (posterior sulcal): not visible even in protruding tongue

II. Features on Dorsal Surface of Tongue (Fig. 2.17A)

A. **Central groove** of tongue
B. **Taste buds**: sensory organs of taste, scattered over mucous membrane of mouth and tongue and especially numerous on and around vallate papillae; found in epithelium of lingual papillae
C. **Lingual papillae**: lie on oral part of dorsum of tongue and at lateral margins; each papilla has connective tissue core and an epithelial covering with many sensory nerve endings in core of filiform papillae; covered with taste buds
  1. **Filiform papillae**: long, numerous and provide roughness of surface; cover 2/3 and are white in color; have no taste buds but are sensitive to touch
  2. **Fungiform papillae**: are less numerous and are scattered on sides and apex between filiform; larger and redder and have a few taste buds; raised 0.5–1.5 mm above surface
  3. **Foliate papillae**: small lateral transverse foldings of mucosa at posterior lateral tongue margin; their epithelium contains taste buds with irrigating glands that open at depth of folds
  4. **Circumvallate** (**vallate**) **papillae**
    a. 7–12 large, round, flat-topped papillae with a diameter of 1–3 mm
    b. Project only a little over tongue surface; lie posteriorly on oral part of dorsum of tongue and form a V-shaped row in front of sulcus terminalis
    c. Each papilla surrounded by depression
      i. Epithelium lining depression contains taste buds along entire height of both sides of depression
      ii. Serous glands (of Ebner) open into depression and their secretion washes away taste-stimulating substances
D. **Sulcus terminalis**: V-shaped groove immediately behind vallate papillae, separating anterior 2/3 (oral part) from posterior 1/3 (pharyngeal part) of tongue
E. **Foramen cecum**: small blind pit that indicates point of origin of thyroglossal duct (which forms thyroid); located in midline in sulcus terminalis
F. **Lingual tonsils**: lie beneath mucous membrane on pharyngeal part of dorsum of tongue, giving pitted appearance
G. Pharyngeal part of tongue: connected to epiglottis by median ridge of mucous membrane, the **median glossoepiglottic fold**; laterally there are 2 similar folds, the **lateral glossoepiglottic folds**
H. **Lingual glands**
  1. **Posterior lingual glands**: mucous glands at base and at posterolateral margins of tongue
  2. **Serous gustatory glands**: of vallate and foliate papillae
  3. **Anterior lingual glands** (**Blandin-Nuhn's glands**): paired, mixed salivary glands found in tongue muscles at inferior side of tongue apex and open on both sides of frenulum

III. Features of Ventral or Sublingual Surface and Floor of Mouth

A. **Sublingual fold** (**plicae**): overlying sublingual gland and supported by mylohyoid muscle; sublingual glands open via multiple small ducts along folds
B. **Sublingual caruncle**: swelling on either side of lingual frenulum for opening of submandibular duct

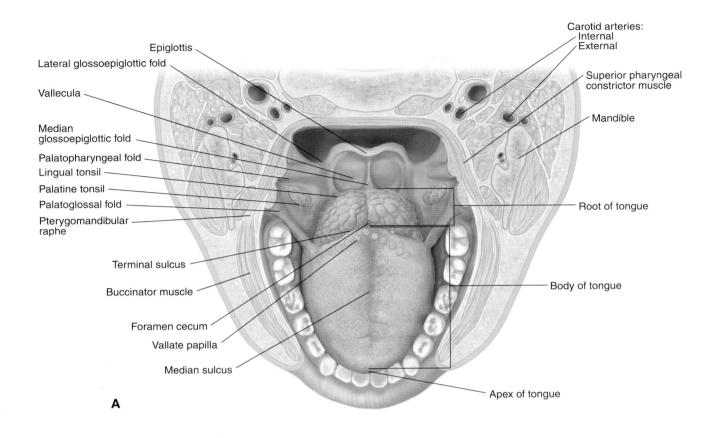

A

Epiglottis

Lateral glossoepiglottic fold

Vallecula

Median glossoepiglottic fold

Palatopharyngeal fold

Lingual tonsil

Palatine tonsil

Palatoglossal fold

Pterygomandibular raphe

Terminal sulcus

Buccinator muscle

Foramen cecum

Vallate papilla

Median sulcus

Carotid arteries:
 Internal
 External

Superior pharyngeal constrictor muscle

Mandible

Root of tongue

Body of tongue

Apex of tongue

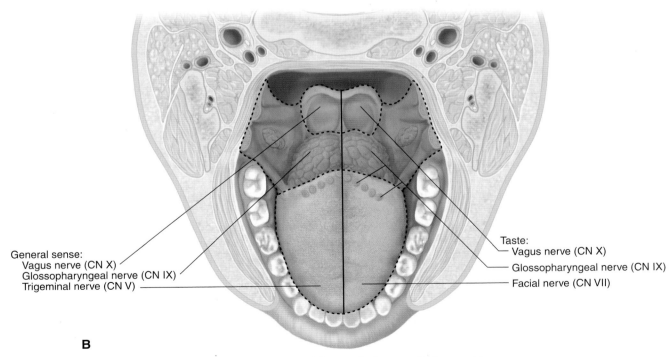

B

General sense:
 Vagus nerve (CN X)
 Glossopharyngeal nerve (CN IX)
 Trigeminal nerve (CN V)

Taste:
 Vagus nerve (CN X)

Glossopharyngeal nerve (CN IX)

Facial nerve (CN VII)

Figure 2.17A,B. Dorsum of Tongue. **A.** Features. **B.** Sensory Nerves.

C. **Lingual frenulum**: midline fold of mucous membrane between tongue and floor

D. **Deep lingual (ranine) vein and deep lingual artery**: can be seen through mucous membrane on lateral side of frenulum

IV. Neurovascular Supply of Tongue (Fig. 2.17B)

A. Sensory innervation of tongue
   1. General sensation
      a. Anterior 2/3 via lingual nerve from mandibular nerve (CN V$_3$) with cell bodies in trigeminal ganglion
      b. Posterior 1/3 via glossopharyngeal nerve (CN IX)
      c. Root of tongue near epiglottis: superior laryngeal branch of vagus nerve (CN X)
   2. Taste
      a. Anterior 2/3 via chorda tympani (CN VII) with cell bodies in geniculate ganglion
      b. Posterior 1/3 via glossopharyngeal nerve (CN IX)
      c. Root of tongue near epiglottis: superior laryngeal branch of vagus nerve (CN X)
      d. Qualities of taste: sweet, sour, bitter and salty; formerly, these were thought to be preferentially perceived at different parts of tongue, however this has been shown to be an overstatement, and currently taste qualities are thought to be fairly equally distributed on tongue

B. Motor innervation of tongue (Fig. 2.17C)
   1. Intrinsic and extrinsic muscles innervated by CN XII
   2. Palatoglossus is innervated by vagus nerve (CN X)

C. Arteries of tongue (Fig. 2.17D)
   1. **Lingual artery**
      a. 2nd anterior branch from external carotid artery
      b. Passes above greater horn of hyoid and medial to hyoglossus muscle to enter tongue
      c. 3 major branches
         i. **Dorsal lingual**: supplies posterior 1/3
         ii. **Deep lingual**: supplies anterior tongue to tip
         iii. **Sublingual**: supplies muscles anteriorly below floor of mouth

D. Veins of tongue
   1. **Lingual**: from dorsum, sides, and undersurface to internal jugular vein
   2. **Vena comitans of hypoglossal nerve** (ranine): begins near apex and runs with hypoglossal nerve to terminate in lingual or common facial veins; usually larger than lingual vein

E. Lymphatics of tongue: 4 main drainage areas
   1. Tip of tongue drains into submental nodes and submandibular nodes
   2. Remainder of anterior 2/3 drains into submandibular and deep cervical nodes on both sides
   3. Lymph from posterior 1/3 drains into upper deep cervical and retropharyngeal nodes
   4. Lateral (margins) drain to submandibular and superior deep cervical nodes
   5. From tip and posterior 1/3, lymph passes to both sides (crossover to contralateral side) and to ipsilateral side
   6. From central part of tongue, in contrast to those from margin, lymph may drain to same and opposite side
   7. Lymphatic network of both sides contains extensive anastomoses across midline so metastatic spread of tongue carcinoma can occur to opposite side

V. Muscles of the Tongue (Fig. 2.17E)

A. **Genioglossus**
   1. Origin: mental spine on inner aspect of symphysis of mandible; lies immediately above geniohyoid muscle
   2. Insertion: entire length of dorsum of tongue and body of hyoid
   3. Action: protrude tongue (pulls it forward and downward) and may depress it if acting together with hypoglossi; pull hyoid bone forward; through action of its anterior fibers, they can retract tip of protruded tongue
   4. Innervation: hypoglossal nerve (CN XII)

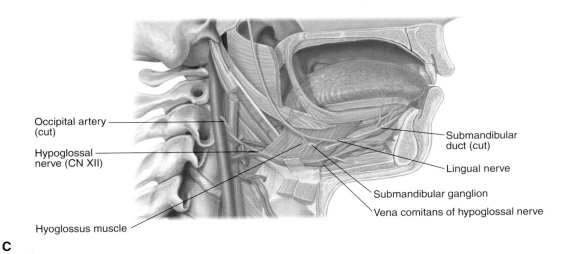

Occipital artery (cut)

Hypoglossal nerve (CN XII)

Hyoglossus muscle

Submandibular duct (cut)

Lingual nerve

Submandibular ganglion

Vena comitans of hypoglossal nerve

C

Dorsal lingual artery and vein

External carotid artery (cut)

Occipital artery (cut)

Facial artery (cut)

Lingual vein and artery

Common facial vein

Internal jugular vein

Superior thyroid artery and vein

Superior laryngeal vein and artery

Hyoglossus muscle (cut)

Submandibular duct (cut)

Sublingual vein and artery

Deep lingual vein and artery

Vena comitans of hypoglossal nerve

D

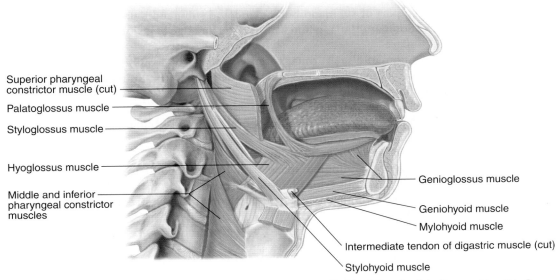

Superior pharyngeal constrictor muscle (cut)

Palatoglossus muscle

Styloglossus muscle

Hyoglossus muscle

Middle and inferior pharyngeal constrictor muscles

Genioglossus muscle

Geniohyoid muscle

Mylohyoid muscle

Intermediate tendon of digastric muscle (cut)

Stylohyoid muscle

E

Figure 2.17C–E. C. Nerves of the Tongue, Mandible Removed, Lateral View. **D.** Blood Supply of the Tongue, Mandible Removed, Lateral View. **E.** Muscles of the Tongue, Mandible Removed, Lateral View.

B. Hyoglossus
  1. Origin: upper surface of greater horn and body of hyoid
  2. Insertion: side of tongue
  3. Action: depresses side of tongue (flattens it) and pulls it back (acting together with styloglossi)
  4. Innervation: hypoglossal nerve (CN XII)

C. Styloglossus
  1. Origin: styloid process of temporal bone
  2. Insertion: side of tongue with fibers directed toward tongue tip
  3. Action: retracts and elevates tongue
  4. Innervation: hypoglossal nerve (CN XII)

D. Palatoglossus
  1. Origin: oral surface of palatine aponeurosis
  2. Insertion: side and dorsum of tongue
  3. Action: elevates tongue, depresses soft palate
  4. Innervation: vagus nerve (CN X)

E. Intrinsic muscles: allow fine control of shape
  1. Superior and inferior longitudinal
  2. Transverse linguae
  3. Verticalis

F. Muscular support of tongue
  1. Consists of mylohyoid, geniohyoid, and digastric muscles
  2. These suprahyoid muscles are opposed to infrahyoid muscles and together help to fix hyoid bone in place to provide stable platform for tongue muscles
  3. Stylohyoid belongs to suprahyoid muscles and with them influences position and state of tension of floor of mouth
  4. Mylohyoid muscles of both sides form so-called **diaphragma oris**

VI. Paralingual Space (Fig. 2.17F,G)

A. General features
  1. Space beneath floor of mouth
  2. Lies between mandible and tongue

B. Boundaries
  1. Roof: oral mucosa of floor of mouth
  2. Laterally: mandible and mylohyoid muscle
  3. Medially: hyoglossus and genioglossus muscles
  4. Inferiorly: hyoglossus and mylohyoid muscles

C. Contents
  1. **Deep part of submandibular gland** and **submandibular duct**
     a. Submandibular gland wraps posterior edge of mylohyoid muscle to enter paralingual space
     b. Submandibular duct extends anteriorly from deep part of gland, medial to sublingual gland, to empty beside lingual frenulum at sublingual caruncle
  2. **Sublingual gland**
     a. Flattened between mandible and side of tongue
     b. Upper margin raises fold of oral mucosa, sublingual plica, onto which its multiple small ducts open
  3. **Lingual nerve** (from mandibular nerve, CN V$_3$)
     a. Enters paralingual space from infratemporal fossa by passing beneath inferior margin of superior pharyngeal constrictor muscle
     b. **Submandibular ganglion**: hangs from lingual nerve near deep part of submandibular gland
        i. Receives presynaptic fibers from chorda tympani fibers (from facial nerve) traveling within lingual nerve
        ii. Postsynaptic fibers descend to enter submandibular gland, or rejoin lingual nerve to travel forward to reach sublingual gland
     c. Lingual nerve passes beneath submandibular duct laterally to medially to enter side of tongue

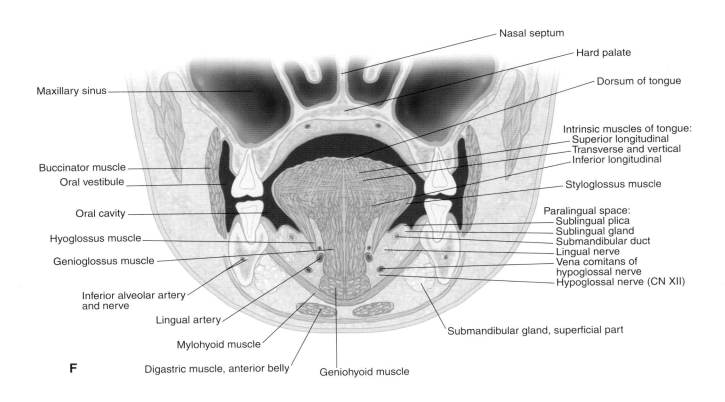

Nasal septum

Hard palate

Dorsum of tongue

Maxillary sinus

Intrinsic muscles of tongue:
Superior longitudinal
Transverse and vertical
Inferior longitudinal

Buccinator muscle
Oral vestibule

Styloglossus muscle

Oral cavity

Paralingual space:
Sublingual plica
Sublingual gland
Submandibular duct
Lingual nerve
Vena comitans of
hypoglossal nerve
Hypoglossal nerve (CN XII)

Hyoglossus muscle

Genioglossus muscle

Inferior alveolar artery
and nerve

Lingual artery

Submandibular gland, superficial part

Mylohyoid muscle

Digastric muscle, anterior belly

Geniohyoid muscle

F

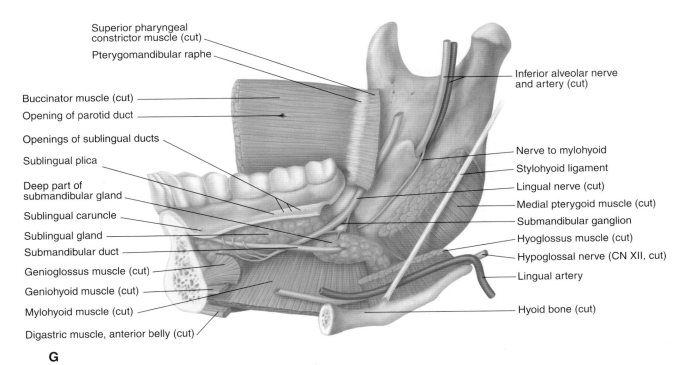

Superior pharyngeal
constrictor muscle (cut)

Pterygomandibular raphe

Inferior alveolar nerve
and artery (cut)

Buccinator muscle (cut)

Opening of parotid duct

Openings of sublingual ducts

Nerve to mylohyoid

Sublingual plica

Stylohyoid ligament

Deep part of
submandibular gland

Lingual nerve (cut)

Medial pterygoid muscle (cut)

Sublingual caruncle

Submandibular ganglion

Sublingual gland

Hyoglossus muscle (cut)

Submandibular duct

Hypoglossal nerve (CN XII, cut)

Genioglossus muscle (cut)

Lingual artery

Geniohyoid muscle (cut)

Mylohyoid muscle (cut)

Hyoid bone (cut)

Digastric muscle, anterior belly (cut)

G

Figure 2.17F,G. Paralingual Space. **F.** Coronal Sectional View. **G.** Paralingual Space, Tongue Removed, Medial View.

d. Provides general sensation to anterior 2/3 of tongue, and taste sensation via chorda tympani fibers

4. Hypoglossal nerve (CN XII)

a. Lies in lowest part of paralingual space, wedged between mylohyoid and hyoglossus muscles

b. Passes into tongue to innervate all of muscles of tongue

c. Accompanied by venae commitans of hypoglossal nerve, which drain to internal jugular vein

VII. Submandibular and Sublingual Glands (Fig. 2.17H)

A. Submandibular gland

1. Size: 2nd largest of major salivary glands, size of walnut, approximately 1/2 size of parotid

2. Type: compound, tubuloalveolar; mixed serous and mucous

3. Location and relations: primarily within submandibular triangle, extending into paralingual space

a. Superficial surface: lies against inner surface of mandibular border, covered by skin, platysma, facial vein, and superficial layer of deep cervical fascia, which forms loose capsule around gland

b. Deep surface: lies on mylohyoid muscle, nerve to mylohyoid, and facial artery

c. Deep portion: projection wrapping posterior margin of mylohyoid muscle to enter paralingual space; medially, by hyoglossus and styloglossus muscles; above, by lingual nerve and submandibular ganglion; below by hypoglossal nerve

4. Submandibular duct (Wharton's): extends anteriorly from deep portion of gland, between mylohyoid and sublingual gland laterally and hyoglossus and genioglossus muscles medially; opens at sublingual caruncle at side of lingual frenulum; lingual nerve passes beneath it

5. Submandibular lymph nodes lie on gland and along border of mandible

B. Sublingual gland

1. Size: smallest of 3 major salivary glands

2. Type: compound, tubuloalveolar; mixed serous and mucous (predominantly mucous)

3. Location and relations: beneath mucous membrane of floor of mouth

a. Above: floor of mouth

b. Below: mylohyoid muscle

c. Behind: deep part of submandibular gland

d. Laterally: sublingual depression of mandible

e. Medially: submandibular duct, lingual nerve, and genioglossus muscle

4. Sublingual ducts

a. Small (of Rivinus): some join submandibular duct, others (10–12) open separately in floor of mouth, forming linear series along top of sublingual fold

b. Large (Bartholin): 1 or 2 duct branches join submandibular duct

C. Innervation of both glands

1. Presynaptic parasympathetic fibers: from superior salivatory nucleus through nervus intermedius of facial nerve, travel via chorda tympani to lingual nerve to synapse in submandibular ganglion

2. Postsynaptic parasympathetic fibers: travel from ganglion to reach both glands

3. Vasoconstrictive postsynaptic sympathetic fibers from superior cervical ganglion

D. Vessels

1. Arteries

a. Submandibular gland: branches of facial artery

b. Sublingual gland: sublingual branch of lingual artery

2. Veins follow arteries

3. Lymphatic drainage to submandibular nodes

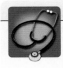

VII. Clinical Considerations

A. Submandibular gland cannot be moved forward because its deep part wraps posterior margin of mylohyoid muscle

B. Submandibular gland can produce stones or calculi that block duct and cause painful gland swelling; submandibular duct can be felt in floor of mouth, medial to sublingual fold

C. Ranula: cystic swellings of opening of salivary gland ducts in mouth due to obstruction; stones may also form within salivary gland ducts, requiring surgical removal

D. Carcinoma of tongue affects males chiefly, and edges of tongue are most commonly affected; tumor is epidermoid carcinoma and may be of any degree of malignancy; metastasis is usually slow, involving lymph nodes of neck; rarely, there may be rapid, widespread metastases; "principal" node is single constant node of deep cervical group, lying at bifurcation of common carotid artery, which receives large number of vessels from tongue

   1. Malignant tumors of posterior part of tongue metastasize to superior deep cervical lymph nodes on both sides

   2. Tumors of apex and anterolateral parts usually do not metastasize to inferior deep cervical nodes

E. Radical neck dissection (block dissection of neck): surgical procedure to remove such metastatic lesions of tongue; as result of extensive lymphatic drainage of tongue, metastatic carcinoma from tongue may be widely disseminated through submental and submandibular regions and along internal jugular vein

F. Hypoglossal nerve paralysis: diagnosed by having patient protrude tongue as far as possible; tongue deviates to side that is paralyzed

(Continued)

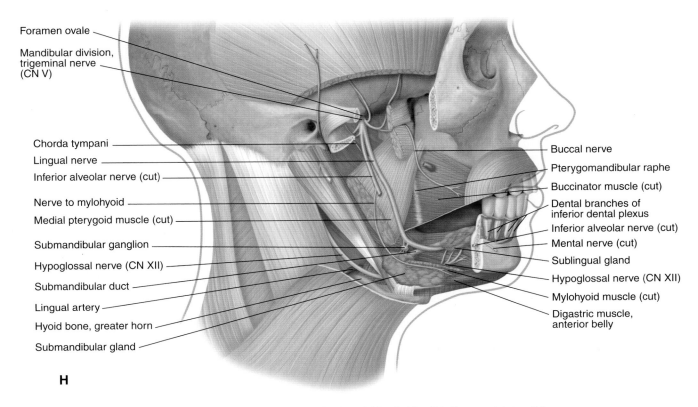

Figure 2.17H. Submandibular and Sublingual Glands, Mandible Removed, Lateral View.

G. **Frenectomy**: enlarged frenulum of tongue may interfere with tongue movements, resulting in "tongue tie"; surgical procedure is used to free tongue

H. Tongue anomalies and variations
   1. **Bifid tongue**: midline cleft
   2. **Black hairy tongue**: papillae are either brown or black
   3. **Geographic tongue**: benign migratory glossitis
   4. **Raspberry tongue**: red, uncoated tongue, with elevated papillae, as seen a few days after onset of rash of scarlet fever
   5. **Coated tongue**: whitish or yellowish coating consisting of desquamated epithelium, debris, bacteria, fungi, etc.

I. **Lingual tonsil**, **thyroglossal cysts**, and **ectopic thyroid tissue**: if thyroid gland fails to migrate from back of tongue to lower neck, thyroid tissue or cystic remnants may occur anywhere along its usual pathway of migration, or even on dorsum of tongue itself

J. Paralysis of genioglossus muscle: tongue mass has tendency to shift posteriorly, blocking airway with risk of suffocation; total relaxation of muscles is seen in general anesthesia and, tongue must be prevented from relapsing by inserting an airway

K. Gag reflex: patient is able to touch anterior part of tongue without discomfort, but when posterior part is touched, patient usually "gags"; CN IX and CN X are responsible for muscular contraction of each side of pharynx (Note: CN IX provides afferent portion of gag reflex; CN X, motor part)

L. Drug absorption: for quick absorption of a drug (e.g., nitroglycerin is used as vasodilator in angina pectoris), spray or pill is placed under tongue where it dissolves rapidly and enters deep lingual veins

M. Sialography of submandibular ducts: means of examining submandibular glands and ducts by injecting contrast medium into their ducts; sublingual gland ducts tend to be too small for this procedure

Palate and Palatine Tonsil

I. General Features of the Palate (Fig. 2.18A)

A. Forms arched (dome-shaped) roof of mouth and floor of nasal cavities

 1. Separates oral cavity from nasal cavities and nasopharynx (part of pharynx superior to soft palate)

 2. Nasal surface covered by respiratory mucosa; oro- and nasopharyngeal surface by oral mucosa (heavy with glands)

B. 2 parts

 1. Hard palate: immovable, anterior 2/3

 2. Soft palate: movable in order to close off nasopharynx during swallowing or phonation

C. Sensory nerve supply: **greater palatine nerve** for sensory supply to gingivae and hard palate and **lesser palatine nerve** to soft palate; anteriormost part of hard palate receives sensory branches of nasopalatine

D. Motor nerve supply: all muscles of soft palate are supplied by vagus nerve (CN X) through pharyngeal plexus of nerves, except tensor veli palatini (supplied by CN V_3)

E. Parasympathetic nerve supply

 1. Presynaptic fibers: in greater petrosal branch of facial nerve (CN VII), through nerve of pterygoid canal, to pterygopalatine ganglion

 2. Postsynaptic fibers: travel with sensory nerves to mucous glands of hard and soft palate

F. Arteries: **descending palatine artery**, a terminal branch of maxillary artery, sends lesser and greater palatine branches to supply soft and hard palate; ascending palatine branch of facial artery also helps

G. Veins: tributaries of pterygoid venous plexus

II. Hard Palate

A. Consists of palatine process of maxillary bones anteriorly and horizontal part of palatine bones

B. Covered by mucous membrane, which is immovably fixed to periosteum with no submucosa layer

C. **Palatine glands**: large mucous glands embedded in mucosa of posterior part of hard palate

III. Soft Palate

A. Location: moveable fibromuscular fold forming posterior projection from hard palate as far as posterior pharyngeal wall

B. Composition: skeletal muscles and aponeurosis covered by mucous membrane containing palatine glands

 1. **Palatine aponeurosis**: fibrous sheet extending posteriorly from caudal edge of palatine bone into soft palate to support and give attachment to muscles of that structure

 2. **Tensor veli palatini**: pulls lateral wall of auditory tube inferiorly, opening tube; innervated by branch of mandibular nerve (CN V_3)

 3. **Levator veli palatini**: elevates soft palate to bring it into contact with posterior pharyngeal wall; innervated by branches of vagus nerve (CN X)

 4. **Musculus uvulae**: helps to close off nasopharynx from oropharynx; **uvula**: paired muscles beside midline are covered by mucous membrane and contains many mucous (palatine) glands in its submucosa; innervated by branches of vagus nerve (CN X)

 5. **Palatoglossus muscle**: within palatoglossal fold to sides of tongue; closes off opening of oropharynx by pulling tongue up and tensing palate innervated by branches of vagus nerve (CN X)

 6. **Palatopharyngeus muscle**: within palatopharyngeal fold in lateral wall of pharynx; lifts larynx during swallowing; innervated by branches of vagus nerve (CN X)

IV. Muscles of the Soft Palate (Fig. 2.18B)

Muscle	Origin	Insertion	Action	Nerve
Levator veli palatini	Petrous bone; medial wall of auditory tube	Decussate with fibers of other side and palatine aponeurosis	Raises soft palate during swallowing or phonation	Pharyngeal plexus (CN X)
Tensor veli palatini	Lateral wall of auditory tube; scaphoid fossa; angular spine of sphenoid bone	Aponeurosis of palate after passing around pterygoid hamulus	Tenses soft palate; opens auditory tube	Trigeminal (CN V$_3$)
Musculus uvulae	Posterior nasal spine; palatine aponeurosis	Mucosa of uvula	Raises and shortens uvula	Pharyngeal plexus (CN X)
Palatopharyngeus	Hard palate and palatine aponeurosis	Lateral posterior pharynx; posterior thyroid cartilage	Pulls walls of pharynx superiorly, anteriorly and medially during swallowing, helps close nasopharynx	Pharyngeal plexus (CN X)
Palatoglossus	Anterior soft palate	Dorsolateral tongue	Raises posterior part of tongue and draws soft palate toward tongue	Pharyngeal plexus (CN X)

V. Palatine Tonsil (Fig. 2.18C)

A. Location
 1. Within tonsillar fossa (bed of palatine tonsil) posterior to palatoglossal fold and anterior to palatopharyngeal fold
 2. Not actually within oral cavity but in lateral wall of anteriormost portion of oropharynx; palatoglossal arch marks boundary between oral cavity and oropharynx (space between is called *isthmus of fauces* and palatoglossal and palatopharyngeal folds are called *anterior* and *posterior pillars of fauces*)
B. Features
 1. Covered by keratinized stratified squamous epithelium and substrate of lymphatic tissue (1–2 mm thick); surface has pit-like invaginations or **tonsillar crypts**; latter may be invaded by lymphocytes and granulocytes, desquamated cells, bacteria, etc. and form whitish **tonsillar thrombi**
 2. Arteries
  a. Ascending palatine and tonsillar branches of facial artery
  b. Palatine branch of ascending pharyngeal artery
  c. Tonsillar branches of dorsal lingual artery
  d. Tonsillar branch of descending palatine artery
 3. Veins: tonsillar veins drain into pharyngeal plexus
 4. Lymph: to superior deep cervical nodes, especially jugulodigastric node
 5. Sensory nerves: branches of glossopharyngeal nerve (CN IX) and lesser palatine branch of maxillary nerve (CN V$_2$) to upper portion

VI. Tonsillar Ring (Waldeyer's) of Lymphatic Tissue

A. Said to "guard" openings into respiratory and digestive systems
B. Composed of lingual tonsil, palatine tonsils, and pharyngeal tonsil (adenoid)

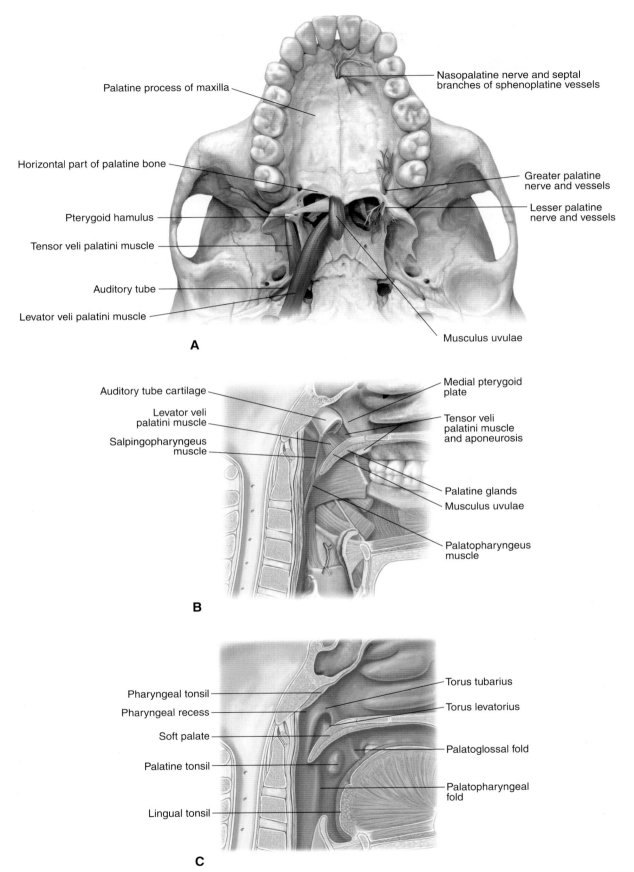

Nasopalatine nerve and septal branches of sphenoplatine vessels

Palatine process of maxilla

Horizontal part of palatine bone

Greater palatine nerve and vessels

Lesser palatine nerve and vessels

Pterygoid hamulus

Tensor veli palatini muscle

Auditory tube

Levator veli palatini muscle

Musculus uvulae

A

Auditory tube cartilage

Levator veli palatini muscle

Salpingopharyngeus muscle

Medial pterygoid plate

Tensor veli palatini muscle and aponeurosis

Palatine glands

Musculus uvulae

Palatopharyngeus muscle

B

Pharyngeal tonsil

Pharyngeal recess

Soft palate

Palatine tonsil

Lingual tonsil

Torus tubarius

Torus levatorius

Palatoglossal fold

Palatopharyngeal fold

C

Figure 2.18A–C. A. Palate, Inferior View. **B.** Muscles of the Palate, Sagittal Section, Medial View. **C.** Palate, Sagittal Section, Medial View.

VII. Clinical Considerations

A. **Cleft lip** (**"harelip"**): congenital anomaly; can occur independently or accompany cleft palate

    1. Seen in 1–2 per 300 live births; 60%–80% are male

    2. Usually affects upper lip; may be unilateral or bilateral and clefts vary from small notches in transitional lip and red border to cleft extending through lip into nose

B. **Cleft palate**: congenital anomaly in which midline fusion of palatine processes of maxillae or palatine bones fails to occur

    1. Cleft may also lie between premaxillary and maxillary portions of hard palate

    2. Permits air, liquids, or solids to pass from nose to mouth or vice versa, which can lead to sucking and swallowing problems in newborn and to speech difficulties in later years

C. **Uranoplasty**: repair of cleft in hard palate; congenital cleft palates may be repaired by using prominent mucoperiosteum on the inferior side of palate as a flap

D. **Palatopharyngeal incompetency**

    1. Occurs when soft palate does not extend far enough posterior to form good seal with pharynx

    2. Commonly associated with cleft palate and can cause problems with speech and swallowing

E. **Jugulodigastric node**: because of inaccessibility of posterior 1/3 of tongue and tonsil; sometimes 1st positive sign of carcinoma in these regions will be swelling of this node, sometimes called "main gland of tonsil"

F. Tonsils and adenoids

    1. Palatine tonsils are subject to infection as result of numerous crypts on their surface

    2. Tend to hypertrophy most commonly in childhood due to a general lymphatic hyperplasia; adenoid hypertrophy can block nasopharynx, creating problems in breathing

    3. Because of tremendous vascular supply of palatine tonsils, extreme care must be used in tonsillectomy

    4. Because of thin lateral wall behind which lie many major vessels, excision must be done with great care

    5. On lateral surface of palatine tonsil, fascia of superior pharyngeal constrictor muscle forms connective tissue capsule in which tonsil may be surgically entirely removed; large vessels and nerves in parapharyngeal space are separated from tonsil by superior constrictor, and are usually relatively protected during surgery

G. **Nasopalatine block**: nasopalatine nerves can be anesthetized by injecting anesthetic into incisive fossa in hard palate

    1. Needle inserted just posterior to incisive papilla; both nerves are anesthetized where they emerge from fossa

    2. Tissues affected are anterior hard palate and mucosa, lingual gingivae, and alveolar bone of 6 anterior maxillary teeth

Nose, Nasal Cavity, and Paranasal Sinuses

I. Nose and Nasal Cavity

A. Part of respiratory tract above hard palate; containing organ of smell

B. External nose

  1. Varies in size and shape, mainly due to differences in cartilages

  2. Pyramidal in shape; has **a root** (inferior to forehead) and an **apex** (at free end)

  3. Nostrils (nares): anterior openings separated by **septum**

  4. Coarse hairs (vibrissae) protect opening of nares and prevent foreign matter from entering nasal cavity

  5. Nose has lateral surfaces and dorsum

   a. Superior part of dorsum is made up of 2 nasal bones and is called the **bridge** of the nose

   b. Lateral surfaces end inferiorly in a rounded portion, **ala nasi**

  6. Nose framework **(Fig. 2.19A,B)**

   a. Consists of bones superiorly and laterally (nasal bones on bridge and frontal process of maxillary bones), and cartilage and fatty tissue, inferiorly

   b. **Septal cartilage** makes up approximately 1/2 of nasal septum and lateral cartilages are seen on either side of septal cartilage

   c. Distal end of nose contains **greater alar cartilage** and several **lesser alar cartilages,** which provide rigid support for nasal alae (wings) and septum

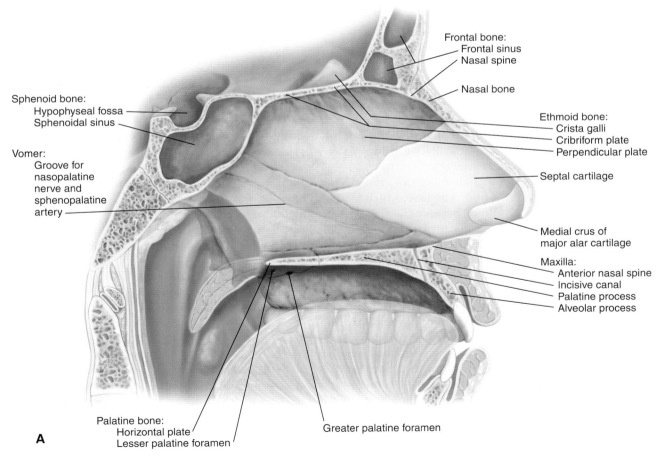

Figure 2.19A. A. Bones of the Nasal Septum and Hard Palate.

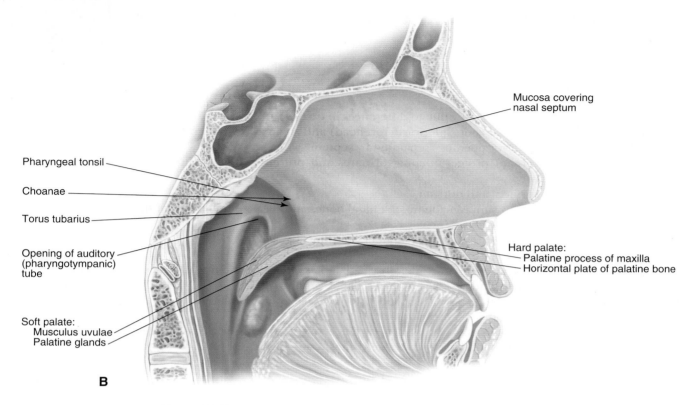

Mucosa covering nasal septum

Pharyngeal tonsil

Choanae

Torus tubarius

Opening of auditory (pharyngotympanic) tube

Soft palate:
 Musculus uvulae
 Palatine glands

Hard palate:
 Palatine process of maxilla
 Horizontal plate of palatine bone

B

Figure 2.19B. B. Mucous Membranes of the Nasal Septum and Hard Palate.

7. Nerves
  a. Muscles: branches of facial nerve (CN VII)
  b. Sensory: infratrochlear nerve and external nasal branch of nasociliary branch of ophthalmic division of CN V to bridge of nose; nasal branches of infraorbital branch of maxillary division of CN V to sides of nose
C. Nasal cavity **(Fig. 2.19C,D)**
  1. Lies below anterior cranial fossa and extends from nares anteriorly to posterior opening of nose, **choanae,** which lead into nasopharynx
  2. Filters, moistens, and warms air; functions as a resonator for speech
  3. Entrance into nasal cavity is called **vestibule (**enclosed laterally by alae of nose, medially by cartilaginous and connective tissue end of nasal septum, and lined by slightly modified facial skin)
  4. Limen nasi: curved mucosal ridge marking border to nasal cavity
  5. Stratified squamous epithelium of epidermis is continuous with pseudostratified, ciliated columnar (respiratory) epithelium at limen nasi
  6. Nasal septum: divides 2 cavities
    a. Anterior part: septal cartilage
    b. Posterior part: bony nasal septum
      i. Upper part: **perpendicular plate of ethmoid bone**
      ii. Lower part: **vomer** plus crests of bone from maxillary and palatine
    c. Covered by mucous membrane, of which an upper posterior part, just below cribriform plate of ethmoid, is olfactory
  7. Lateral wall of nasal cavity: exhibits 3 shelves, **conchae or turbinates**, which are bony projections covered by mucous membrane and increase respiratory surface of nose; conchae cover spaces called inferior, middle, and superior **nasal meatuses**
    a. Inferior concha: separate bone connected to maxilla; covers **inferior meatus** into which opens nasolacrimal duct from lacrimal sac, conducting tears into nasal cavity

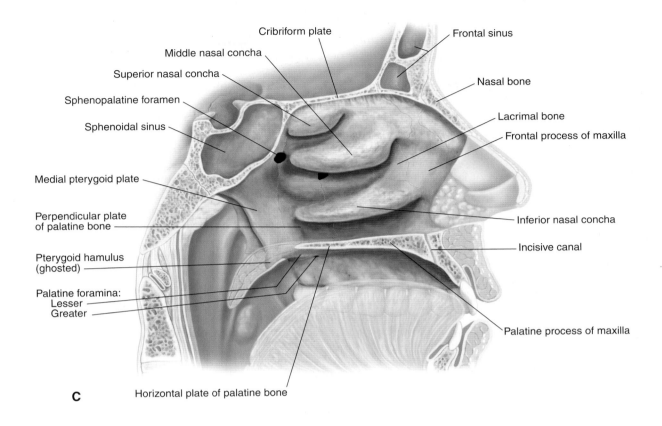

Cribriform plate

Middle nasal concha

Superior nasal concha

Sphenopalatine foramen

Sphenoidal sinus

Medial pterygoid plate

Perpendicular plate of palatine bone

Pterygoid hamulus (ghosted)

Palatine foramina:
Lesser
Greater

Frontal sinus

Nasal bone

Lacrimal bone

Frontal process of maxilla

Inferior nasal concha

Incisive canal

Palatine process of maxilla

Horizontal plate of palatine bone

C

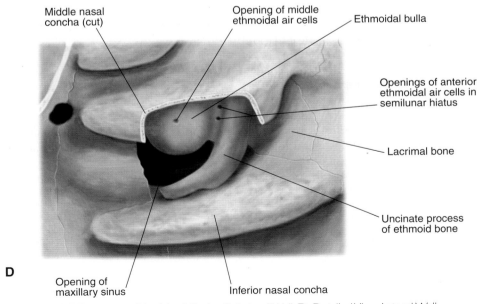

Middle nasal concha (cut)

Opening of middle ethmoidal air cells

Ethmoidal bulla

Openings of anterior ethmoidal air cells in semilunar hiatus

Lacrimal bone

Uncinate process of ethmoid bone

Opening of maxillary sinus

Inferior nasal concha

D

Figure 2.19C,D. Bones of the Nasal Cavity. **C.** Lateral Wall. **D.** Detailed View, Lateral Wall.

    b. **Middle concha**: covers **middle meatus**
        i. **Bulla ethmoidalis**: bulge formed by ethmoid air cells; middle ethmoidal air cells drain onto its eminence
        ii. **Uncinate process**: thin process of ethmoid bone below bulla supporting mucous membrane forming semilunar hiatus
        iii. **Semilunar hiatus**: groove anteroinferior to bulla ethmoidalis; receives ducts of nasal sinuses
            a) **Frontal sinus**: drains into highest portion of semilunar hiatus, called *infundibulum*
            b) **Anterior ethmoidal air cells**: several air cells drain into hiatus near its midpoint
            c) **Maxillary sinus**: drains into lowest portion of hiatus
    c. **Superior concha**: small (1/2 length of middle concha and lies above posterior 1/2 of latter) and rounded with **sphenoethmoidal recess** above it and **superior meatus** below it; receives 1–2 openings from posterior ethmoidal air cells
    d. Roof of nasal cavity: curved and narrow, except posteriorly where hollow body of sphenoid forms roof; formed, anterior to posterior, by nasal and frontal bones, cribriform plate of ethmoid, and body of sphenoid
    e. Floor of nasal cavity: is wider than roof; formed by hard palate (palatine process of maxilla and horizontal process of palatine bone)
8. Mucosa of nasal cavity: begins at border of nasal vestibule (Fig. 2.19E,F)
    a. **Olfactory region**
        i. Mucosa is an area of approximately 10 cm² and up to 100 micrometers thick with slightly brownish coloration and with olfactory chemoreceptors to form olfactory organ
        ii. Covers superior concha, corresponding parts of roof of nasal cavity and nasal septum
        iii. Thicker than respiratory mucosa
        iv. Contains pseudostratified columnar epithelium with supporting and basal cells and olfactory cells (bipolar neurons with long, nonmotile cilia that respond to odoriferous substances and basal processes which form axons of olfactory nerves)
        v. Lamina propria of this mucosa also contains serous olfactory glands
            a) Secretion of mixed glands moistens air and begins preliminary movement to pharynx by ciliary action of respiratory epithelium purification; any matter adhering to nasal secretion is moved to pharynx by ciliary action of respiratory epithelium
            b) Olfactory organ and sensory nerves of nasal mucosa control respiratory air for chemical impurities and can elicit "nasal reflex," or sneeze
    b. **Respiratory region**
        i. Contains pseudostratified, ciliated columnar epithelium with goblet cells and cilia that beat toward pharynx
        ii. Many seromucous nasal glands produce thin liquid secretion containing mucus
        iii. Covers middle and inferior conchae and remaining parts of wall, together with mucosa of paranasal sinuses
        iv. Most inspired air passes through region of middle and inferior meatuses

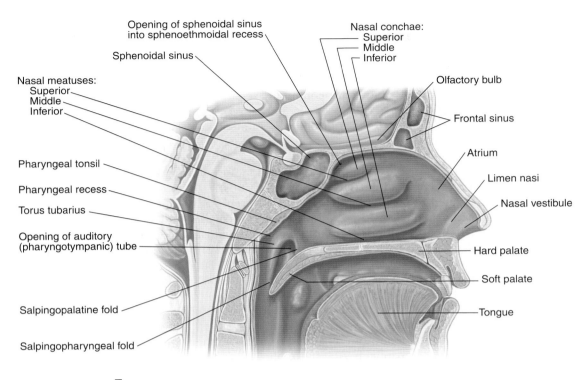

E

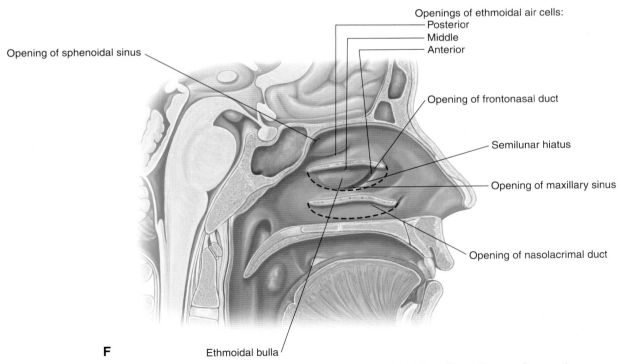

F

Figure 2.19E,F. E. Lateral Wall of the Nasal Cavity. **F.** Lateral Wall of the Nasal Cavity, Conchae Removed.

II. Paranasal Sinuses (Fig. 2.19G–I)

A. Air-filled diverticula of nasal cavity

B. 3 large paired sinuses and collection of air cells

   1. Frontal sinuses

      a. Appear in approximately 7th year of life (may be earlier)

      b. Lie posterior to superciliary arches between outer and inner tables of frontal bone, vary in size, are commonly asymmetrically formed

      c. Both frontal sinuses are commonly separated by a septum, which is usually not straight

      d. Open into anterosuperior end of semilunar hiatus at ethmoidal infundibulum via **frontonasal duct**

   2. Maxillary sinus

      a. Appears in fetus at approximately 4th month of pregnancy

      b. Very large in adults (largest paranasal sinus)

      c. Related to orbit above; to molar and premolar teeth below; to lower 1/2 of nasal cavity medially; and posteriorly to pterygopalatine and infratemporal fossae

      d. Drains at its superior end into semilunar hiatus of middle meatus

      e. Deepest part of sinus lies above roots of 2nd premolar and 1st molar teeth; canine tooth is not usually topographically closely related

      f. Infraorbital canal, with its infraorbital nerve (CN V_2) and vessels, lies in its superior wall

      g. Opening of sinus is poorly situated for good drainage because it lies near roof

   3. Sphenoidal sinuses

      a. In sphenoid bone and separated from each other by asymmetric septum

      b. Occur approximately 7th year of life

      c. Nasal cavity and ethmoid air cells are anterior; layer of bone is posterior; nasopharynx and nasal cavity are inferior; brain, optic chiasma, intercavernous sinus, and hypophysis are superior; and laterally optic nerve, cavernous sinus, and its contents

      d. Open into sphenoethmoidal recess of nasal cavity

      e. Occasionally extends into basal part of occipital bone

   4. Ethmoidal air cells

      a. Begin to form in fetus during 2nd 1/2 of pregnancy

      b. Numerous, small, thin-walled sacs, which communicate with each other

      c. Contained entirely in ethmoid labyrinth

      d. Medially are superior and middle meatuses; laterally is orbit; anteriorly is frontal process of maxillary bone; and posteriorly is sphenoid sinus

      e. Anterior air cells open into middle meatus into semilunar hiatus; middle set open into middle meatus on bulla ethmoidalis; posterior set open into superior meatus

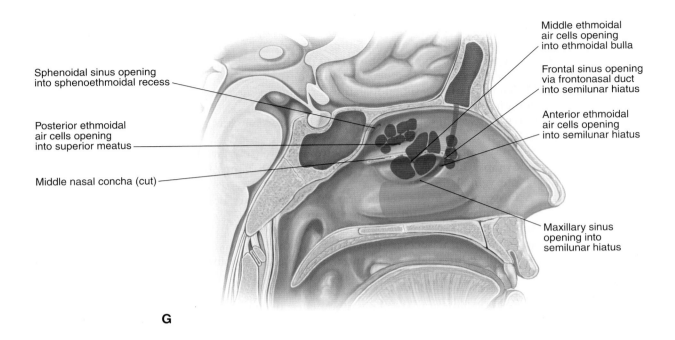

Sphenoidal sinus opening into sphenoethmoidal recess

Posterior ethmoidal air cells opening into superior meatus

Middle nasal concha (cut)

Middle ethmoidal air cells opening into ethmoidal bulla

Frontal sinus opening via frontonasal duct into semilunar hiatus

Anterior ethmoidal air cells opening into semilunar hiatus

Maxillary sinus opening into semilunar hiatus

G

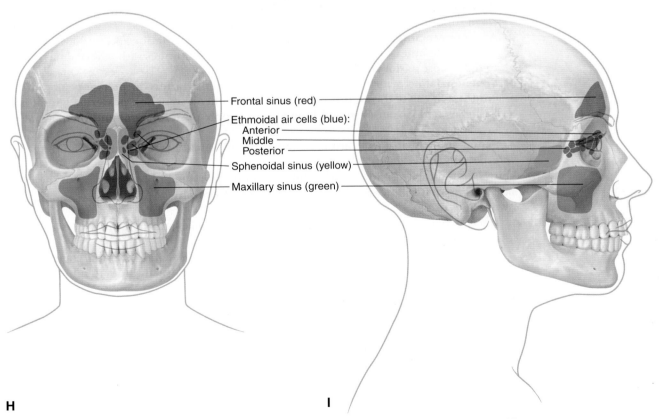

Frontal sinus (red)

Ethmoidal air cells (blue):
Anterior
Middle
Posterior

Sphenoidal sinus (yellow)

Maxillary sinus (green)

H

I

Figure 2.19G–I. Paranasal Sinuses. **G.** Medial View. **H.** Anterior View. **I.** Lateral View.

III. Nerves, Vessels, and Lymphatics of Nasal Cavity (Fig. 2.19J,K)

A. **Olfactory nerves**
1. Concerned with smell only; arise from cells in uppermost part of nasal mucosa (mostly over superior concha and adjoining septum)
2. Penetrate cribriform plate and end in overlying olfactory bulb

B. General sensory nerves to mucous membranes
1. Most enter cavity via sphenopalatine foramen, in lateral nasal wall behind posterior end of middle concha
2. Carry postsynaptic parasympathetic fibers for mucous glands from pterygopalatine ganglion
   a. Presynaptic fibers: via greater petrosal nerve from facial nerve (CN VII)
   b. Synapse in pterygopalatine ganglion, which hangs below maxillary nerve within pterygopalatine fossa
   c. Postsynaptic fibers: rejoin branches of maxillary nerve to reach nasal cavity (for mucous glands) and orbit (for lacrimal gland)
3. Anterior and posterior ethmoidal nerves
   a. Branches of nasociliary nerve from ophthalmic nerve (CN V_1)
   b. Supply ethmoidal air cells and walls of nasal cavity anteriorly
4. Branches of maxillary nerve to nasal cavity
   a. Posterior superior lateral nasal branches
   b. Posterior inferior lateral nasal branches: from greater palatine nerve as it descends
   c. Nasopalatine nerve: to nasal septum; ends on anterior hard palate by passing through incisive canal
5. Maxillary sinus receives innervation from anterior, middle and posterior superior alveolar branches of maxillary nerve (CN V_2)

C. Blood supply of nasal cavity: branches of ophthalmic, maxillary and facial arteries (Fig. 2.19L,M)
1. **Posterior ethmoidal artery**: from ophthalmic artery to posterior ethmoidal air cells and small superior parts of lateral wall and septum
2. **Anterior ethmoidal artery**: from ophthalmic artery to anterior and middle ethmoidal air cells and anterior lateral wall and nasal septum; continues with external nasal nerve to tip of nose as **dorsal nasal artery**
3. **Sphenopalatine artery**: terminal branch of maxillary artery in pterygopalatine fossa; enter nasal cavity through sphenopalatine foramen; branches: **posterior lateral nasal branches** and **posterior septal branches** to supply posterolateral and medial walls of nasal cavity
4. **Septal branch of facial artery**: from superior labial artery (source of nosebleeds, especially in children)

D. Veins of nasal cavity: follow arteries, but drain into pterygoid plexus, some into cavernous sinus (those that follow ethmoidal arteries) and others into facial vein

E. Lymphatics of nasal cavity and paranasal sinuses
1. Inferior part of nasal cavity drains into submandibular and superficial cervical nodes following facial artery
2. Major portion of cavity drains posteriorly to deep cervical and retropharyngeal nodes
3. Anterior part: communicates with vessels of skin of nose; usually drain to submandibular and superior deep cervical nodes
4. Posterior part: drains into retropharyngeal nodes located in fascia posterior to pharynx; efferents from these go to deep cervical nodes; part of this drainage may go directly to superior deep cervical nodes; a few channels from this same area also may go to subparotid nodes 1st and then to superior deep cervical nodes
5. Paranasal sinuses: drain partly into retropharyngeal and partly by directed paths to superior deep cervical nodes

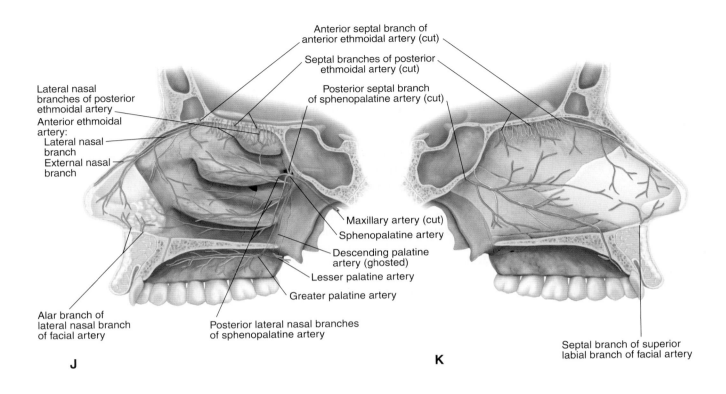

Anterior septal branch of
anterior ethmoidal artery (cut)

Septal branches of posterior
ethmoidal artery (cut)

Posterior septal branch
of sphenopalatine artery (cut)

Lateral nasal
branches of posterior
ethmoidal artery

Anterior ethmoidal
artery:
  Lateral nasal
  branch
  External nasal
  branch

Maxillary artery (cut)

Sphenopalatine artery

Descending palatine
artery (ghosted)

Lesser palatine artery

Greater palatine artery

Alar branch of
lateral nasal branch
of facial artery

Posterior lateral nasal branches
of sphenopalatine artery

Septal branch of superior
labial branch of facial artery

J

K

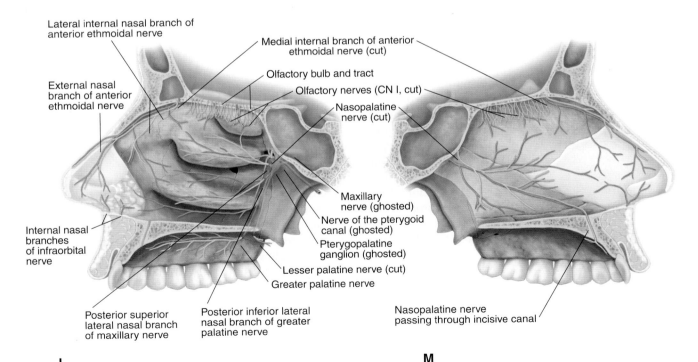

Lateral internal nasal branch of
anterior ethmoidal nerve

Medial internal branch of anterior
ethmoidal nerve (cut)

Olfactory bulb and tract

External nasal
branch of anterior
ethmoidal nerve

Olfactory nerves (CN I, cut)

Nasopalatine
nerve (cut)

Maxillary
nerve (ghosted)

Nerve of the pterygoid
canal (ghosted)

Pterygopalatine
ganglion (ghosted)

Internal nasal
branches
of infraorbital
nerve

Lesser palatine nerve (cut)

Greater palatine nerve

Posterior superior
lateral nasal branch
of maxillary nerve

Posterior inferior lateral
nasal branch of greater
palatine nerve

Nasopalatine nerve
passing through incisive canal

L

M

Figure 2.19J–M. **J.** Blood Supply of the Lateral Wall of the Nasal Cavity. **K.** Blood Supply of the Nasal Septum. **L.** Nerves of the Lateral
Wall of the Nasal Cavity. **M.** Nerves of the Nasal Septum.

IV. Clinical Considerations

A. Kiesselbach's area: anterior part of nasal septum where many septal arteries anastomose and can result in profuse nosebleeds (**epistaxis**) with injury; can typically be controlled by pinching nose between finger and thumb or packing nose

B. Nasal septum is commonly deviated to 1 side or other and, in conjunction with deviation, may present spurs that project still farther into 1 nasal cavity; deviated septum and spur may come in contact with projecting conchae from lateral nasal wall, resulting in partial occlusion of cavity, impaired nasal breathing, or in discomfort as a result of contact; deviation may be result of birth injury, but mostly occurs in adolescence and adulthood from trauma; i.e., sports, fighting, etc.

C. Rhinitis: inflammation of nasal mucous membrane, which becomes swollen and inflamed during severe upper respiratory infection or allergic reactions (e.g., hay fever, poor air quality, etc.)

D. Suppurative infections in sinuses: especially ethmoid and sphenoid, present risk of erosion into cranial cavity and subsequent meningitis

E. Inflammation of maxillary sinus: may produce dental symptoms, because nerves innervating upper jaw teeth lie in floor of maxillary sinus

F. Any process producing **obstruction to flow of mucus from paranasal sinuses** into nose may predispose to chronic infection in sinuses, which may range from allergic inflammation of nasal mucosa to deviation of nasal septum

G. Fracture of nose: common and usually transverse

   1. If caused by direct blow, horizontal plate of ethmoid is commonly fractured; potentially dangerous because bacteria-rich nasal mucosa may inoculate interior of skull through fractured bone

   2. Commonly accompanied by CSF **rhinorrhea** (profuse watery discharge from nose)

H. Because maxillary sinus opens below frontal sinus, infectious material formed in frontal sinus easily spreads to it; discharge of any inflammatory exudate from maxillary sinus is quite difficult due to high location of its opening

I. Hypophysis can be surgically approached via nasal cavity and sphenoidal sinus

J. Anosmia (loss of sense of smell): not serious handicap and can occur with aging

K. Nasal polyp: focal submucosal thickening due to edema, which is pinkish gray and edematous and may attain a remarkably large size; must be distinguished from a meningocele (removal of latter can lead to CSF leakage)

L. Rhinoplasty: reparative or plastic surgery of nose

M. Transillumination of sinuses

   1. Maxillary sinus: done in dark room; bright light is placed in patient's mouth on 1 side of hard palate or firmly against cheek; light passes through sinus and appears as crescent-shaped, dull glow below orbit; if excess fluid or mass or thickened mucosa are present, glow is decreased

   2. Frontal sinus: light is directed superiorly under medial aspect of eyebrow; normal condition produces a glow above orbit

N. Rhinorrhea: discharge from nose; CSF rhinorrhea: from fracture of cribriform plate and tearing of meninges

Eyelid and Lacrimal Apparatus

I. General Features of Eyelid and Anterior Eyeball

A. Anterior eyeball: pupil (black) and iris (colored) are seen through transparent cornea, which is continuous with sclera or white outer fibrous coat of eye

B. Eyelids (superior and inferior palpebrae): moveable folds covering eyeball anteriorly (Fig. 2.20A)

  1. Palpebral fissure: space between eyelids (palpebrae)

  2. Medial and lateral commissures (canthi): where lids meet at corners or angles

    a. Lacus lacrimalis (lacrimal lake): space in medial angle (canthus or corner) between lids, occupied by lacrimal caruncle (small, fleshy hillock)

    b. Semilunar fold (plica semilunaris): vertical curved fold of conjunctiva lateral to lacrimal caruncle; remnant of nictitating membrane seen in some animals

    c. Medially on each lid is an elevation, **lacrimal papilla**, surmounted with small opening, **lacrimal punctum**

  3. Cilia or eyelashes

    a. Short hairs set in double or triple rows

    b. Ciliary glands (of Zeis): sebaceous glands associated with eyelashes

    c. Between hair follicles are apocrine type sweat glands (glands of Moll)

    d. Tarsal (Meibomian) glands: embedded in tarsal plates; open along border of lid, behind cilia and glands in a single row; their fatty secretion floats on tear layer, helping prevent evaporation; also waterproofs edges of eyelids to prevent tears from seeping onto skin

II. Structure of Eyelids (Fig. 2.20B)

A. Function: protect eye from drying, shield eye from environmental challenges

B. Layers from outside to inside

  1. Skin: very thin, continuous with conjunctiva at margins, no hairs, little fat

  2. Loose connective tissue: without fat

  3. Orbicularis oculi muscle (palpebral portion): lines eyelids to form sphincter together with orbital portion surrounding orbit

  4. Tarsal plates and orbital septum

    a. Tarsal plates: thin plates of fibrous connective tissue in each lid, upper being larger; attached to palpebral ligaments laterally and medially and to orbital septum

    b. Orbital septum (palpebral fascia): fibrous membrane attached to margins of bony orbit where it is continuous with periorbita (periosteum); attached to superior and inferior tarsal plates; in upper lid, tendinous fibers of levator palpebrae muscle penetrate orbital septum to attach to skin of eyelid, whereas deep, smooth muscle part (superior tarsal muscle) attaches to superior tarsus; pierced by vessels and nerves

    c. Tarsal (Meibomian) glands: embedded in tarsal plates; yellow streaks seen through conjunctiva; secrete lipids that float on lacrimal fluid, retarding evaporation, and waterproof edges of lids to prevent overflow of tears

  5. Conjunctiva: mucous membrane deep to tarsi and orbital septum and lines inside of eyelids

    a. Palpebral portion: thick, red, very vascular, lines inside of eyelids

      i. Continuous with skin at lid margin; forms semilunar fold at medial angle

      ii. Reflects from lid onto anterior surface of eyeball at superior and inferior **conjunctival fornices**

    b. Bulbar (ocular) portion: thin, transparent, slightly vascular over sclera; on cornea only epithelial part is present; attaches loosely to anterior of eyeball and is also loose and wrinkled over sclera where it contains small, visible blood vessels; adherent to periphery of cornea

    c. Conjunctival sac: space between palpebral conjunctiva of eyelid and bulbar conjunctiva on eyeball

III. Levator Palpebrae Superioris Muscle (Fig. 2.20C)

A. Origin: bone above optic foramen at apex of orbit

B. Inserts

1. Superficial portion: most fibers insert via aponeurotic fibers penetrating orbital septum to reach anterior surface of superior tarsus, mingle with orbicularis oculi muscle, and skin of upper lid

2. Deep portion: smooth muscle (**superior tarsal muscle**) attaching to upper edge of superior tarsal plate

C. Innervation

1. Superficial portion: superior division of oculomotor nerve (CN III)

2. Deep portion (superior tarsal muscle): sympathetic fibers from superior cervical ganglion via internal carotid plexus; interruption of sympathetics causes ptosis (drooping) of eyelids, also pupil constriction, flushing of face, and anhidrosis (lack of sweating), known as Horner's syndrome

IV. Neurovasculature of Eyelids

A. Motor nerves

1. Zygomatic branch of facial nerve to orbicularis oculi

2. Oculomotor nerve (CN III) to levator palpebrae superioris

3. Sympathetics to superior tarsal muscle

B. Sensory nerves

1. Upper eyelid: palpebral branches of supraorbital, supratrochlear, infratrochlear and lacrimal branches of ophthalmic nerve (CN V_1)

2. Lower eyelid: palpebral branch of infraorbital nerve from maxillary nerve (CN V_2)

C. Blood vessels: palpebral branches of lacrimal and ophthalmic arteries; veins drain to inferior and superior ophthalmic veins

D. Lymphatics

1. Upper lid: drain to superficial parotid and superficial cervical nodes

2. Lower lid: tends to drain to submandibular nodes

V. Lacrimal Apparatus (Fig. 2.20D)

A. Consists of lacrimal gland and its ducts, conjunctiva, lacrimal papilla, puncta, and canaliculi, lacrimal lake and sac, and nasolacrimal duct

B. **Lacrimal gland**

1. Location: lies in lacrimal fossa on superior lateral aspect of roof of orbit; levator palpebrae superioris muscle indents gland to divide it into orbital and palpebral portion; in structure, resembles serous salivary gland; 3–9 excretory ducts open into superior fornix of conjunctival sac

2. Blood supply: lacrimal branches of ophthalmic artery

3. Nerve supply: secretomotor parasympathetic fibers from facial nerve (CN VII)

   a. Presynaptic parasympathetic fibers: via greater petrosal nerve arising from facial nerve at geniculate ganglion; unites with deep petrosal (sympathetic) nerve to form nerve of pterygoid canal; reaches pterygopalatine ganglion within pterygopalatine fossa to synapse

   b. Postsynaptic parasympathetic fibers: leave pterygopalatine ganglion to join zygomatic nerve from maxillary nerve, passes into orbit and through zygomaticotemporal branch and communicating branch to reach lacrimal nerve and lacrimal gland

   c. Postsynaptic sympathetic fibers (vasoconstrictive): from superior cervical ganglion via internal carotid plexus and deep petrosal nerve join parasympathetic fibers to form nerve of pterygoid canal and traverse pterygopalatine ganglion; travel with parasympathetic fibers to reach blood vessels within gland

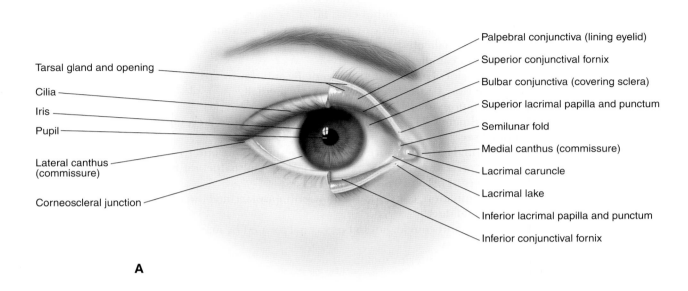

Tarsal gland and opening

Cilia

Iris

Pupil

Lateral canthus (commissure)

Corneoscleral junction

Palpebral conjunctiva (lining eyelid)

Superior conjunctival fornix

Bulbar conjunctiva (covering sclera)

Superior lacrimal papilla and punctum

Semilunar fold

Medial canthus (commissure)

Lacrimal caruncle

Lacrimal lake

Inferior lacrimal papilla and punctum

Inferior conjunctival fornix

A

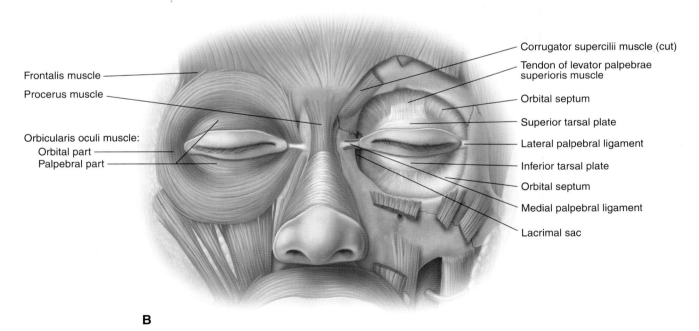

Frontalis muscle

Procerus muscle

Orbicularis oculi muscle:
  Orbital part
  Palpebral part

Corrugator supercilii muscle (cut)

Tendon of levator palpebrae superioris muscle

Orbital septum

Superior tarsal plate

Lateral palpebral ligament

Inferior tarsal plate

Orbital septum

Medial palpebral ligament

Lacrimal sac

B

Figure 2.20A,B. A. Eyelids, Anterior View. **B.** Facial Muscles Surrounding Orbit, Anterior View.

   C. Lacus lacrimalis (**lacrimal lake**): an area of medial corner of eye

     1. Floor of lake is occupied by **lacrimal caruncle** (small, reddish elevation of modified skin) where sebaceous glands secrete whitish secretion into medial angle

     2. Lacrimal fluid from lacrimal gland arrives at conjunctival sac after irrigating cornea and collects in lacrimal lake

  D. Lacrimal papillae, puncta, and canaliculi

     1. Location: at medial end of each lid

     2. Origin: lacrimal puncta or pores open on summit of lacrimal papilla, leading into lacrimal canaliculi

     3. Course of canaliculi

       a. Superior: 1st upward, then medially and downward

       b. Inferior: 1st descends, then directly medially

     4. Termination: in lacrimal sac

     5. approximately 75% of fluid is drained away with each eyeblink

  E. Lacrimal sac

     1. Location: lacrimal groove formed by lacrimal bone and frontal process of maxillary

       a. Covered anteriorly by expansion of medial palpebral ligament and posteriorly by fibers of orbicularis oculi muscle

       b. Termination: continuous below with nasolacrimal duct

  F. Nasolacrimal duct

     1. Location and course: lies in bony canal formed by maxilla, lacrimal bone, and inferior nasal concha

     2. Termination: inferior meatus of nose

  G. Function

     1. Prevent drying of eyeball; wash out foreign bodies that might damage eyeball

     2. Mechanism: blinking of eye by contraction of orbicularis oculi muscles helps to spread secretion throughout conjunctival sac; also, orbicularis oculi, because of attachment to lateral surface of lacrimal sac, "pumps" tears into duct system by creating vacuum

VI. Clinical Considerations

  A. Anomalies of eyelids

     1. Ablepharon: eyelids absent, and eyes are exposed

     2. Ankyloblepharon: eyelids fused

     3. Cryptophthalmos: eyes hidden by overlying skin; no indication of any lid formation present

     4. Coloboma: vertical fissure of 1 or both upper lids

     5. Ectropion (eversion) or **entropion** (inversion): of lids; quite rare

     6. Epicanthus: fold of skin covering inner or, rarely, outer canthus; common in Asian populations at inner canthus but occurs abnormally in Down's syndrome

     7. Distichiasis: presence of accessory row of eyelashes

  B. Inflammation of eyelids and conjunctiva

     1. Dermatitis of eyelids: common, usually allergic in origin and may be caused by medications used or chemicals present in eyelash dyes and cosmetics, and poison ivy

     2. Blepharitis: inflammation of lid margin due to infection of sebaceous glands

       a. Usually chronic with acute exacerbations

       b. Photophobia, excessive lacrimation, itching, loss of lashes, lid margin is red and scaly; possible edema, congestion, perifollicular abscesses, and lymphocytic infiltration

(Continued)

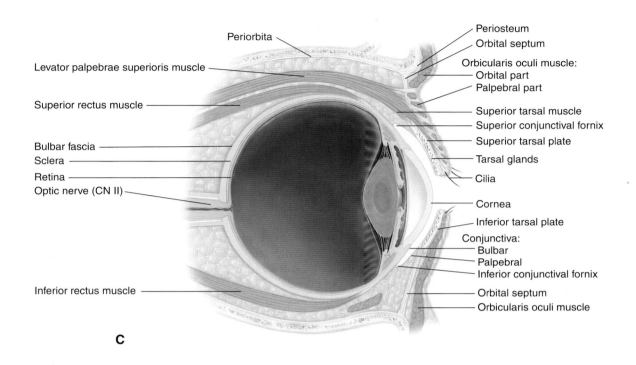

Periorbita

Levator palpebrae superioris muscle

Superior rectus muscle

Bulbar fascia
Sclera
Retina
Optic nerve (CN II)

Inferior rectus muscle

Periosteum
Orbital septum
Orbicularis oculi muscle:
Orbital part
Palpebral part
Superior tarsal muscle
Superior conjunctival fornix
Superior tarsal plate
Tarsal glands
Cilia
Cornea
Inferior tarsal plate
Conjunctiva:
Bulbar
Palpebral
Inferior conjunctival fornix
Orbital septum
Orbicularis oculi muscle

C

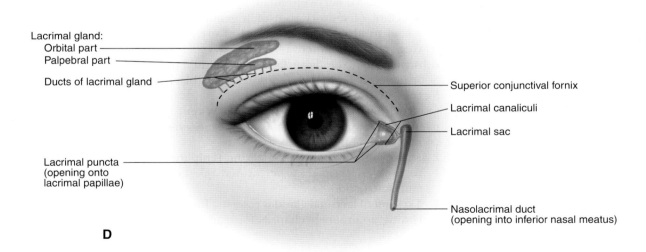

Lacrimal gland:
Orbital part
Palpebral part
Ducts of lacrimal gland

Superior conjunctival fornix
Lacrimal canaliculi
Lacrimal sac

Lacrimal puncta
(opening onto
lacrimal papillae)

Nasolacrimal duct
(opening into inferior nasal meatus)

D

Figure 2.20C,D. C. Eyelid and Eyeball, Parasagittal Sectional View. **D.** Lacrimal Apparatus, Anterior View.

3. **Hordeolum** (sty): an acute, circumscribed, suppurative inflammation of gland of Zeis or Moll (external hordeolum) or Meibomian gland (acute chalazion or internal hordeolum)
   a. Usually caused by *Staphylococcus aureus*
   b. Common in children
   c. Reddish swelling near eyelash roots which can develop into an abscess, which not uncommonly may rupture spontaneously
4. **Chalazion**: chronic granuloma of eyelid due to infection and obstruction of Meibomian gland or its duct; oval or round mass of a few mm develops in lid and causes no symptoms except for a feeling of pressure
5. **Conjunctivitis**
   a. Acute type (pinkeye): inflammation of bulbar and palpebral conjunctiva and may be caused by several organisms; children affected more often than adults
   b. Chronic type: may be caused by bacteria, irritating fumes, or allergies.; moderate conjunctival thickening, reddening, and itching in allergic cases
6. Hyperemia of conjunctiva: conjunctiva is usually colorless, except when its vessels are dilated and congested ("blood-shot") eyes; hyperemia is caused by local irritation (e.g., smoke, dust, etc.)

C. Mechanical injuries of eyelids
1. Subcutaneous hemorrhage into eyelids (black eye, shiner): caused by blunt force injury; hemorrhage is slowly resorbed
2. Mechanical injury is most common form of eye disease and may be produced by contusion, concussion, penetrating wound, or perforating wound of eye

D. Neoplasms: skin of eyelids is common site for epithelial neoplasms
1. Squamous papilloma: develops at lid margin and on palpebral conjunctiva
2. **Seborrheic keratosis**: not true neoplasm; appears commonly on lid skin
3. Basal cell carcinoma: most common malignant neoplasm of eyelids with 80% developing at inner canthus or on lower lid margin
4. Neoplasms arising in eyelid adnexa are uncommon

E. Drooping of eyelid (ptosis): may be due to lesion of oculomotor nerve or sympathetic supply

F. Lesions of facial nerve eliminate blink reflex

G. Destruction of sensory root of trigeminal nerve or its ophthalmic division may lead to ulcerations of cornea of eye because of loss of afferent limb of tearing reflex; conjunctiva becomes dry and is constantly irritated by foreign substances that abrade surface as eye and lid move

H. Subcutaneous hemorrhage into eyelids (black eye, shiner) caused by blunt force injury

I. Obstruction of lacrimal drainage system predisposes to infection or **dacrocystitis**; appears as redness, tenderness and swelling near medial canthus; common in young children

J. Excessive and uncomfortable tearing (**epiphora**)
1. Removal of lacrimal sac performed as last resort in persistent inflammation and obstruction
2. Excision of lacrimal gland is reserved for cases where sac has been removed, leaving no drainage channel for tears and excessive "watering" of eye

Bony Orbit

I. General Features of Bony Orbit (Fig. 2.21A)

A. Pyramidal shaped, consisting of margin anteriorly; apex posteromedially; and 4 walls (lateral, medial, roof, and floor)

B. Distance from orbital margin to optic canal is approximately 40–50 mm in adult

C. Walls of orbit are very thin in regions of paranasal sinuses (especially medially and inferiorly) and may allow disease processes to spread into orbit from these sites

D. Related to frontal sinus above, maxillary sinus below, and ethmoid air cells and sphenoid sinus medially

E. Contain and protect eyeballs and their muscles, nerves, and vessels, along with most of lacrimal apparatus; orbital fat fills space not occupied by structures

II. Components of Bony Orbit (Fig. 2.21B)

A. Orbital margin
1. Superiorly: supraorbital margin formed by frontal bone; **supraorbital notch** or **foramen** medially for neurovascular bundle
2. Inferiorly: infraorbital margin formed by maxilla and orbital process of zygomatic bone
3. Medially: frontal bone meets maxilla
4. Laterally: frontal bone meets zygomatic bone

B. Lateral wall
1. Orbital process of zygomatic bone anteriorly and greater wing of sphenoid posteriorly
2. Small foramina for zygomaticofacial and zygomaticotemporal branches of zygomatic nerve from maxillary nerve (CN V_2)
3. Lateral wall separates orbit from infratemporal fossa and temporalis muscle and middle cranial fossa posteriorly (temporal lobe of brain)

C. Medial wall
1. From anterior to posterior: frontal process of maxilla, lacrimal bone (houses lacrimal sac), **lamina papyracea** (orbital plate) of ethmoid, small part of body of sphenoid, and root of lesser wing of sphenoid
2. Superior edge of orbital plate of ethmoid is perforated by **anterior and posterior ethmoidal foramina** for anterior and posterior ethmoidal nerves and vessels
3. Medial wall is very thin over ethmoidal air cells; it is related to nasal cavity and posteriorly to sphenoidal sinus
4. Anterior lacrimal crest of maxilla and posterior lacrimal crest of lacrimal bone border **fossa for lacrimal sac**, which continues downward into nasolacrimal canal (for nasolacrimal duct)

D. Roof
1. **Orbital plate of frontal bone** anteriorly and lesser wing of sphenoid posteriorly
2. Superior orbital fissure between greater and lesser wings of sphenoid lies at boundary of roof and lateral wall of orbit; transmits CNs III, IV, V_1, and VI; superior ophthalmic vein; and sympathetic fibers
3. Anteromedially: trochlear fovea for pulley of superior oblique muscle
4. Laterally: under roof, **lacrimal fossa** for lacrimal gland
5. Superior to orbit: anterior cranial fossa with frontal lobe of brain and olfactory bulbs and tract

E. Floor
1. From anterior to posterior: mostly by orbital surface of maxilla (anteromedially), and orbital process of zygomatic and small orbital process of palatine bone (at posteromedial angle)
2. Medially near junction of floor and medial wall is fossa for lacrimal sac and opening of nasolacrimal duct
3. Between floor and lateral wall is inferior orbital fissure, which transmits infraorbital nerve (from CN V_2) and artery into infraorbital groove, which becomes infraorbital canal anteriorly, and exits onto face via infraorbital foramen; fissure also transmits connections of inferior ophthalmic vein with pterygoid plexus
4. Maxillary sinus and maxillary infraorbital nerve lie below floor

F. Apex: opening of optic canal for optic nerve (CN II) and ophthalmic artery; ringed by frontal, sphenoid, and ethmoid bones

III. Fascia of Orbit

A. Orbital septum: continuous with periorbita (periosteum of bony orbit) at margins of orbit; attaches to tarsal plates

B. Dura mater: continuous into orbit on optic nerve and blends with outer layer of eyeball (sclera); note: arachnoid and pia also continue onto optic nerve and end where nerve meets eyeball

C. Fascia bulbi (Tenon's capsule)

1. Thin membrane enveloping eyeball from optic nerve to level of ciliary muscle; surrounded by periorbital fat

2. Separated from sclera by episcleral space; continuous with subdural and subarachnoid spaces

3. Fuses with sheath of optic nerve and with sclera at entrance of this nerve

4. Fuses with bulbar conjunctiva

5. Represents deep fascia of extrinsic eye muscles reflecting onto eyeball at their insertions

6. Special fascial extensions

   a. From superior rectus muscle, unites with tendon of levator palpebrae superioris muscle; prevents eye from being raised too far superiorly

   b. From inferior rectus muscle, joins inferior tarsus

   c. From medial and lateral rectus muscles, fascia extends to lacrimal and zygomatic bones; these are strong and known as **medial** and **lateral check ligaments** for they are thought to check action of respective muscles

   d. Fascia of inferior oblique and inferior rectus muscle form a sling, suspensory ligament of eyeball

IV. Clinical Considerations

A. Orbital fractures

1. Blow-out fracture: pressure within orbit can rise enough to cause fracture of thin walls; most commonly affects orbital floor and causes orbital fat to bulge down into maxillary sinus

2. Blow to eye may fracture orbital walls, due to thinness of medial and inferior orbital walls, whereas margins remain intact

3. Superior wall stronger than medial and inferior walls, but thin enough to be translucent and can be easily penetrated; object can pass into frontal lobe of brain

4. Orbital fractures commonly result in intraorbital bleeding, which exerts pressure on eyeball and can cause exophthalmos (eyeball protrusion)

5. With strong impact on bony brim, fractures usually take place at sutures between bones forming orbital margin

B. Orbital tumors: usually produce exophthalmos; malignant tumor in sphenoidal and posterior ethmoidal air cells can erode bony orbital wall and compress orbital contents

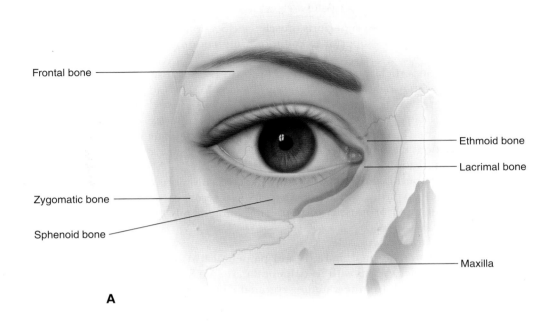

Frontal bone

Ethmoid bone

Lacrimal bone

Zygomatic bone

Sphenoid bone

Maxilla

A

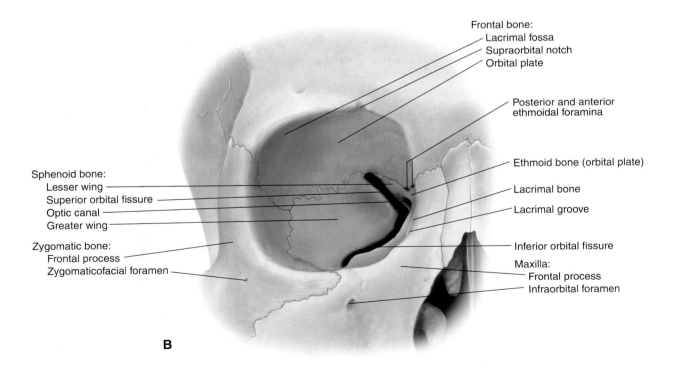

Frontal bone:
Lacrimal fossa
Supraorbital notch
Orbital plate

Posterior and anterior
ethmoidal foramina

Ethmoid bone (orbital plate)

Sphenoid bone:
Lesser wing
Superior orbital fissure
Optic canal
Greater wing

Lacrimal bone

Lacrimal groove

Zygomatic bone:
Frontal process
Zygomaticofacial foramen

Inferior orbital fissure

Maxilla:
Frontal process
Infraorbital foramen

B

Figure 2.21A,B. Bony Orbit. **A.** Surface Relations, Anterior View. **B.** Anterior View.

Extrinsic Muscles of the Eye

I. Muscles Controlling Eyelids (Fig. 2.22A)

A. **Levator palpebrae superioris muscle** (see Section 2.20)
   1. Origin: arises superior to common ring tendon, from orbital roof near apex
   2. Insertion
      a. Superficial part: main aponeurotic insertion passes through orbital septum to mingle with orbicularis oculi fibers and attach to skin and anterior surface of superior tarsal plate
      b. Deep part (superior tarsal muscle or Muller's): descends below aponeurosis to attach onto superior edge of superior tarsal plate; smooth muscle
   3. Action: elevates upper eyelid
   4. Innervation
      a. Superficial part: superior division of oculomotor nerve (CN III)
      b. Deep part: sympathetic fibers from internal carotid plexus
   5. Most superior muscle in orbit, lying immediately below periorbita of roof and frontal nerve
B. Orbicularis oculi muscle
   1. Surrounds orbital margins and palpebral fissure in ring form, extending into upper and lower eyelids with its palpebral part (see Section 2.20)
   2. Closes eyelids; innervated by zygomatic branch of facial nerve (CN VII)

II. Extraocular Muscles of Eye (Fig. 2.22B)

A. 6 pairs of muscles that move eyeball (levator palpebrae superioris is considered an extraocular muscle, but does not move eyeball)
   1. 4 rectus muscles: superior, inferior, medial, and lateral
   2. 2 oblique muscles: superior and inferior
B. 2 eyeballs functionally linked to system for conjugate eye movements, which is regulated by nuclei of oculomotor nerves in midbrain and in superior colliculus of mesencephalic tectum
C. **Common ring tendon** (anulus tendineus communis) (Fig. 2.22C)
   1. Surrounds optic canal at apex of orbit and attached to body and lesser wing of sphenoid and below optic canal
   2. Encloses optic canal and medial part of superior orbital fissure within ring
   3. Neurovascular relations to ring
      a. Above ring: frontal, lacrimal, and trochlear nerves pass through superior orbital fissure
      b. Within ring: optic nerve and ophthalmic artery emerge from optic canal, and superior and inferior divisions of oculomotor nerve, abducent nerve, nasociliary nerve, and superior ophthalmic vein pass through lower medial portion of superior orbital fissure to lie within ring
   4. All 4 rectus muscles arise from common ring tendon

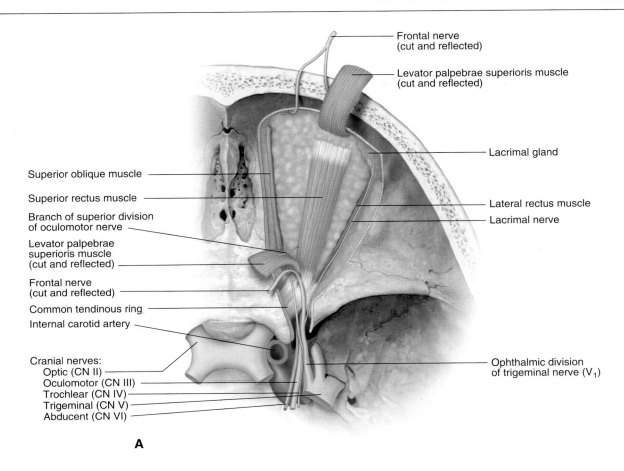

Frontal nerve
(cut and reflected)

Levator palpebrae superioris muscle
(cut and reflected)

Lacrimal gland

Lateral rectus muscle

Lacrimal nerve

Superior oblique muscle

Superior rectus muscle

Branch of superior division
of oculomotor nerve

Levator palpebrae
superioris muscle
(cut and reflected)

Frontal nerve
(cut and reflected)

Common tendinous ring

Internal carotid artery

Ophthalmic division
of trigeminal nerve (V$_1$)

Cranial nerves:
Optic (CN II)
Oculomotor (CN III)
Trochlear (CN IV)
Trigeminal (CN V)
Abducent (CN VI)

A

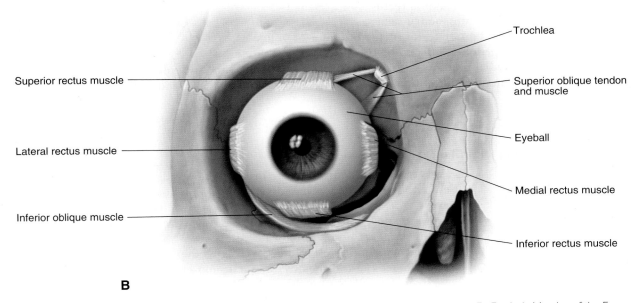

Trochlea

Superior oblique tendon
and muscle

Superior rectus muscle

Eyeball

Lateral rectus muscle

Medial rectus muscle

Inferior oblique muscle

Inferior rectus muscle

B

Figure 2.22A,B. A. Levator Palpebrae Superioris and Superior Recuts Muscles, Superior View. **B.** Extrinsic Muscles of the Eye, Anterior View.

D. Rectus muscles **(Fig. 2.22D–G)**

　　1. All insert via broad aponeuroses into sclera on anterior 1/2 of eyeball, approximately 6 mm behind corneal margin

　　2. Actions of rectus muscles

　　　　a. **Superior rectus**: directs pupil upward and medially; rotates eyeball medially (intorsion)

　　　　b. **Medial rectus**: directs pupil medially (adducts)

　　　　c. **Lateral rectus**: directs pupil laterally (abducts)

　　　　d. **Inferior rectus**: directs pupil down and medially; rotates eyeball laterally (extorsion)

　　3. Innervations of rectus muscles

　　　　a. Superior rectus: superior division of oculomotor nerve (CN III)

　　　　b. Medial rectus: inferior division of oculomotor nerve (CN III)

　　　　c. Lateral rectus: abducent nerve (CN VI)

　　　　d. Inferior rectus: inferior division of oculomotor nerve (CN III)

E. Oblique muscles

　　1. Both insert onto posterior 1/2 of eyeball

　　2. Origins and insertions of oblique muscles

　　　　a. **Superior oblique**: arises above common ring tendon, passes forward to medial corner of orbit to pass through fibrocartilaginous pulley, trochlea, to insert via an aponeurosis into sclera on posterolateral superior surface of eyeball

　　　　b. **Inferior oblique**: arises from maxilla beside lacrimal sac, passes posterolaterally to insert into sclera on undersurface of eyeball posterolaterally

　　3. Actions of oblique muscles

　　　　a. Superior oblique: directs pupil down and laterally; rotates eyeball medially (intorsion)

　　　　b. Inferior oblique: directs pupil up and laterally; rotates eyeball laterally (extorsion)

　　4. Innervations of oblique muscles

　　　　a. Superior oblique: trochlear nerve (CN IV)

　　　　b. Inferior oblique: inferior division of oculomotor nerve (CN III)

F. Summary of eyeball muscle action

　　1. Abduction: lateral rectus

　　2. Adduction: medial rectus

　　3. Elevation: superior rectus and inferior oblique

　　4. Depression: inferior rectus and superior oblique

　　5. Medial rotation (intorsion): superior rectus and superior oblique

　　6. Lateral rotation (extorsion): inferior rectus and inferior oblique

III. Clinical Considerations

　　A. Lesions of nerves controlling eye movements results in abnormal deviations of eye and faulty eye movements (e.g., if oculomotor nerve (III) is destroyed whereas trochlear (IV) and abducent (VI) are functional, eye will look lateralward and downward because these muscles are now unopposed by those normally supplied by oculomotor nerve)

　　B. Under normal conditions both eyes work together (**conjugate movement**)

　　C. Just before deep fascial sheaths of 4 rectus muscles blend with bulbar sheath, they expand laterally to fuse with each other, forming what is called *intermuscular membrane*; tumors or other masses lying internal to this membrane and rectus muscles may not be visible unless space among muscles is explored; therefore, orbit is commonly described as being subdivided into 2 spaces, 1 within and 1 outside muscle cone

　　D. Paralysis of 1 or more ocular muscles, due to nerve injury, results in **diplopia** (double vision)

(Continued)

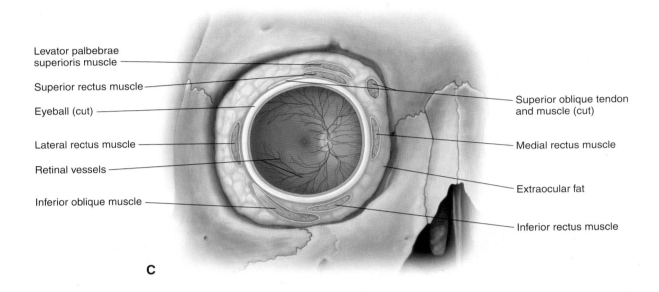

Levator palbebrae
superioris muscle

Superior rectus muscle

Eyeball (cut)

Lateral rectus muscle

Retinal vessels

Inferior oblique muscle

Superior oblique tendon
and muscle (cut)

Medial rectus muscle

Extraocular fat

Inferior rectus muscle

C

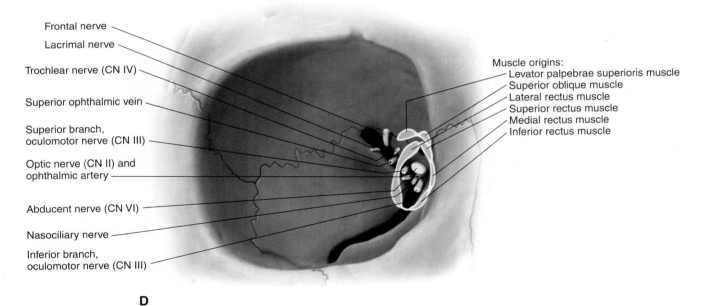

Frontal nerve

Lacrimal nerve

Trochlear nerve (CN IV)

Superior ophthalmic vein

Superior branch,
oculomotor nerve (CN III)

Optic nerve (CN II) and
ophthalmic artery

Abducent nerve (CN VI)

Nasociliary nerve

Inferior branch,
oculomotor nerve (CN III)

Muscle origins:
Levator palpebrae superioris muscle
Superior oblique muscle
Lateral rectus muscle
Superior rectus muscle
Medial rectus muscle
Inferior rectus muscle

D

Figure 2.22C,D. C. Common Ring Tendon, Anterior View. **D.** Extrinsic Muscles of the Eye, Coronal Section, Anterior View.

E. For clinical testing, each muscle is examined in its position of greatest efficiency (i.e., when its action is at a right angle to axis around which it moves eyeball)

    1. Medial and lateral rectus have simple actions: abduction or adduction; compare movements of both eyes to detect impairment

    2. Other 4 extraocular muscles have 2 actions, so to isolate 1 pair to test other, perform 1 of their actions

        a. Based on principle of bent leg situps: psoas muscle can flex thigh or flex trunk; when performing 1 of its actions, the other cannot be done, so situps are done with thigh flexed so that abdominal muscles are used to flex trunk

        b. Superior and inferior rectus move eye inward and upward or inward and downward; when patient looks inward, superior and inferior rectus muscles cannot perform other actions of elevation or depression, but superior and inferior oblique can do these actions; so, to test superior and inferior oblique, ask patient to look toward the nose and then either up (testing inferior oblique) or down (testing superior oblique)

        c. Superior and inferior oblique move eyes laterally and down or laterally and up; so ask patient to look out away from the nose, then up (testing superior rectus) or down (testing inferior rectus)

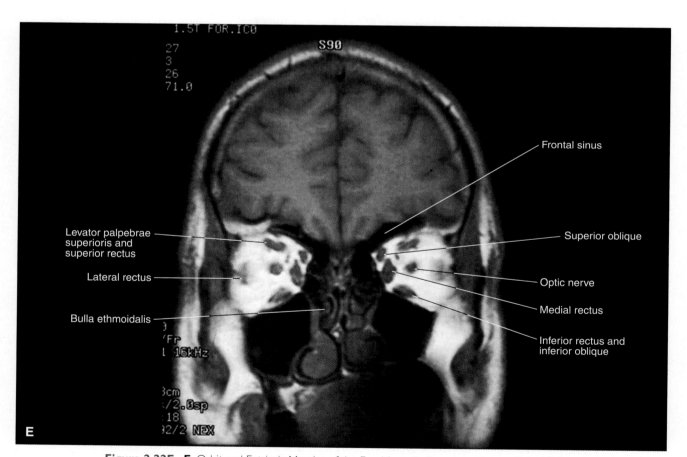

Figure 2.22E. E. Orbit and Extrinsic Muscles of the Eye, Magnetic Resonance Image, Coronal View.

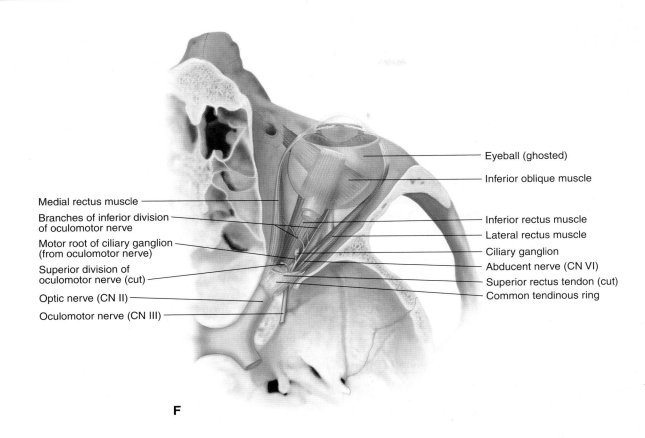

Eyeball (ghosted)

Inferior oblique muscle

Medial rectus muscle

Branches of inferior division
of oculomotor nerve

Motor root of ciliary ganglion
(from oculomotor nerve)

Superior division of
oculomotor nerve (cut)

Optic nerve (CN II)

Oculomotor nerve (CN III)

Inferior rectus muscle

Lateral rectus muscle

Ciliary ganglion

Abducent nerve (CN VI)

Superior rectus tendon (cut)

Common tendinous ring

F

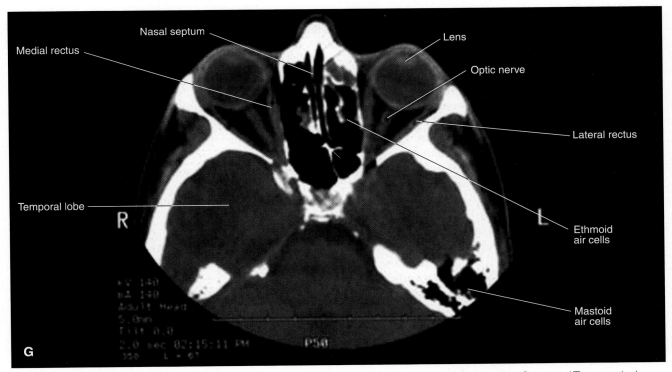

Nasal septum

Lens

Medial rectus

Optic nerve

Lateral rectus

Temporal lobe

Ethmoid
air cells

Mastoid
air cells

G

Figure 2.22F,G. **F.** Extrinsic Muscles of the Eye, Superior View. **G.** Orbit and Extrinsic Muscles of the Eye, Computed Tomography Image,
Transverse View.

Structure of the Eyeball

I. General Features of the Eyeball (Fig. 2.23)

A. Spheroid located in anterior part of orbit; approximately 1 inch in diameter

B. Anterior and posterior parts

   1. Posterior 4/5 of eyeball is occupied by a transparent jelly-like material, **vitreous body**

   2. Anterior part

      a. Lens: transparent, biconvex, and circular structure found on anterior surface of vitreous body and posterior to iris and pupil; held in position by **suspensory ligaments**

      b. Anterior chamber: between cornea and iris; contains **aqueous humor**

      c. Posterior chamber: between iris and lens, communicates with anterior chamber through pupil

C. 3 layers

   1. Outer layer

      a. Sclera: posterior part; tough connective tissue layer

      b. Cornea: anterior part; transparent

   2. Middle or **vascular layer: choroid layer**; continuous anteriorly with **ciliary body**, and then colored part of eye, **iris**

   3. Inner layer: retina; sensory layer with and optical part in its posterior 1/2

II. Layers of the Eyeball (Bulbus Oculi)

A. Outer fibrous coat consists of a white, opaque posterior 5/6, sclera, and transparent anterior 1/6, cornea

   1. Sclera

      a. Made up of densely packed collagenous fibers; loosely attached to choroid layer; pierced by optic nerve and ciliary nerves and vessels

      b. Lamina cribrosa sclerae: circular posterior area of sclera, which is perforated by fibers of optic nerve

   2. Corneoscleral junction (**limbus**): where cornea and sclera meet; contains small canal, sinus venosus sclerae (**canal of Schlemm**) encircles eye and is important connection between anterior chamber and venous system; apparatus for outflow of aqueous humor

   3. Cornea

      a. Avascular, transparent anterior covering of eyeball; highly sensitive to touch

      b. 5 layers, from superficial to deep

         i. Superficial noncornified stratified squamous epithelial layer directly continuous with conjunctiva

         ii. Acellular basement membrane or **anterior limiting lamina** called *Bowman's membrane*

         iii. Connective tissue stroma (substantia propria, consisting of 90% collagenous lamellae)

         iv. Acellular **posterior limiting lamina** (Descemet's membrane)

         v. Posterior epithelium or endothelium

B. Middle or vascular coat: consists of choroid, ciliary body, and iris

   1. Choroid

      a. Dark reddish-brown membrane between retina and sclera; posterior 2/3 of middle coat, which ends anteriorly in ciliary body

      b. Contains venous plexuses and capillaries (capillary lamina or choriocapillaries) for nutrition and oxygenation of retina; engorged with blood in life (highest perfusion rate per gram of tissue of all vascular beds in body and responsible for "red eye" reflection seen in flash photography)

      c. Firmly attached to retina, but easily stripped from sclera

   2. Ciliary body

      a. Connects choroid with circumference of iris

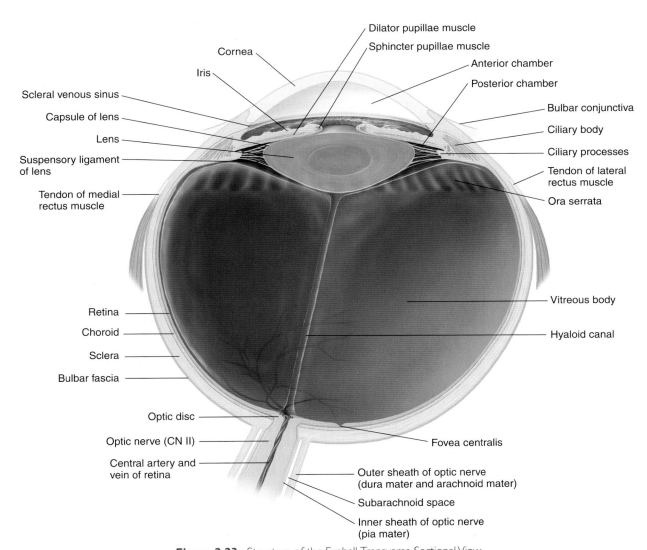

Figure 2.23. Structure of the Eyeball, Transverse Sectional View.

        b. **Ciliary processes**
- i. Folds on inner surface that secrete aqueous humor; fills anterior segment of eyeball
- ii. Anchor **suspensory ligaments of lens or ciliary zonule** (**of Zinn**)

        c. **Ciliary muscle**
- i. Circularly arranged smooth muscle fibers in outer portion of ciliary body
- ii. Contracts to relax suspensory ligament of lens, allowing lens to bulge, called **accommodation**; innervated by parasympathetic fibers

3. Iris
- a. Heavily pigmented colored part of eye; contractile diaphragm in front of lens with central opening, pupil
- b. Found between cornea and lens, attached radially to ciliary body and cornea by short pectinate ligaments
- c. Contains 2 groups of smooth muscle that regulate amount of light entering eye
  - i. **Dilator pupillae**: radial group for enlargement of pupil; innervated by sympathetic fibers
  - ii. **Sphincter pupillae**: circular group to constrict pupil; innervated by parasympathetic fibers
- d. Eye color depends on pigment distribution in iris
  - i. Blue eyes: pigment limited to posterior surface of iris
  - ii. Brown eyes: pigment scattered throughout iris

C. Retina

1. Internal coat, divisible into pars optica (visual part) and pars ceca (nonvisual part)

2. Ora serrata: near edge of ciliary body, is junction point of retina where pars optica transforms to pars ceca

        a. Pars optica
- i. Light sensitive; consists of 2 layers
  - a) **Pars pigmentosa**: outer pigmented layer that extends from optic nerve exit to pupillary margin; consists of simple layer of polygonal cuboidal cells whose cytoplasm contains brown melanin pigment granules; villous processes from apices of these cells, which project between ends of rods and cones of deeper pars nervosa
  - b) **Pars nervosa**: internal, transparent, pale red layer (in living); consists of 3 cell layers representing 3 serially connected neurons present in developing retina
    - i) **Layer of photoreceptors:** turned toward pigment epithelium and away from light because light must penetrate inner layers of retina before it reaches receptors, which consist of rods (for night and twilight vision) and cones (for color, acute, and daylight vision); receptors are formed essentially alike but differ in their receptor structure; approximately 75–120 million rods and 4–6 million cones
    - ii) **Layer of bipolar cells**
    - iii) **Layer of ganglion cells:** axons of retinal ganglion cells unite to form optic nerve, which some consider to correspond to a central tract
- ii. **Optic disc**: circular, depressed white area posterior at optic fundus where optic nerve fibers leave eyeball and retinal vessels also enter and leave; contains no photoreceptors and is insensitive to light, thus called "blind spot"
- iii. **Macula lutea**: small, oval, yellow area lateral to optic disc
- iv. **Fovea centralis**: central depressed area in macula; area of most acute vision

        b. **Pars ceca**
- i. Nonvisual part lying anterior to ora serrata
- ii. 2 parts
  - a) **Pars ciliaris**: part of retina covering ciliary body posteriorly
  - b) **Pars iridica**: retinal pigmented cells covering posterior surface of iris

III. Divisions of the Eyeball

A. Ocular chamber
   1. Anterior to lens and suspensory ligament; contains aqueous humor
   2. Divided into anterior and posterior chamber by iris
      a. **Anterior chamber:** lies behind cornea and in front of iris and pupil; chamber angle (iridocorneal or filtration angle) is formed by cornea and iris laterally; lined by connective tissue network (pectinate ligament or trabecular network) through which aqueous humor arrives in sinus venosus sclerae (canal of Schlemm) which is a wide ring-shaped vein at border of cornea and sclera (limbus) and is responsible for aqueous fluid drainage back to bloodstream
      b. **Posterior chamber:** extends from posterior surface of iris and ciliary body to anterior surface of vitreous body; communicates with anterior chamber via pupil

B. **Vitreous chamber**
   1. Lies behind lens (between lens and retina)
   2. Contains vitreous body

IV. Refractive Media of the Eyeball

A. Cornea: transparent, strongly curved, anterior continuation of sclera
B. Aqueous humor
   1. Clear, watery fluid of anterior and posterior chambers
   2. Maintains intraocular pressure and nourishes lens and cornea
   3. Formed by epithelium of ciliary body and is secreted into posterior chamber, passes through pupil, and is absorbed from anterior chamber in area of iridocorneal angle, draining through specialized trabecular network into sinus venosus sclerae; final drainage is into venous system
C. Lens: crystalline, biconvex, composed of elastic capsule containing lens fibers; suspended from ciliary processes by suspensory ligament (ciliary zonule)
D. **Vitreous body**
   1. Colorless, transparent jelly mass in space between lens and retina
   2. Contained in thin, vitreous membrane, which thickens anteriorly and fuses with lens capsule to form suspensory ligament of lens
   3. Contains hyaloid canal: embryonic channel from optic nerve to lens for hyaloid artery
   4. **Hyaloid fossa:** anteriorly, in which lens rests

V. Innervation of Muscles of the Eyeball

A. **Ciliary muscle** and **sphincter pupillae muscle**
   1. Parasympathetically innervated
   2. Presynaptic parasympatic fibers: from inferior division of oculomotor nerve (CN III) to **ciliary ganglion**, which lies on lateral surface of optic nerve near apex of orbit
   3. Postsynaptic parasympathetic fibers: leave ciliary ganglion in **short ciliary nerves** traveling anteriorly parallel to optic nerve, penetrate sclera at back of eyeball, pass through choroid to reach ciliary muscle and sphincter pupillae muscle
B. **Dilatator pupillae muscle**
   1. Sympathetically innervated
   2. Presynaptic sympathetic fibers: from T1 through sympathetic trunk to superior cervical ganglion
   3. Postsynaptic sympathetic fibers: leave superior cervical ganglion in internal carotid nerve, pass through internal carotid plexus to superior orbital fissure, pass through ciliary ganglion and short ciliary nerves to penetrate sclera at back of eyeball and run forward through choroid to reach dilatator pupillae muscle

VI. Clinical Considerations

A. Glaucoma: group of eye diseases characterized by increase in intraocular pressure due to imbalance in production and absorption of aqueous humor, causing pathological changes in optic disc and typical visual field defects; almost always due to tissue changes which decrease outflow of aqueous humor from eyes

  1. Blindness can result from compression of inner layer of eyeball (retina)

  2. Retinal arteries are not reduced in order to help maintain normal intraocular pressure

B. Formation and circulation of aqueous humor: fluid leaves capillary net in ciliary processes of posterior chamber, flows medially to edge of pupil, and enters anterior chamber; here it flows laterally to iridocorneal angle to enter meshwork of spaces (Fontana) of angle; from these, fluid enters scleral venous sinus (canal of Schlemm) and drains via aqueous veins into scleral plexuses

C. Cataract and **presbyopia**: opacity of crystalline lens of eye or its capsule in response to certain infections (e.g., rubella) or simply as a part of aging

  1. Presbyopia: with aging, lenses become harder and more flattened, which reduces focusing power of lenses

  2. Cataract extraction combined with intraocular lens implant has become common procedure

  3. Extraocular capsular cataract extraction involves removing lens capsule, but leaving capsule to receive implant; recent procedure consists of lasering lens to clear lens opacity

D. Accomodation: refractive power of lens increased to focus near objects on retina; brought about by changes in lens shape

  1. For near vision, requires: a convergence of eyes; increase in thickness of lens; and pupil constriction

  2. For far vision: because eye at rest is adjusted for distant vision, thickening of lens is not necessary

E. Emmetropia (sight in proper measure): normal refraction in eye where parallel rays of light are focused on retina without use of accommodation

F. Ametropia: images fail to come to proper focus on retina, due to discrepancy between size and refractive powers of eye

G. Astigmatism: distorted vision caused by a variation in refractive power along different meridians of eye; most due to irregularities in corneal shape

H. Choked disc or papilledema: because optic nerve surrounded by meningeal sheaths of central nervous system (CNS), increased intracranial pressure can be transmitted through CNS to subarachnoid space around CN II; central vein passes out of retina through optic nerve and passes through meningeal sheaths; increased subarachnoid pressure leads to interference of normal venous flow leading to edema or abnormal swelling of optic nerve head on surface of retina; disc is elevated and retinal veins are dilated

I. Hyperopia or **hypermetropia** (**farsightedness**): visual defect in which parallel light rays reaching eye come to focus behind retina; there is too little refracting power for length of eyeball; vision is better for far objects than for near

J. Myopia (**nearsightedness**): parallel rays of light come to focus in front of retina because refractive power for eyeball length is too great; vision is better for near objects than for far

K. Diplopia: perception of 2 images of single object due to failure to align both eyes properly; may result from strabismus or from other abnormalities

L. Esotropia and exotropia: abnormal inward or outward gazes, respectively

M. Entropion: outward turning of palpebral surface of eyelid

N. Visual field: area within which objects are distinctly seen by eye in fixed position

O. Photophobia: abnormal sensitivity of eyes to light

P. Retinal detachment: separation of sensory (neural) from pigment layer of retina; may follow blow to eye and usually results from seepage of fluid between neural and pigment layers of retina, sometimes days or weeks after eye trauma; patient complains commonly of "flashes of light" or "black specks" floating in front of eye

Q. Kayser-Fleischer ring: pigmented ring of variable color (usually green or brown) just inside limbus; sign of hepatolenticular degeneration (Wilson's disease)

R. Corneal pathology

  1. Opaque cornea: corneal fibers lose transparency

  2. Keratitis: inflammation of cornea (may be ulcerative)

  3. Arcus senilis: benign peripheral corneal degeneration

  4. Pterygium: wing-like plaque usually lying across nasal 1/2 of conjunctiva and cornea due to repeated exposure to wind and dust and hot, dry climates

  5. Corneal injury: foreign objects can produce corneal abrasions that result in sudden stabbing pain in eyeball and excessive tearing

S. Uveitis: inflammation of vascular layer of eyeball (uvea); may progress to severe visual impairment and blindness if not treated

T. Artifical eye: socket for artificial eye formed (after eye enucliation) by fascial sheath of eyeball; postsurgically, eye muscles cannot retract too far due to their fascial sheaths and remain attached to eyeball sheath; thus some coordinated movement of well placed artificial eye is possible

U. Corneal reflex: if examiner lightly touches cornea (typically using cotton wisp), normal positive response is a blink; absence of a blink suggests lesion of CN V_1, lesion of CN VII (motor nerve to orbicularis oculi) may also impair reflex (Note: presence of cataract can interfere with reflex response)

V. Coloboma: any eye defect

Blood Vessels and Nerves of Orbit and Eye

I. Blood Vessels of Orbit (Fig. 2.24A–C)

A. Ophthalmic artery

1. Supplies eyeball, extrinsic muscles, and orbital tissues
2. From internal carotid artery after it leaves cavernous sinus
3. Enters optic canal inferior to optic nerve; as it enters orbit, is 1st on lateral side of optic nerve, then usually crosses superior to optic nerve and passes anteriorly on medial side of orbit, to finally terminate by dividing into **dorsal nasal** and **supratrochlear branches**
4. Branches
   a. **Central retinal artery** (Fig. 2.24D)
      i. Enters optic nerve posterolaterally, distal to optic canal approximately 1cm behind eyeball; passes forward within nerve to enter retina at optic disc
      ii. Has superior and inferior branches that then divide into nasal and temporal branches, supplying retina to ora serrata
      iii. End arteries that do not anastomose with any other vessel; sole supply of retina; if occluded, blindness results
   b. **Meningeal artery**: enters middle cranial fossa by turning posteriorly and exiting orbit via superior orbital fissure
   c. **Ciliary arteries**
      i. **Short posterior ciliary**: 6–12, pierce sclera around entrance of optic nerve; to choroid and ciliary processes; long posterior ciliaries proceed anteriorly to supply ciliary body
      ii. **Long posterior ciliary**: 2 enter sclera on either side of optic nerve; run between choroid and sclera to ciliary body, where their branches form anterior major arterial circle
      iii. **Anterior ciliary**: from muscular branches running with tendons of recti muscles to form vascular zone under conjunctiva; pierce sclera to join major circle
   d. **Lacrimal artery**: proceeds anterolaterally above upper edge of lateral rectus muscle and terminates by dividing into **glandular branches** to lacrimal gland and **palpebral branches** to upper eyelid laterally; give off anterior ciliary artery to eyeball
   e. **Supraorbital artery**: passes anteriorly through supraorbital notch or foramen to supply scalp as far as vertex
   f. **Posterior ethmoidal artery**: passes through posterior ethmoidal foramen to supply mucous membrane of ethmoid air cells, frontal sinuses, and nasal cavity
   g. **Anterior ethmoidal artery**: passes through anterior ethmoidal foramen, enters cranial cavity and gives off **anterior meningeal branch**; enters nasal cavity giving off nasal branches to septum and lateral wall and terminates as **external (or dorsal) nasal artery** (follows external nasal nerve)
   h. **Muscular branches**: come off at intervals to supply orbital muscles; give rise to **anterior ciliary branches** to eyeball
   i. **Medial palpebral branches**: to medial side of upper and lower eyelids
   j. **Dorsal nasal branch**: terminal branch of ophthalmic artery supplying bridge of nose
   k. **Supratrochlear artery**: terminal branch of ophthalmic artery; leaves orbit on its medial side to course superiorly on forehead with supratrochlear nerve

B. Veins of orbit

1. Venous drainage of eyeball
   a. **Central vein of retina**
      i. Retina drains by veins that accompany central artery and branches
      ii. Empty independently into cavernous sinus, but usually has branch to superior ophthalmic vein
   b. **Vorticose veins**
      i. Drain outer coats in outer layer of choroid
      ii. Converge into 4–5 veins, pierce sclera between optic nerve and corneoscleral junction to drain into superior ophthalmic vein

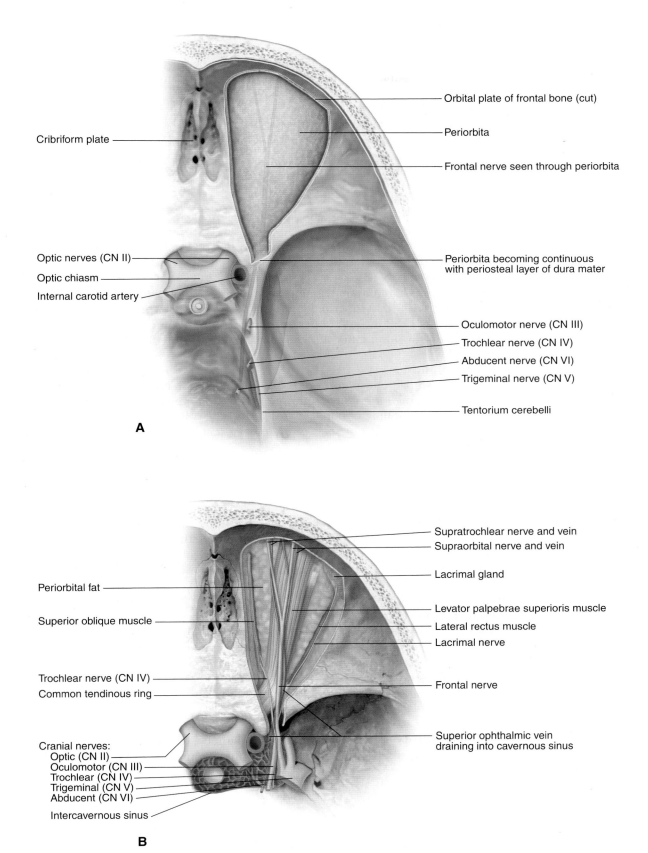

Orbital plate of frontal bone (cut)

Periorbita

Frontal nerve seen through periorbita

Cribriform plate

Optic nerves (CN II)

Optic chiasm

Internal carotid artery

Periorbita becoming continuous
with periosteal layer of dura mater

Oculomotor nerve (CN III)

Trochlear nerve (CN IV)

Abducent nerve (CN VI)

Trigeminal nerve (CN V)

Tentorium cerebelli

A

Supratrochlear nerve and vein

Supraorbital nerve and vein

Lacrimal gland

Periorbital fat

Levator palpebrae superioris muscle

Superior oblique muscle

Lateral rectus muscle

Lacrimal nerve

Trochlear nerve (CN IV)

Common tendinous ring

Frontal nerve

Superior ophthalmic vein
draining into cavernous sinus

Cranial nerves:
  Optic (CN II)
  Oculomotor (CN III)
  Trochlear (CN IV)
  Trigeminal (CN V)
  Abducent (CN VI)

Intercavernous sinus

B

Figure 2.24A,B. Contents of the Orbit. **A.** Superficial Dissection, Superior View. **B.** Intermediate Dissection, Superior View.

    2. Ophthalmic veins

        a. Drain extraocular muscles, periorbital fat, vorticose veins of eyeball, eyelids, and forehead

        b. **Inferior ophthalmic vein**: small; usually joins superior ophthalmic vein

        c. **Superior ophthalmic vein**: empties into cavernous sinus through superior orbital fissure

        d. Communications

            i. Pterygoid plexus through inferior orbital veins

            ii. Angular vein (becoming facial vein)

II. Nerves of Orbit (Fig. 2.24E)

A. Optic nerve (**CN II**)

    1. Direct continuation of axons of cells in retina

    2. Passes through common ring tendon and optic canal ensheathed by meninges

    3. Ends as optic chiasma; optic tracts carry axons to CNS

    4. Provides vision (special afferent fibers) and reflex pathway for response to light

    5. Actually not true nerve but tract of CNS

B. Oculomotor nerve (**CN III**)

    1. Origin: nucleus in midbrain tegmentum; appears in interpeduncular fossa

    2. Passes anteriorly within superior lateral wall of cavernous sinus; its superior and inferior divisions enter orbit through superior orbital fissure within common ring tendon

        a. Superior division: innervates levator palpebrae superioris and superior rectus muscles

        b. Inferior division

            i. Parasympathetic motor root (GVE) carries presynaptic parasympathetic fibers to ciliary ganglion; postsynaptic neurons pass to eyeball via **short ciliary nerves** to innervate sphincter pupillae muscle and ciliary muscle, related to lens thickness

            ii. Innervates (GSE) medial rectus, inferior rectus, and inferior oblique muscles

C. Trochlear nerve (**CN IV**)

    1. Origin: nucleus in midbrain tegmentum; leave CNS through anterior medullary velum dorsally (only cranial nerve from posterior surface of brainstem), cross to opposite side, pass anteroinferiorly to enter dura beneath anterior attachment of tentorium cerebelli to petrous ridge

    2. Passes anteriorly within lateral wall of cavernous sinus between oculomotor and ophthalmic nerves, crosses oculomotor, and passes through superior orbital fissure above common ring tendon

    3. Innervates (GSE and GSA) superior oblique muscle; enters muscle superolaterally near apex

D. Ophthalmic nerve (**CN V$_1$**)

    1. Origin: cell bodies in trigeminal (semilunar) ganglion

    2. Passes anteriorly within lateral wall of cavernous sinus, below oculomotor and trochlear nerves, gives meningeal branch to tentorium cerebelli then divides into 3 orbital branches and enters orbit through superior orbital fissure

        a. **Lacrimal nerve**

            i. Enters orbit above common ring tendon; passes anterolaterally above upper edge of lateral rectus muscle

            ii. Receives communicating branch of zygomaticotemporal nerve containing secretory fibers (postsynaptic parasympathetic, GVE) for lacrimal gland

            iii. Also carries sensory innervation to gland, conjunctiva and skin of lateral upper eyelid

            iv. Smallest branch of ophthalmic nerve

        b. **Frontal nerve**

            i. Largest branch of ophthalmic nerve

            ii. Passes through superior orbital fissure superior to common ring tendon to become most superior structure in orbit, passing superior to orbital muscles

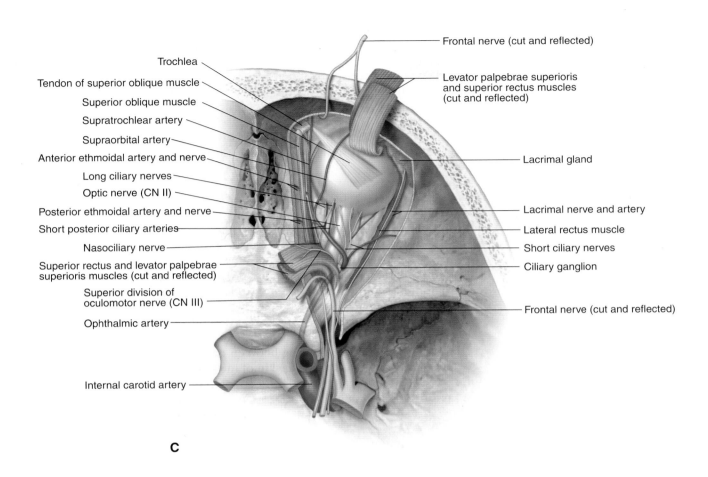

Frontal nerve (cut and reflected)

Trochlea

Tendon of superior oblique muscle

Superior oblique muscle

Supratrochlear artery

Supraorbital artery

Anterior ethmoidal artery and nerve

Long ciliary nerves

Optic nerve (CN II)

Posterior ethmoidal artery and nerve

Short posterior ciliary arteries

Nasociliary nerve

Superior rectus and levator palpebrae superioris muscles (cut and reflected)

Superior division of oculomotor nerve (CN III)

Ophthalmic artery

Internal carotid artery

Levator palpebrae superioris and superior rectus muscles (cut and reflected)

Lacrimal gland

Lacrimal nerve and artery

Lateral rectus muscle

Short ciliary nerves

Ciliary ganglion

Frontal nerve (cut and reflected)

C

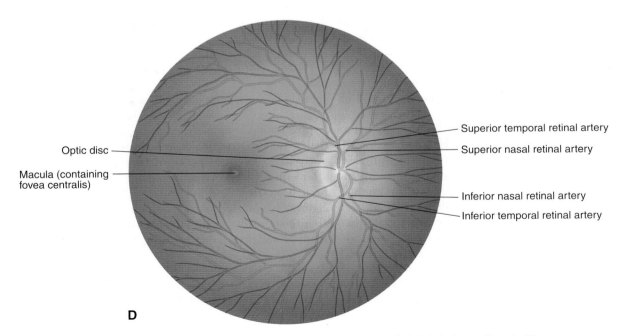

Optic disc

Macula (containing fovea centralis)

Superior temporal retinal artery

Superior nasal retinal artery

Inferior nasal retinal artery

Inferior temporal retinal artery

D

Figure 2.24C,D. **C.** Contents of the Orbit, Deeper Dissection, Ophthalmic Artery, Superior View. **D.** Central Retinal Artery Branches, Anterior View.

iii. 2 branches

    a) **Supraorbital nerve**: passes through supraorbital notch or foramen to skin and conjunctiva of upper eyelid and to scalp to its vertex; also branches to mucous membrane of frontal sinus

    b) **Supratrochlear nerve**: runs superior to trochlea of superior oblique muscle; leaves orbit after giving off branches to medial side of upper eyelid and conjunctiva and root of nose; supplies scalp on medial side of forehead

  c. **Nasociliary nerve**

    i. Enter orbit through common ring tendon between 2 divisions of CN III, passes anteromedially between superior rectus muscle and optic nerve

    ii. Branches

      a) **Sensory root of ciliary ganglion**

      b) **Long ciliary nerves**: enter posterior part of eyeball and are sensory to eyeball, especially cornea

      c) **Posterior ethmoidal nerve**: passes medially between superior oblique and medial rectus to enter posterior ethmoidal foramen; carries sensory fibers from ethmoid air cells and sphenoid sinus

      d) **Anterior ethmoidal nerve**: terminal branch of nasociliary nerve; passes medially between superior oblique and medial rectus to enter anterior ethmoidal foramen; enters cranial cavity at side of cribriform plate of ethmoid, continues anteriorly on plate giving off a meningeal branch; leaves cranium to enter nasal cavity giving branches to septum and lateral wall of nasal cavity and finally emerging between nasal bone and nasal cartilages as **external nasal branch**, supplying skin of lower 1/2 of nose

      e) **Infratrochlear nerve**: terminal branch of nasociliary nerve; leaves orbit superior to medial angle of eye to supply eyelids and conjunctiva medially, upper 1/2 of nose, and lacrimal sac

E. Abducent nerve (CN VI)

  1. Origin: nucleus in tegmentum of pons; leaves CNS in groove between medulla and pons

  2. Penetrates dura covering inferior petrosal sinus, passes anteriorly within cavernous sinus, crosses internal carotid artery laterally to enter orbit through superior orbital fissure

  3. Innervates (GSE and GSA for proprioception) lateral rectus muscle; enters medial surface of muscle near apex

F. Autonomic nerves of orbit

  1. Lacrimal gland

    a. Presynaptic parasympathetic fibers

      i. Arise from cells in superior salivatory nucleus to run in nervus intermedius of facial nerve

      ii. Greater petrosal nerve: given off at geniculate ganglion, leaves petrous temporal bone at hiatus of greater petrosal nerve, passes across middle cranial fossa to unite with deep petrosal to become nerve of pterygoid canal and reach pterygopalatine ganglion within pterygopalatine fossa

    b. Postsynaptic parasympathetic fibers

      i. From pterygopalatine ganglion, join zygomatic branch of maxillary nerve; pass anterolaterally through inferior orbital fissure to enter orbit; pass superiorly with zygomaticotemporal branch and its communicating branch to reach lacrimal nerve and lacrimal gland

    c. Sympathetic fibers: postsynaptic sympathetic fibers from superior cervical ganglion travel through internal carotid plexus and deep petrosal nerve to join parasympathetic fibers within nerve of pterygoid canal

  2. Sphincter pupillae and ciliary muscles

    a. Presynaptic parasympathetic fibers

      i. Arise in Edinger-Westphal nucleus of midbrain, travel through oculomotor nerve

      ii. Pass in motor root from inferior division of oculomotor nerve to ciliary ganglion, located on lateral surface of optic nerve near apex of orbit

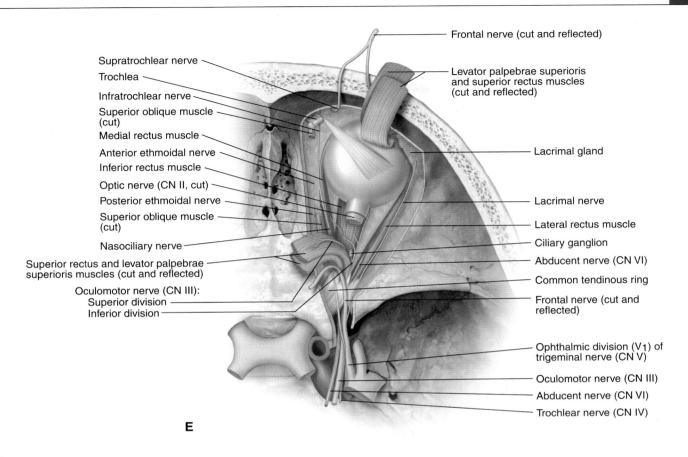

Frontal nerve (cut and reflected)

Supratrochlear nerve

Trochlea

Infratrochlear nerve

Superior oblique muscle (cut)

Medial rectus muscle

Anterior ethmoidal nerve

Inferior rectus muscle

Optic nerve (CN II, cut)

Posterior ethmoidal nerve

Superior oblique muscle (cut)

Nasociliary nerve

Superior rectus and levator palpebrae superioris muscles (cut and reflected)

Oculomotor nerve (CN III):
Superior division
Inferior division

Levator palpebrae superioris and superior rectus muscles (cut and reflected)

Lacrimal gland

Lacrimal nerve

Lateral rectus muscle

Ciliary ganglion

Abducent nerve (CN VI)

Common tendinous ring

Frontal nerve (cut and reflected)

Ophthalmic division (V$_1$) of trigeminal nerve (CN V)

Oculomotor nerve (CN III)

Abducent nerve (CN VI)

Trochlear nerve (CN IV)

E

Figure 2.24E. Contents of the Orbit, Deepest Dissection, Superior View.

    b. Postsynaptic parasympathetic fibers
       i. Pass anteriorly within short ciliary nerves to reach back of eyeball
      ii. Penetrate sclera to pass through choroid to reach muscles
     iii. Innervate sphincter pupillae muscle (circularly arranged smooth muscle fibers within iris) and ciliary muscle (circularly arranged smooth muscle fibers within ciliary body); sphincter pupillae closes pupil to limit light entering eyeball; ciliary muscle relaxes suspensory ligament of lens to allow lens to bulge, resulting in accommodation

3. Dilator pupillae muscle
    a. Sympathetic innervation from superior cervical ganglion via internal carotid plexus and sympathetic root of ciliary ganglion
    b. Pass within short ciliary nerves to back of eyeball, penetrate sclera, travel forward within choroid to reach muscle
    c. Smooth muscle fibers are radially arranged to enlarge pupil, allowing more light to reach retina and increasing peripheral vision

4. Superior tarsal muscle: see Section 2.20

III. Clinical Considerations

    A. Eyegrounds (fundus of eye as seen with ophthalmoscope): appearance of retinal arteries as observed by ophthalmoscopic examination can indicate various health issues

    B. Pathology in cavernous sinus: tumors or aneurysms of carotid artery in this location may encroach upon all nerves passing through sinus, such as in IV and VI, thus causing complete paralysis of all ocular muscles

C. Cornea is sensitive to pain and touch and is innervated by ciliary twigs from nasociliary nerve

D. **Horner's syndrome**: characterized by constriction of pupil, partial drooping of upper eyelid, sinking in of eyeball, warmth of facial skin due to vasodilation, and lack of sweating; can result from any lesion in sympathetic pathway

E. **Argyll Robertson pupil**: pupil does not constrict for light but will constrict for near vision; usually caused by lesion in pretectal zone of midbrain, center for light reflexes

F. In loss of parasympathetic innervation to eye, pupillary dilators are unopposed and pupil dilates (mydriasis) more than normal and pupillary light reflex is also absent

G. CN III (oculomotor) injury: ptosis of upper lid; abduction of pupil (due to unopposed CN VI); slight depression in direction of pupil (due to intact CN IV); dilation of pupil (due to intact sympathetics); accomodation is abolished; and patient cannot adduct pupil (medial rectus muscle is "out")

H. CN IV paralysis: eye looks up nasally due to CN III dominance

I. CN VI paralysis: eye looks downward and medially due to CN III dominance

J. **Strabismus**: an abnormal deviation of eye so that gaze is not conjugate

K. **Nystagmus**: repetitive, involuntary movement (horizontal, vertical, rotatory, or mixed) of 1 or both eyes

L. **Light reflex**: light shines into eye and is picked up by retina and impulses are carried via optic nerve to brain centers; there is direct connection between these centers and nucleus of CN III; presynaptic parasympathetic cells are stimulated and impulses pass along CN III to ciliary ganglion; after synapse, postsynaptic fibers travel to sphincter pupillae muscle to constrict pupil as a response to bright light

M. **Night blindness (nyctalopia)**: encountered in people with vitamin A deficiency, whereby total amount of visual pigment is reduced, thus decreasing sensitivity to light of both rods and cones; this reduction does not interfere with bright light or daylight vision, but does significantly affect dim light or night vision

N. **Color blindness**: due to a deficiency in or lack of particular color cone
   1. Most are red-green blind (with a preponderance of green-color blindness)
   2. Inherited by an X-linked recessive gene; thus more males affected than females
   3. Minority are blue-blind, inherited through an autosomal gene

O. Blindness: visual acuity less than 20/200 with limitation of visual field to an angle of 20°

P. **Diabetic retinopathy**: small, fatty retinal deposits and petechiae are seen; common in patients who have had diabetes for over 15 years

Q. **Exophthalmos (proptosis)**: abnormal protrusion of eyeball (seen in Graves' disease)

R. **Presbyopia**: diminution of accomodation of lens of eye occurring normally with aging

S. **Miosis**: contraction (constriction) of pupil

T. **Mydriasis**: pupillary dilation

U. Blockage of central vein of retina: vein enters cavernous sinus and can lead to thrombophlebitis of sinus; this can also lead to thrombus passing to central retinal vein and producing blockage of small retinal veins, resulting in slow, painless loss of vision

V. Blockage of central artery of retina: terminal branches of retinal central artery are end arteries; thus, obstruction by an embolus can lead to instant and total blindness; usually unilateral and seen most commonly in elderly people

Visual Pathway

I. Summary of Visual Pathways (Fig. 2.25)

A. Begins in retina: 1st- and 2nd-order neurons and cell body (perikarya) of 3rd neuron of visual pathway are found in retina; axons of 3rd-order neuron (retinal ganglion axons) gather at optic disc to form **optic nerve**

B. In humans and mammals with binocular vision: approximately 1/2 of optic nerve fibers cross in **optic chiasma** with decussating fibers coming from nasal (medial) halves of both retinas and passing in an arc to opposite side; nondecussating fibers come from temporal (lateral) halves

    1. Thus, fibers from both eyes pass in **optic tracts** to visual center (striate area of each side)

    2. Fibers from **macula lutea** (areas of retina with most acute vision) pass as unbroken **papillomacular bundle** found directly behind eyeball at lateral side of optic nerve; bundle then passes to center of optic nerve (at 10 mm from eyeball) with its fiber organization corresponding to retinal topography; macular fibers lie in lateral margin of optic chiasma

C. In optic tracts: medial part carries fibers from both upper retinal quadrants; lateral part carries fibers from lower retinal quadrants; papillomacular tract, again is found centrally

D. **Lateral geniculate body** or **nucleus** (**LGN**): dorsally situated major nucleus that contains all optic nerve fibers and a small ventral accessory nucleus belonging to subthalamic regions

    1. Point-to-point connection exists between retina (ganglion cell axons) and LGN

    2. Most optic nerve fibers end in LGN

        a. Some fibers do bypass LGN and end in superior colliculus or pretectal area of midbrain

        b. A few fibers actually bifurcate and end in both LGN and midbrain

    3. Number of fibers in optic tracts and cell bodies in LGN = ~16

    4. **Papillomacular bundle** forms wedge, found in middle region of LGN, that is bordered medially by fibers from upper retinal quadrant and laterally by fibers from lower retinal quadrant

    5. **Main nucleus:** consists of 6 cell layers separated by thin zones of white matter (optic nerve fibers); layers 1 and 2 have large cells, whereas 3 and 6 have polymorphic neurons of small and medium size cells; cell bodies of 4th-order neurons of geniculate nucleus lie under each another in "projection column" within LGN

    6. Fibers from corresponding regions of corresponding retinal halves of both eyes end in different layers of geniculate body (i.e., uncrossed fibers from temporal 1/2 of retina end at 4th-order neurons of layers 2, 3, and 5, whereas decussated fibers from nasal halves of retina terminate in layers 1, 4, and 6 of LGN)

E. **Optic radiations** (**geniculocalcarine tracts**): 4th-order axons from neurons of LGN project to visual cortex, where they also end as columns; projections from corresponding regions are not aligned beneath, but rather beside each other, in columns of ocular dominance approximately 0.3–0.5 mm wide; efferent fibers of layers 3–6 form **optic radiations or geniculocalcarine tract** and give off collaterals to thalamic pulvinar; efferents from layers 1 and 2 also enter optic radiations, and their collaterals pass to superior colliculus in midbrain tectum; retrograde corticogenicular fibers from striate area go back to LGN

    1. Tracts from upper retinal quadrants course directly backwards around lateral ventricles in inferior part part of parietal lobe and end in striate area #17, above calcarine sulcus; those of lower quadrants, course forward toward tip of temporal horn of lateral ventricle and then loop backward (**Meyer's or Flechsig or Achambault's loop**) in temporal lobe to reach visual cortex below calcarine sulcus

    2. Though site of most acute vision (macular) is small in retina, its representation in visual cortex involves greatest part of striate area

    3. Peripheral retinal parts project to a small, rostrally situated visual cortical area

F. Reflex collaterals of efferent fibers: from LGN and some collaterals from optic nerve fibers, which pass by LGN, reach superior colliculus of midbrain tectum, rostrally adjoining pretectal area and tegmentum; pupillary reflex is mediated via pretectal nuclei and Edinger-Westphal nucleus; efferent limb of reflex path passes by way of ciliary ganglion; reflex eye movements involve participation of cerebral cortex, which can also take over role of reflex center

G. In addition to classic geniculostriate visual pathways that end in primary striate visual cortex, a 2nd visual pathway has been described: **retinocolliculopulvinar–cortical pathway**, which terminates in extrastriate cortical areas such as areas 18 and 19 and temporal lobe; these pathways are important for processing highly abstracted visual perceptions, whereas classic pathways are concerned with object identification

II. Clinical Considerations

A. Severance of optic nerve results in blindness in affected eye

B. Loss of optic tract leads to failure of corresponding visual halves of both eyes (i.e., **homonymous hemianopsia [hemianopia]**)

C. Destruction of central portion of chiasma leads to a loss of all decussating fibers: **bitemporal hemianopsia**; loss of both nasal halves of retina also results in loss of both temporal visual field halves

D. Destruction of lateral parts of chiasma, as result of "processes" spreading from wall of internal carotid artery, leads to **binasal hemianopsia**; loss of uncrossed fibers from temporal parts of both retinas also leads to loss of nasal visual fields

E. Lesions of geniculocalcarine tract: give rise to **contralateral homonymous hemianopsia** similar to that seen with lesions of optic tract; due to spread of tract fibers in parietal and temporal lobes, lesion involving part of this fiber system at these sites produces **contralateral quadrantic visual field defect** (upper, if temporal fibers are affected; lower if parietal fibers are affected)

F. Lesion destroying entire visual cortex on 1 side produces **contralateral homonymous hemianopia**

G. Lesion destroying upper or lower calcarine gyrus produces **contralateral lower** or **upper quadrantic visual field defect**

H. Vascular lesions in occipital cortex tend to spare macular area because of its 2 sources of blood supply (posterior and middle cerebral arteries)

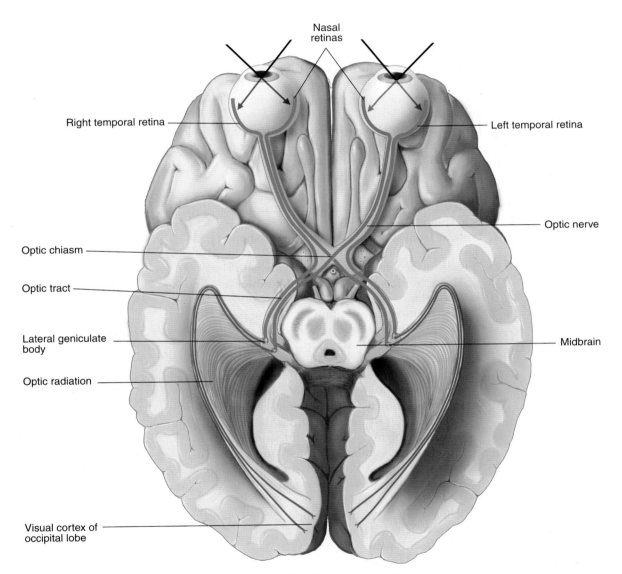

Nasal retinas

Right temporal retina

Left temporal retina

Optic nerve

Optic chiasm

Optic tract

Lateral geniculate body

Midbrain

Optic radiation

Visual cortex of occipital lobe

Figure 2.25. Visual Pathway, Inferior View.

Ear

I. General Features of the Ear (Fig. 2.26A)

A. Divided into 3 parts: external, middle, and internal ear
   1. External ear: from auricle to tympanic membrane
   2. Middle ear: from tympanic membrane to cochlea; connects to nasopharynx via auditory (pharyngotympanic) tube
   3. Inner ear: organ of hearing and balance

B. Embryology of ear
   1. **External ear** and **external acoustic meatus**: form from 1st pharyngeal arch surrounding 1st pharyngeal cleft
   2. **Middle ear cavity**: forms from tubotympanic recess of endoderm from 1st pharyngeal pouch
   3. **Ear ossicles**: form from cartilages of 1st pharyngal arch (malleus and incus) and 2nd arch (stapes)
   4. **Inner ear**: **membranous labyrinth** with receptor fields for both organs arise from single anlage, ectodermal otic (auditory) placode, that forms otic vesicle or otocyst with further differentiation into upper part for equilibrium (semicircular canals) and lower part for hearing (cochlea)

II. External Ear (Fig. 2.26B)

A. **Auricle** (**pinna**)
   1. Projects from side of head; irregularly shaped plate of elastic cartilage covered by thin skin
   2. Lateral surface: irregular and concave with crests and grooves
      a. **Helix** (rim): with small **auricular tubercle**
      b. **Antihelix**
         i. Elevation anterior and parallel to helix
         ii. Splits into 2 crura, which bound triangular fossa
      c. **Scapha**: groove between helix and antihelix
      d. **Concha**: deep concavity anterior to and bordered by anthelix
      e. **Tragus**: posterior projection, anterior to concha and over meatus
      f. **Antitragus**: posterior tubercle opposite tragus
      g. **Intertragic notch**: lies between tragus and antitragus
      h. **Lobule**: inferior part of pinna, below antitragus and notch; non-cartilaginous; consisting of fibrous tissue, fat, and blood vessels; easily pierced for taking small blood samples and also for inserting earrings
   3. Medial surface: shows 2 eminences, corresponding to depressions of lateral surface
   4. Internal structure: basic framework of elastic cartilage and dense fibrous tissue to which thin skin is firmly attached
   5. Auricular muscles (anterior, superior, and posterior; see Section 2.9): innervated by facial nerve (CN VII)

B. **External acoustic meatus** (Fig. 2.26C)
   1. Extent: from bottom of concha to tympanic membrane, approximately 2.4 cm
   2. Course: S shaped, at 1st being convex upward and convex backward
   3. Form: cylindrical, with 2 constrictions, 1 near outer end; other, the isthmus, located deeper

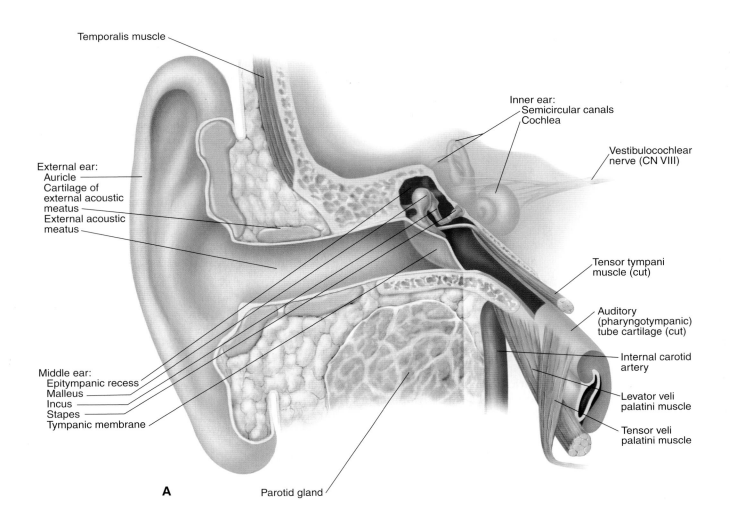

Temporalis muscle

Inner ear:
Semicircular canals
Cochlea

Vestibulocochlear
nerve (CN VIII)

External ear:
Auricle
Cartilage of
external acoustic
meatus
External acoustic
meatus

Tensor tympani
muscle (cut)

Auditory
(pharyngotympanic)
tube cartilage (cut)

Internal carotid
artery

Middle ear:
Epitympanic recess
Malleus
Incus
Stapes
Tympanic membrane

Levator veli
palatini muscle

Tensor veli
palatini muscle

A

Parotid gland

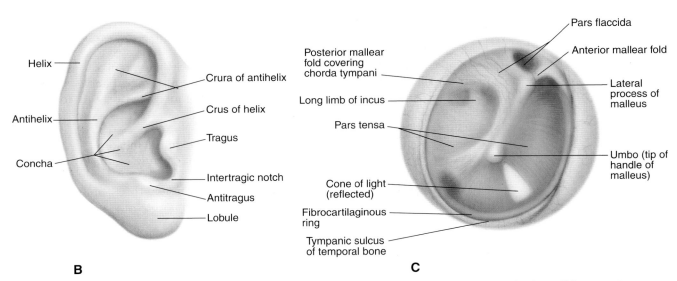

Helix

Crura of antihelix

Crus of helix

Antihelix

Tragus

Concha

Intertragic notch

Antitragus

Lobule

B

Posterior mallear
fold covering
chorda tympani

Pars flaccida

Anterior mallear fold

Lateral
process of
malleus

Long limb of incus

Pars tensa

Umbo (tip of
handle of
malleus)

Cone of light
(reflected)

Fibrocartilaginous
ring

Tympanic sulcus
of temporal bone

C

Figure 2.26A–C. A. General Features of the Ear, Anterior Schematic View. **B.** External Ear, Lateral View.
C. Tympanic Membrane, Lateral View.

4. **Tympanic membrane**: at medial end, set obliquely, so that floor and anterior wall are longer than roof and posterior wall
   a. Covered with thin skin externally and mucous membrane of middle ear internally
   b. Via otoscope, has concavity toward external acoustic meatus with shallow, cone-shaped central depression, which peaks at **umbo**
   c. Central axis of membrane passes perpendicular through umbo, running anteriorly and inferiorly as it turns laterally
   d. Membrane is thin (flaccid part, or pars flaccida) above lateral process of malleus and lacks radial circular fibers seen in rest of membrane (tense part, or pars tensa); flaccid part forms lateral wall of superior recess of epitympanic cavity
5. Parts
   a. Cartilaginous: approximately 8.0 mm long and continuous with cartilage of pinna; firmly attached to auricular process of temporal bone
   b. Osseous: approximately 16 mm long, narrower than cartilaginous part, inner end narrower than outer; tympanic sulcus: narrow groove to which periphery of tympanic membrane is attached
6. Canal lined with skin (epidermis continuing onto tympanic membrane) with hairs and modified sweat glands that give rise to cerumen or earwax (ceruminous glands)

C. Relations of external ear
   1. Anteriorly: condyle of mandible and parotid gland
   2. Posteriorly: mastoid air cells
D. Neurovascular supply
   1. Arteries: branches of posterior auricular of external carotid artery, anterior auricular from superficial temporal artery, and deep auricular branch of maxillary artery
   2. Lymphatic drainage: to superficial parotid nodes (lateral surface of superior 1/2 of auricle), mastoid and deep cervical nodes (medial surface of upper 1/2 of auricle) and superficial cervical lymph nodes (lower 1/2 of auricle)
   3. Nerves: auricular branch of vagus and auriculotemporal of mandibular nerve (CN V_3); auricle supplied by great auricular and lesser occipital nerves of cervical plexus

III. Middle Ear (Fig. 2.26D)

A. **Tympanic cavity** proper: narrow, air-filled chamber with concave sides located in petrous part of temporal, opposite tympanic membrane
B. **Epitympanic recess**: above level of membrane
C. Form: commonly described as box with roof, floor, lateral, medial, posterior, and anterior walls, but more closely resembles narrow cleft obliquely situated between anterolateral and posteromedial walls, continuous with mastoid air cells posterolaterally and auditory tube anteromedially
   1. Roof (tegmental) wall: formed by **tegmen tympani**, bony plate between cranial and tympanic cavities
   2. Floor (jugular) wall: plate of bone between tympanic cavity and jugular fossa; inferior tympanic canaliculus transmits tympanic branch of glossopharyngeal nerve
   3. Lateral (membranous) wall: formed by tympanic membrane; superiorly it is formed by lateral bony wall of epitympanic recess (Fig. 2.26E)
      a. Structure and relations
         i. Set obliquely, forming angle of 53° with floor of external meatus
         ii. Periphery, where attached to bone in tympanic sulcus, is fibrocartilaginous (anulus)
         iii. Where tympanic sulcus is lacking at tympanic notch (of Rivinus) 2 bands, anterior and posterior malleolar folds, extend from notch to lateral process of malleus
         iv. Triangular area between (and superior to) folds is pars flaccida of membrane

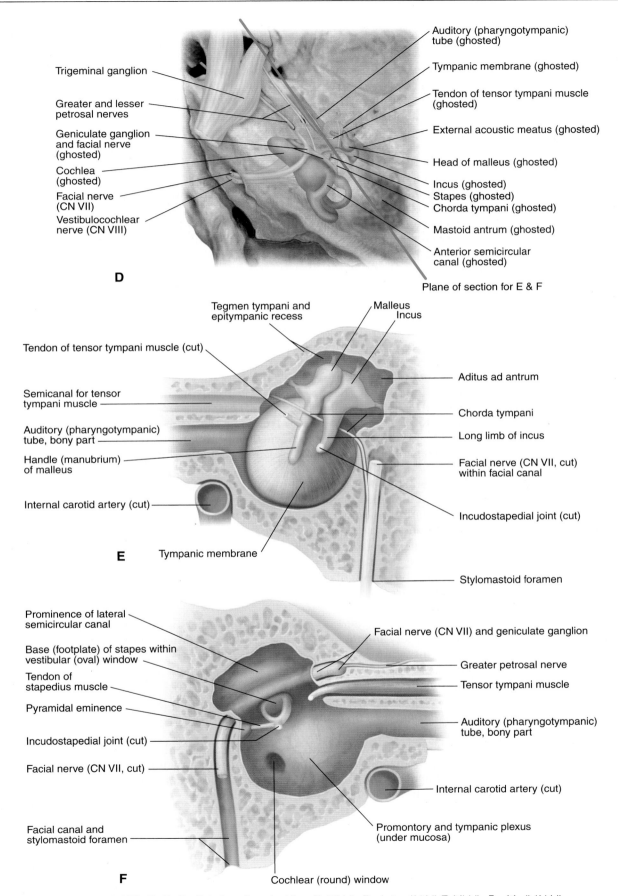

Trigeminal ganglion

Greater and lesser petrosal nerves

Geniculate ganglion and facial nerve (ghosted)

Cochlea (ghosted)

Facial nerve (CN VII)

Vestibulocochlear nerve (CN VIII)

Auditory (pharyngotympanic) tube (ghosted)

Tympanic membrane (ghosted)

Tendon of tensor tympani muscle (ghosted)

External acoustic meatus (ghosted)

Head of malleus (ghosted)

Incus (ghosted)

Stapes (ghosted)

Chorda tympani (ghosted)

Mastoid antrum (ghosted)

Anterior semicircular canal (ghosted)

Plane of section for E & F

D

Tendon of tensor tympani muscle (cut)

Semicanal for tensor tympani muscle

Auditory (pharyngotympanic) tube, bony part

Handle (manubrium) of malleus

Internal carotid artery (cut)

Tegmen tympani and epitympanic recess

Malleus
Incus

Aditus ad antrum

Chorda tympani

Long limb of incus

Facial nerve (CN VII, cut) within facial canal

Incudostapedial joint (cut)

Tympanic membrane

Stylomastoid foramen

E

Prominence of lateral semicircular canal

Base (footplate) of stapes within vestibular (oval) window

Tendon of stapedius muscle

Pyramidal eminence

Incudostapedial joint (cut)

Facial nerve (CN VII, cut)

Facial canal and stylomastoid foramen

Facial nerve (CN VII) and geniculate ganglion

Greater petrosal nerve

Tensor tympani muscle

Auditory (pharyngotympanic) tube, bony part

Internal carotid artery (cut)

Promontory and tympanic plexus (under mucosa)

Cochlear (round) window

F

Figure 2.26D–F. D. Ear Relations, Superior View. **E.** Middle Ear, Lateral Wall. **F.** Middle Ear, Medial Wall.

      b. Manubrium of malleus is firmly fixed to membrane at its middle; umbo: depression at inferior end of manubrium, where membrane is concave

      c. Chorda tympani nerve runs between handle of malleus and incus

      d. **Epitympanic recess**: small space above tympanic membrane for head of malleus

      e. Special features

         i. Notch of Rivinus: deficiency in bony rim

         ii. Iter chordae anterius and posterius

         iii. **Petrotympanic fissure**: for inferior passage of chorda tympani

         iv. Sensitive to pain; innervated on outer surface by auriculotemporal nerve (CN V_3) and auricular branch of CN X; its inner surface innervated by tympanic branch of CN IX

D. Medial (labyrinthic) wall: bone between middle and inner ear (Fig. 2.26F)

    1. **Vestibular (oval) window**: with long axis horizontal

    2. **Cochlear (round) window**: contains secondary tympanic membrane

    3. **Promontory**: rounded eminence between oval and round windows

    4. **Facial canal**: above oval window, then curves downward along posterior wall

    5. **Prominence of lateral semicircular canal**: above facial canal

E. Posterior (mastoid) wall

    1. Entrance (aditus) to mastoid antrum, actually from epitympanic recess to mastoid air cells; antrum and mastoid air cells lined by mucous membrane continuous with lining of middle ear cavity

    2. **Pyramidal eminence**: penetrated at its apex by tendon of stapedius muscle passing to stapes

    3. Fossa of incus

F. Anterior (carotid) wall: bone separating cavity from internal carotid artery

    1. Perforated by tympanic branch of internal carotid artery and sympathetic nerves

    2. **Auditory tube** and **canal for tensor tympani** (Fig. 2.26G)

      a. **Auditory (Eustachian or pharyngotympanic) tube**: has a wide, funnel-shaped pharyngeal opening into posterolateral wall of nasopharynx near choanae of nasal cavity

      b. approximately 4 cm long; passes obliquely anteromedially and downward at 45° angle with median plane

      c. Wall reinforced with cartilage in its medial, longer part (which in cross section appears hook shaped with swollen and thickened margins to form torus tubarius) and its lateral, terminal part lies in temporal bone bordering carotid canal medially

      d. Lumen of cartilaginous part always open in its upper part (like entire osseous portion), but in rest of cartilaginous portion of tube, it is normally pressed together to form narrow slit, which can be dilated by tensor veli palatini muscle by act of swallowing

      e. Arteries of tube: derived from ascending pharyngeal artery, branch of external carotid srtery and middle meningeal artery and artery of pterygoid canal, branches of maxillary artery

      f. Veins of tube: drain into pterygoid venous plexus

      g. Lymphatics: drain to deep cervical lymph nodes

      h. Nerves: arise from tympanic plexus, which is formed by fibers of CN IX; also receives fibers from pterygopalatine ganglion, anteriorly

IV. Auditory Ossicles (Fig. 2.26H–L)

A. **Malleus**: handle attaches to tympanic membrane with tip at umbo; head lies in epitympanic recess and articulates with incus, neck connects to handle and anterior and lateral processes

B. **Incus**: located between malleus and stapes and articulates with them; has large body that lies in epitympanic recess, where it articulates with head of malleus, short crus, and long crus; long crus lies parallel to handle of malleus and lower end articulates with stapes by lenticular process

C. **Stapes**: articulates with incus with head, neck splits into 2 crura attached to foot plate, whose base fits into oval window on medial wall of tympanic cavity

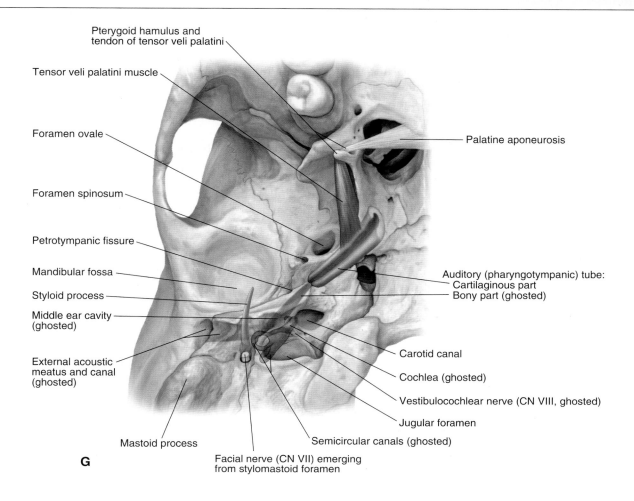

Pterygoid hamulus and tendon of tensor veli palatini

Tensor veli palatini muscle

Foramen ovale

Foramen spinosum

Petrotympanic fissure

Mandibular fossa

Styloid process

Middle ear cavity (ghosted)

External acoustic meatus and canal (ghosted)

Mastoid process

Facial nerve (CN VII) emerging from stylomastoid foramen

Palatine aponeurosis

Auditory (pharyngotympanic) tube:
Cartilaginous part
Bony part (ghosted)

Carotid canal

Cochlea (ghosted)

Vestibulocochlear nerve (CN VIII, ghosted)

Jugular foramen

Semicircular canals (ghosted)

G

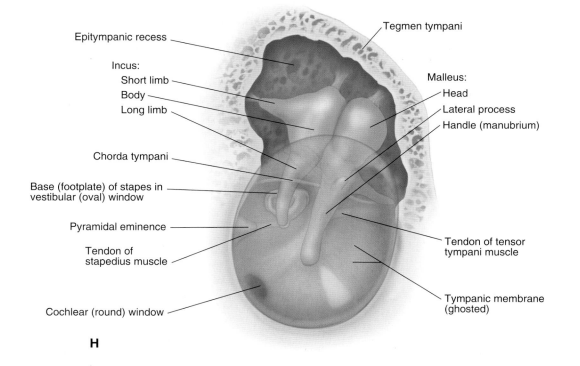

Epitympanic recess

Incus:
Short limb
Body
Long limb

Chorda tympani

Base (footplate) of stapes in vestibular (oval) window

Pyramidal eminence

Tendon of stapedius muscle

Cochlear (round) window

Tegmen tympani

Malleus:
Head
Lateral process
Handle (manubrium)

Tendon of tensor tympani muscle

Tympanic membrane (ghosted)

H

Figure 2.26G,H. **G.** Auditory Tube, Inferior View. **H.** Auditory Ossicles and Tympanic Membrane, Medial View.

V. Intrinsic Muscles

A. Tensor tympani muscle
   1. Origin: from cartilaginous part of auditory tube and great wing of sphenoid
   2. Insertion: handle of malleus
   3. Action: tenses membrane
   4. Innervation: mandibular nerve (CN V_3)

B. Stapedius muscle
   1. Origin: inner wall of pyramidal eminence (hollow, cone-shaped prominence on posterior wall of tympanic cavity)
   2. Insertion: neck of stapes
   3. Action: draws stapes posteriorly and tilts its base in oval window tightening anular ligament and reducing oscillatory range
   4. Innervation: facial nerve (CN VII)

VI. Inner Ear (Labyrinth) (Fig. 2.26M–O)

A. Contains vestibulocochlear organs concerned with sound reception and maintenance of balance

B. Osseous labyrinth: cavities in otic capsule of petrous bone; 3 parts, lined with periosteum; filled with perilymph
   1. **Vestibule**: central part of labyrinth
      a. In lateral wall: oval window
      b. In medial wall: perforations for nerves and opening for endolymphatic duct (vestibular aqueduct)
      c. Posteriorly: 5 openings for semicanals
      d. Anteriorly: opening for cochlea
   2. **Semicircular canals**: 3 in number
      a. Anterior (superior): lateral end has dilation, the **ampulla**, which opens into vestibule; medial end joins posterior canal, forming **common crus**
      b. Posterior: caudal end has an ampulla, which opens into vestibule
      c. Lateral has ampulla, which opens into vestibule at lateral end; other end opens into posterior part of vestibule
   3. **Cochlea**: has apex and base; apex directed anteriorly and laterally; base faces posteromedially and lies at bottom of internal acoustic meatus
      a. **Modiolus**: bony, central conical pillar
      b. Bony canal makes 21/2 turns around modiolus; lower end diverging from modiolus has openings for round window; at apex, canal called **helicotrema**
      c. **Osseous spiral lamina**: bony shelf projecting from modiolus; with **basilar membrane**, it divides an upper **scala vestibuli** and lower **scala tympani**

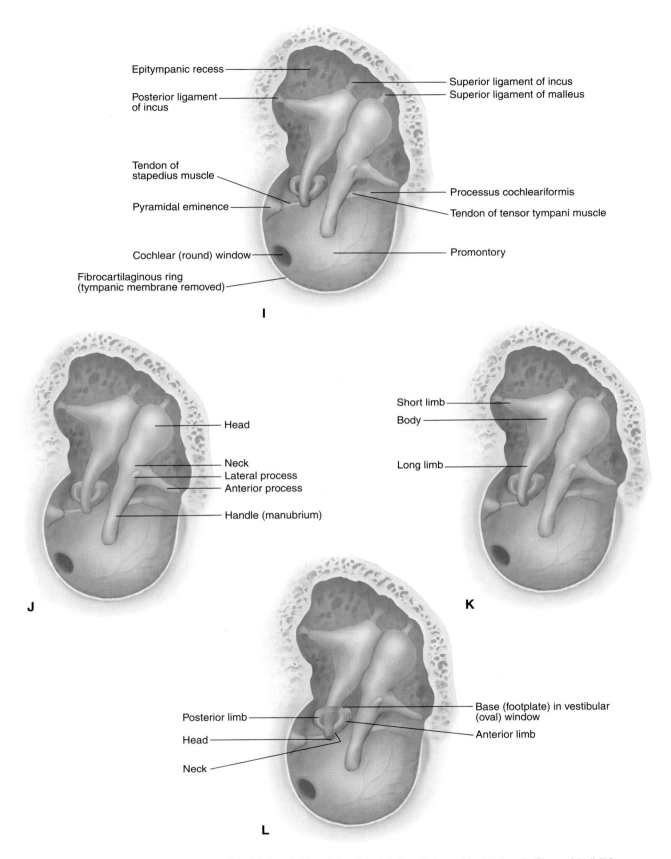

Epitympanic recess

Posterior ligament
of incus

Tendon of
stapedius muscle

Pyramidal eminence

Cochlear (round) window

Fibrocartilaginous ring
(tympanic membrane removed)

Superior ligament of incus
Superior ligament of malleus

Processus cochleariformis

Tendon of tensor tympani muscle

Promontory

I

Head

Neck
Lateral process
Anterior process

Handle (manubrium)

J

Short limb
Body

Long limb

K

Posterior limb

Head

Neck

Base (footplate) in vestibular
(oval) window

Anterior limb

L

Figure 2.26I–L. I. Auditory Ossicles, Medial View. **J.** Manubrium, Medial View. **K.** Incus, Medial View. **L.** Stapes, Medial View.

C. **Membranous labyrinth** (Fig. 2.26P)
  1. Made up of interconnected sacs and tubes (ducts); connective tissue and epithelium, filled with endolymph
  2. **Utricle**: in bony vestibule; has 5 openings for semicircular canals and ductus utriculosaccularis (becomes endolymphatic duct and sac)
  3. **Saccule**: in vestibule; has opening into endolymphatic duct and chochlear duct (ductus reuniens)
  4. Semicircular canals open into utricle, conform to bony labyrinth
  5. **Cochlear duct**: that part of labyrinth separated from scala tympani by basilar membrane and from scala vestibuli by vestibular membrane

VII. Sense Organs

A. For equilibrium: **macula utriculi**, **macula sacculi**, and **cristae ampullaris**
B. For hearing: **spiral organ** (**of Corti**) in floor of cochlear duct

VII. Neurovasculature of Middle and Inner Ear

A. Blood supply of bony labyrinth: anterior tympanic branch of maxillary, stylomastoid branch of posterior auricular, and petrosal branch from middle meningeal
B. Blood supply of membranous labyrinth: **labrynthine artery**, which arises from anterior inferior cerebellar artery or from basilar and travels with CNs VII and VIII through internal auditory meatus; gives off a cochlear branch and 2 vestibular branches
C. Vestibular portion of vestibulocochlear nerve (CN VIII) for equilibrium
  1. Ganglion: vestibular, located in acoustic meatus
  2. Branches of nerve: superior, to macula utriculi and cristae of superior and lateral canals; inferior, to macula sacculi; and posterior, to crista of posterior canal
D. Auditory portion of vestibulocochlear nerve (CN VIII) for hearing
  1. Ganglion: spiral, in spiral canal at center of bony modiolus
  2. Distribution: fibers pass through osseous spiral lamina to organ of Corti
E. Facial nerve (CN VII)
  1. Accompanies CN VIII in internal acoustic meatus until it reaches geniculate ganglion (a sensory ganglion)
  2. Here nerve makes sharp posterior bend in medial wall of middle ear beneath lateral semicircular canal (creating a prominence) and then turns laterally and inferiorly in posterior wall of middle ear to finally exit from stylomastoid foramen
  3. 4 branches within petrous temporal bone
    a. **Greater petrosal**
      i. 1st branch of facial nerve, at geniculate ganglion
      ii. Carries presynaptic parasympathetic fibers and some sensory fibers for taste
      iii. Turns anterior and medial and enters middle cranial fossa through hiatus of greater petrosal nerve on anterior surface of petrous temporal bone
      iv. Crosses foramen lacerum and is joined by deep petrosal nerve (sympathetic, postganglionic); 2 become nerve of pterygoid canal (Vidian)
      v. Nerve of pterygoid canal enters pterygopalatine fossa, where its parasympathetic fibers synapse in pterygopalatine ganglion
      vi. Postsynaptic fibers are distributed to lacrimal gland and mucous membranes and vessels of oral cavity, nasal cavity, pharynx, and other regions
    b. Communication with lesser petrosal: latter is contribution from tympanic plexus and is parasympathetic fibers from CN IX; function of fibers of facial nerve in lesser petrosal is uncertain

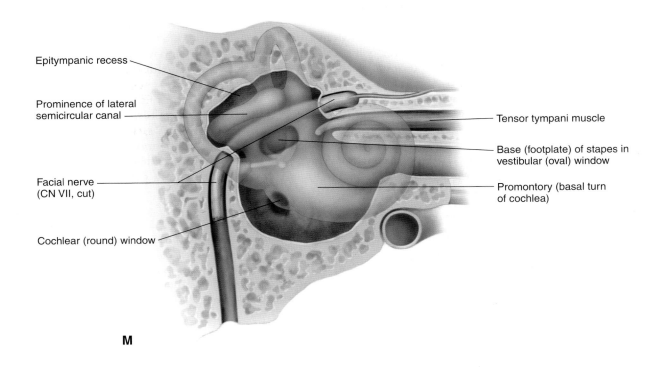

Epitympanic recess

Prominence of lateral
semicircular canal

Facial nerve
(CN VII, cut)

Cochlear (round) window

Tensor tympani muscle

Base (footplate) of stapes in
vestibular (oval) window

Promontory (basal turn
of cochlea)

M

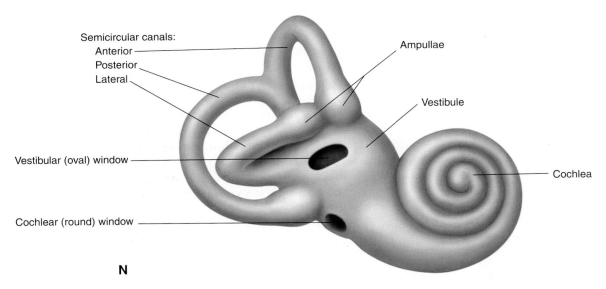

Semicircular canals:
Anterior
Posterior
Lateral

Vestibular (oval) window

Cochlear (round) window

Ampullae

Vestibule

Cochlea

N

Figure 2.26M,N. M. Inner Ear, Relations, Medial View. **N.** Bony Labyrinth, Medial View.

      c. **Nerve to stapedius muscle**

      d. **Chorda tympani**: arises from facial while it is in facial canal posterior to middle ear; courses through middle ear on inner surface of tympanic membrane, exits from petrotympanic fissure to infratemporal fossa to join lingual nerve; contains taste fibers from anterior 2/3 of tongue and secretomotor fibers to submandibular and sublingual glands

    4. Emerging from skull via stylomastoid foramen, it gives off its posterior auricular branch, branch to posterior belly of digastric muscle, and branch to stylohyoid muscle before dividing into terminal branches to face (temporal, zygomatic, buccal, mandibular, and cervical)

F. Tympanic plexus

    1. Tympanic branch of glossopharyngeal nerve passes up through inferior tympanic canaliculus to ramify on promontory

    2. Carries presynaptic parasympathic fibers for otic ganglion and parotid gland

    3. Forms lesser petrosal nerve, which penetrates floor of middle cranial fossa at hiatus of lesser petrosal nerve to run to foramen ovale and reach otic ganglion in infratemporal fossa

IX. Spiral Organ (of Corti)

A. Receptor of auditory stimuli and is situated on basilar membrane and extends from base to apex of cochlea

B. Projects into cochlear duct and is thus bathed by endolymph

C. In transverse section, it is seen to consist of row of inner hair cells and row of outer hair cells, which have hairlike projections into endolymph

    1. These cells are accompanied by various types of supporting cells

    2. Nerves are direct continuation of hair cells

D. Tectorial membrane

    1. Projects into endolymph from osseous spiral lamina and is suspended over hair cells

    2. When hair cell touches membrane, impulse is carried via cochlear nerve to brain and is recognized as sound

E. Base of cochlea is involved with high sounds, whereas low sounds involve area near helicotrema (due to fact that basilar membrane is longer near apex of coil and shorter toward base)

X. Mechanism of Hearing Sound Waves

A. Air waves enter external auditory meatus and cause tympanic membrane to vibrate

B. Vibrations are carried through malleus, incus, and stapes to oval window in vestibule of osseous labyrinth

C. If too loud, reflex stimulation of tensor tympani and stapedius muscles decreases magnitude of vibrations at oval window

D. Vibrations caused by stapes induce vibrations in perilymph of scala vestibuli (and scala tympani across helicotrema)

E. Membrane of round window bulges out as that of oval window bulges in

F. Vibrations pass through vestibular membrane into cochlear duct

G. A theory of hearing states that specific portion of basilar membrane responds to any given frequency of vibration in perilymph and endolymph, and stimulated hair cells send impulses to brain for interpretation

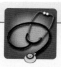

XI. Clinical Considerations

A. Lesions in external acoustic canal: infections or boils in canal may cause nausea and vomiting because general somatic afferent fibers (pain, etc.) from this area are carried in vagus nerve (X), which also carries gag reflex from upper gastrointestinal tract

B. Clinical examination of meatus and tympanic membrane is done with otoscope, which shines light down tapering, hollow speculum; external acoustic meatus

(Continued)

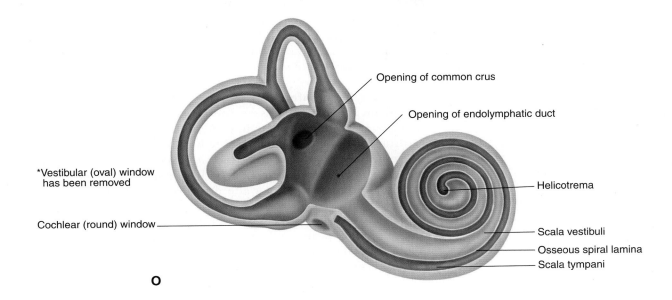

Opening of common crus

Opening of endolymphatic duct

*Vestibular (oval) window has been removed

Helicotrema

Cochlear (round) window

Scala vestibuli

Osseous spiral lamina

Scala tympani

O

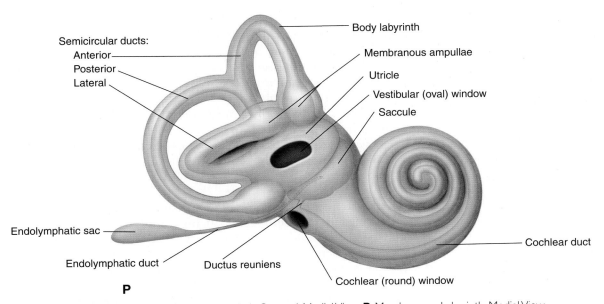

Body labyrinth

Semicircular ducts:
Anterior
Posterior
Lateral

Membranous ampullae

Utricle

Vestibular (oval) window

Saccule

Cochlear duct

Endolymphatic sac

Endolymphatic duct

Ductus reuniens

Cochlear (round) window

P

Figure 2.26O,P. O. Bony Labyrinth Opened, Medial View. **P.** Membranous Labyrinth, Medial View.

is straightened by pulling auricle backward and upward; cone of light seen has its apex at umbo and expands downward and forward; this cone may change in disease, especially middle ear effusion

C. Myringotomy: incision in tympanic membrane; incision heals and does not cause any hearing deficit; used to relieve severe otitis media

D. Tears in tympanic membrane (due to infection, trauma, etc.) usually heal spontaneously and may not produce any effect on hearing unless very large

E. Otitis externa: inflammation of external ear, usually caused by bacterial or fungal infection; may be circumscribed with formation of a furuncle (boil) or diffuse

F. Otitis media (middle ear infection)
 1. Very common in pediatrics; less common in adults
 2. Inflammation and fluid exudate in middle ear cavity, producing pressure on eardrum, commonly with pain and reduction in movement of ossicle
 3. May be serous (secretory) due to obstruction of auditory tube, or suppurative (purulent) due to bacterial infection; both types may involve hearing loss
 4. Inflammation in middle ear may affect chorda tympani and alter sense of taste
 5. Inadequate treatment of recurrent otitis media can produce impaired hearing through repeated inflammation and eventual scarring of ossicles, limiting their ability to vibrate in response to sound waves
 6. **Mastoid infections**: recurrent otitis media commonly leads to mastoiditis, necessitating antibiotic treatment or surgical incision and drainage of mastoid area

G. Cholesteatoma: hole in upper part of tympanic membrane may permit squamous epithelium from external acoustic meatus to grow into interior of middle ear; keratin produced can form cholesteatoma, a mass that can interfere with function of ossicles, erode bone, etc.

H. Inner ear infections: inflammation of inner ear may produce buzzing or ringing sound (tinnitus) when localized in cochlea and vertigo (sense of external world moving) centered in semicircular canals

I. Progressive calcification of stapes-oval window union (otosclerosis) is common cause of hearing loss in middle-aged and elderly patients

J. Conduction deafness: caused by interference with sound waves through outer or middle ear; may include impacted cerum (ear wax), ruptured tympanic membrane, severe middle ear infection, or adhesions of 1 or more auditory ossicles (otosclerosis); can be successfully treated

K. Perceptive (sensorineural) deafness
 1. Results from disorders that affect inner ear, cochlear nerve or nerve pathways, or auditory centers in brain
    a. Ranges in severity from inability to hear certain frequencies to deafness
    b. May be caused by diseases, trauma, and genetic or developmental problems
 2. May be related to old-age changes
    a. Ability to hear high frequency sounds generally affected 1st
    b. Hearing aids may help these patients
 3. This type of deafness is permanent because involves sensory structures that cannot heal themselves through replication or regeneration

L. If stapedius muscle is paralyzed (i.e., cutting CN VII proximal to origin of stapedius muscle exit from pyramid process of middle ear as result of fracture of base of skull or petrous portion of temporal bone) **hyperacusis** develops (hyperacute sense of hearing)

M. At birth, tympanic cavity, ossicles and mastoid antrum are same size as in adult, but bony walls are thinner and spread of infection is therefore greater

N. Deafness can result from damage to organ of Corti, cochlear duct, or vestibulocochlear nerve and its ganglion

O. **Meniere's disease**: combination of loss of balance (vertigo) and ringing in ears (tinnitus) probably caused by disturbance in normal secretion and reabsorption of fluid in inner ear; excessive blood levels of salicylic acid (aspirin) may also produce tinnitus

P. Otic barotrauma: ear injury by imbalance in pressure between surrounding air and air in middle ear; may occur in divers and fliers

Q. High tone deafness: consistant exposure to very loud sounds causes degenerative changes in spiral organ leading to this condition; seen in workers exposed to loud noises, such as those who are not wearning protective gear (e.g., street drillers, those working around jet engines, and even people living in large, noisy cities as compared to those living on a farm or in woods)

R. Blockage of auditory (pharyngotympanic) tube: tube forms route for infection from nasopharynx to tympanic cavity; easily blocked by swelling of mucous membrane, even in mild infection such as common cold; when tube is occluded, reduced air in tympanic cavity usually absorbed into mucosal blood vessels, resulting in decreased pressure in cavity, retraction of tympanic membrane, and interference with free movement; hearing is finally affected

S. Motion sickness: maculae of membranous labyrinth are static organs that have small otoliths (particles) embedded among hair cells; under influence of gravity, otoliths cause hair cells to bend, which stimulates vestibular nerve and allows appreciation of position of head in space; hairs also respond to quick tilting movements, linear acceleration and deceleration; motion sickness occurs from some form of discordance between vestibular and visual stimulation

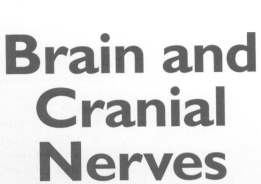

Brain and Cranial Nerves

Meninges of Brain

I. Cranial Meninges (Fig. 3.1A)

A. Fibrous coverings of brain
  1. Located immediately internal to cranium
  2. Protective and nourishing membranes that form supporting framework for brain, its vessels, and venous sinuses
  3. Enclose fluid-filled cerebrospinal fluid (CSF) cavity in which brain floats, reducing effects of gravity and inertia

B. 3 layers
  1. **Dura mater**
     a. Outermost layer: very tough, thick, and fibrous; in contact with arachnoid, separated from arachnoid by potential subdural space
     b. 2 layers
        i. Periosteal layer: adherent to bones as periosteum
        ii. Meningeal layer: inner, smooth, strong, fibrous membrane, with mesothelial layer on inner surface; fused to periosteal layer in most places, but separates from periosteal layer to form dural venous sinuses and partitions and shelves that help support brain
  2. **Arachnoid mater**
     a. Middle layer: thin, delicate, transparent, avascular, cobweblike membrane
     b. Closely applied to dura; lines dura like inner tube within tire
     c. Bound to pia via arachnoid trabeculae: filaments spanning subarachnoid space
     d. Subarachnoid space filled with CSF
     e. **Arachnoid granulations**
        i. Small mushroom- or peg-shaped projections of arachnoid through dura into superior sagittal sinus or venous lacunae; may cause granular pits within inner table of calvaria
        ii. Function to return CSF to venous system
     f. Subarachnoid cisterns: dilated portions of subarachnoid space located in regions where brain contour changes and arachnoid bridges over space
  3. **Pia mater**
     a. Innermost layer, thin, vascular, delicate membrane, intimately related to brain; follows contours of brain and sends extensions into brain along perivascular planes; cannot be dissected from brain; has been likened to sausage casing
     b. Blends with epineurium of cranial nerves (CNs)

C. Dura also called *pachymenix* (Greek = *pachys*, thick + *menix*, membrane); arachnoid and pia together are *leptomeninges* (Greek = *leptos*, slender + *meninges*, membranes)

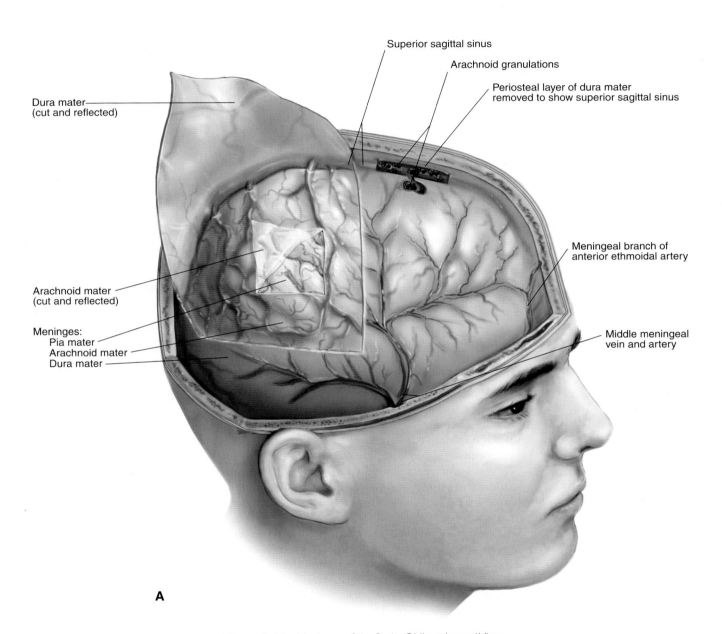

Superior sagittal sinus

Arachnoid granulations

Periosteal layer of dura mater
removed to show superior sagittal sinus

Dura mater
(cut and reflected)

Meningeal branch of
anterior ethmoidal artery

Arachnoid mater
(cut and reflected)

Middle meningeal
vein and artery

Meninges:
Pia mater
Arachnoid mater
Dura mater

A

Figure 3.1A. Meninges of the Brain, Oblique Lateral View.

II. Partitions and Shelves Formed by Meningeal Layer of Dura (Fig. 3.1B)

A. **Falx cerebri**
   1. Sickle-shaped sagittal partition, which hangs between cerebral hemispheres within longitudinal fissure
   2. Attachments
      a. Inner aspect of calvaria from crista galli of ethmoid and frontal crest of frontal bone to internal occipital protuberance, where it joins tentorium cerebelli
      b. Inferior border is free; nearly touches corpus callosum

B. **Tentorium cerebelli**
   1. Forms wide, tent-like partition between cerebellum and cerebrum
   2. Attachments
      a. Posterior and lateral to bone along transverse sinus
      b. Anterior and lateral to ridge of petrous bone and posterior clinoid process
      c. Attached in midline to falx cerebri and falx cerebelli
      d. Free anteromedial margin surrounds cerebral peduncles at opening called **tentorial notch**
   3. Divides cranial cavity into supratentorial and infratentorial compartments

C. **Falx cerebelli**
   1. Small, sagittal crescentic partition; projects between cerebellar hemispheres
   2. Attachments
      a. Internal occipital crest from protuberance to foramen magnum
      b. Tentorium cerebelli in midline superiorly

D. **Diaphragma sellae**
   1. Forms roof of sella turcica; covers pituitary gland
   2. Attachments: clinoid processes; has opening for infundibulum and hypophyseal veins

III. Dural Venous Sinuses (see Section 3.2)

IV. Meningeal Arteries

A. Course between dura and bone; supply dura and calvaria
B. Principal supply
   1. **Anterior meningeal**: branch of anterior ethmoidal artery, which supplies dura on floor of anterior cranial fossa
   2. **Middle meningeal**
      a. Branch of maxillary artery in infratemporal fossa, which enters middle cranial fossa via foramen spinosum
      b. Courses anteriorly, laterally and superiorly in outer layer of dura and divides into anterior (frontal) and posterior (parietal) branches
      c. Supplies 80% of dura; supplies most of supratentorial dura except floor of anterior cranial fossa
      d. **Accessory meningeal**: small branch of middle meningeal or maxillary artery; passes via foramen ovale to supply dura around cavernous sinus
   3. **Posterior meningeal**: usually branches from ascending pharyngeal artery but can come from occipital and vertebral arteries; enters through jugular foramen; limited to posterior cranial fossa
C. Summary of meningeal arteries

Artery	Source	Area	Entry
Meningeal branch	Anterior ethmoid artery	Anterior cranial fossa	Anterior ethmoid canal
Meningeal branch	Posterior ethmoid artery	Anterior cranial fossa	Posterior ethmoid canal
Recurrent branch	Lacrimal artery	Anterior cranial fossa	Superior orbital fissure
Middle meningeal branch	Maxillary artery	Middle cranial fossa	Foramen spinosum
Accessory meningeal branch	Maxillary artery	Middle cranial fossa	Foramen ovale
Meningeal branch	Ascending pharyngeal artery	Middle cranial fossa	Foramen lacerum
Posterior meningeal branch	Ascending pharyngeal artery	Posterior cranial fossa	Jugular foramen
Meningeal branch	Ascending pharyngeal artery	Posterior cranial fossa	Hypoglossal foramen
Meningeal branch	Vertebral artery	Posterior cranial fossa	Foramen magnum

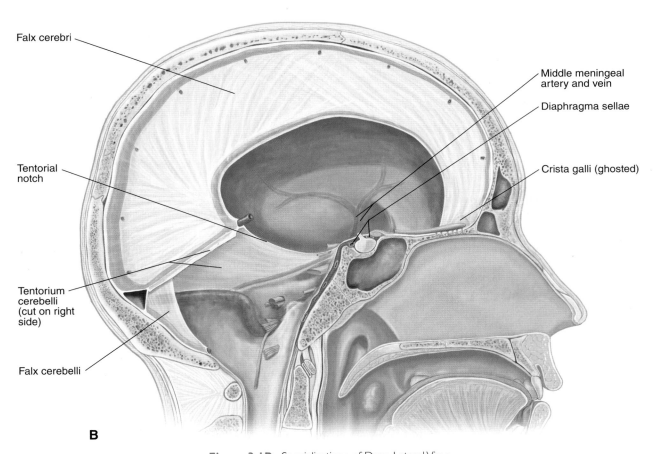

Falx cerebri

Middle meningeal
artery and vein

Diaphragma sellae

Tentorial
notch

Crista galli (ghosted)

Tentorium
cerebelli
(cut on right
side)

Falx cerebelli

B

Figure 3.1B. Specializations of Dura, Lateral View.

V. Meningeal Nerves

A. Sensory nerve supply to the dura is via all 3 divisions of CN V and CN X and from 1st and 2nd cervical nerves

B. Meningeal branches of ethmoidal nerves (from nasociliary) supply anterior cranial fossa and anterior falx cerebri

C. Meningeal branch from ophthalmic nerve (CN V_1) passes back to tentorium cerebelli and posterior part of falx cerebri

D. Meningeal branches of CN V_2 supply middle cranial fossa

E. Meningeal branches of CN V_3 supplies area of middle meningeal artery supply

F. Sensory innervation from C1 and C2 by way of CNs X and XII supply posterior cranial fossa

G. Blood vessels of dura are supplied by autonomic nervous system (as are all vessels of head and neck)

H. Pain from dura can be referred to face

I. Summary of nerves of meninges

Branch	Nerve	Distribution
Meningeal branches	Ethmoidal nerves	Anterior cranial fossa
Meningeal branch	Trigeminal ganglion (V)	Tentorium and middle cranial fossa
Recurrent branch	Ophthalmic (V_1)	Middle cranial fossa
Tentorial branch	Ophthalmic (V_1)	Tentorium
Meningeal branch	Maxillary (V_2)	Middle cranial fossa
Meningeal branch	Mandibular (V_3)	Middle and posterior cranial fossae
Meningeal branches	C1 and C2	Posterior cranial fossa

VI. Meningeal Veins

A. Small, follow arteries; drain to nearest dural sinus

B. Located between dura and skull

C. Communicate with emissary, diploic, and cerebral veins and end in various dural sinuses

D. Middle meningeal vein: communicates with sphenoparietal sinus and drains into the pterygoid plexus of veins in the infratemporal fossa and directly or indirectly into internal jugular vein

VII. Clinical Considerations

A. Meningitis
1. Inflammation of meninges surrounding brain and/or spinal cord
2. May be caused by bacterial, viral, or fungal organisms or by irritating substances that may not be infectious
3. May produce movement-associated headache pain and neck stiffness
4. **Meningismus**: symptoms of meningitis with acute febrile illness or dehydration without infection of meninges

B. Meningiomas
1. Majority of brain tumors are tumors of meningeal tissue, which can cause damage by pressure being exerted on adjacent brain tissue
2. True tumors of neural tissue occur most frequently as abnormal collections of very primitive neuroectodermal tissue

C. Meningoencephalitis: inflammation of brain and meninges

D. Meningocele: hernial protrusion of the meninges through defect in cranium or vertebral column

    E. **Tentorial notch** or **incisure**
- **1.** Curved margin of tentorium cerebelli surrounding upper brainstem as it passes from posterior to middle cranial fossa
- **2.** When intracranial pressure increases, brain can herniate through this incisure
- **3.** Early sign of this herniation is often lateral deviation of eye, because oculomotor nerve, lying against medial surface of temporal lobe, is compressed against edge of tentorial notch, and innervation of lateral rectus muscle by CN VI is unbalanced

  F. All dural sinuses ultimately drain into internal jugular veins

  G. Connections of dural sinuses with veins outside of cranial cavity, via emissary veins, are clinically important because infection can spread from outside to inside via these veins because they have no valves

  H. Injury to meningeal vessels is frequently associated with skull fractures
- **1.** Hemorrhages from these vessels usually occurs outside (**epidural**) the dura mater
- **2.** Epidural hemorrhages produce compression symptoms at brain

  I. Blunt head trauma
- **1.** Can detach periosteal dura from calvaria without fracturing cranial bones
- **2.** Not usually seen in base of skull where 2 layers of dura are firmly attached and hard to separate from bone
- **3.** At skull base, fracture tears dura and causes CSF leakage

  J. Bulging diaphragma sellae: pituitary tumors can extend superiorly through opening in dipahragma sellae or put pressure on it, causing it to bulge
- **1.** Expansion of diaphragma sellae can lead to disturbances in endocrine function (either before or after expansion)
- **2.** Visual disturbances are also possible due to pressure on optic chiasma

  K. Dural headaches: dura is sensitive to pain, especially where related to dural venous sinuses and meningeal arteries
- **1.** Pain can be caused by pulling on arteries at cranial base or veins near vertex, where they pierce the dura
- **2.** Distention of scalp or meningeal vessels (or both) can cause headache (e.g., occurring after lumbar spinal puncture for removal of CSF from stimulation of sensory endings in the dura; patient is generally advised to keep head down after lumbar puncture to minimize stretching of dura and reduce chances of headache)

Dural Venous Sinuses and Venous Drainage of Brain

I. Dural Venous Sinuses (Fig. 3.2A,B)

A. Between periosteal and meningeal dura

B. Large, valveless, rigid-walled, venous channels forming anastomosing system between layers of dura mater, draining cerebral veins, some diploic veins, emissary veins, and meningeal veins into internal jugular vein

C. Major dural venous sinuses

1. **Superior sagittal sinus** (Fig. 3.2C)

   a. Lies in superior part of falx cerebri from foramen cecum (may connect here with veins of nose) and arches posteriorly to end at confluence of sinuses at internal occipital protuberance

   b. Usually turns to right to become right transverse sinus

   c. Drains superior cerebral veins, some dural and diploic veins and communicates with lacunae on either side of this sinus

   d. **Venous lacunae**: variable lateral extensions that receive arachnoid granulations, which also enter sinus directly; arachnoid granulations penetrate meningeal layer of dura to drain CSF into venous system

   e. Important connection with occipital veins via parietal emissary veins passing through parietal foramina

2. **Inferior sagittal sinus** (Fig. 3.2D)

   a. In lower free edge of falx cerebri

   b. Receives veins from falx cerebri and medial side of hemispheres; ends by uniting with great cerebral vein to become straight sinus

3. **Straight sinus**

   a. Along line of attachment of falx cerebri to tentorium cerebelli

   b. Receives inferior sagittal sinus, **great cerebral vein** (of Galen), inferior cerebral and superior cerebellar veins; terminates in confluence of sinuses and drains primarily into left transverse sinus

4. **Occipital sinus**

   a. In attached margin of falx cerebelli; small; begins at foramen magnum, communicates with vertebral veins

   b. Ends at confluence of sinuses

5. **Confluence of sinuses**

   a. At internal occipital protuberance where superior sagittal, straight, and occipital sinuses drain

   b. Drains to transverse sinuses

6. **Transverse sinus** (Fig. 3.2E)

   a. Paired; each begins at confluence of sinuses; passes laterally in attached margin of tentorium anteriorly to petrous temporal bone, then unites with superior petrosal sinus and bends inferiorly to become sigmoid sinus

   b. Receives inferior cerebral and superior cerebellar veins, and diploic veins

7. **Sigmoid sinus**

   a. Paired direct continuations of transverse sinuses, located in posterior cranial fossa behind petrous bone; each becomes continuous with superior bulb of internal jugular vein

   b. Receives veins from cerebellum, and posterior temporal diploic vein; communicates with superficial veins by mastoid and condyloid emissary veins in canals; separated by very thin bone from mastoid air cells

8. **Sphenoparietal sinus**

   a. Paired; located on posterior surface of lesser wings of sphenoid bone

   b. Each receives middle cerebral veins and anterior temporal diploic veins and communicates with meningeal veins

   c. Drains to cavernous sinus

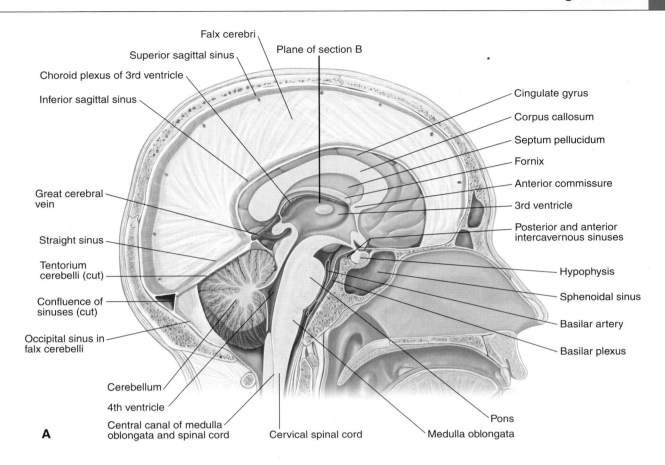

Falx cerebri

Plane of section B

Superior sagittal sinus

Choroid plexus of 3rd ventricle

Inferior sagittal sinus

Cingulate gyrus

Corpus callosum

Septum pellucidum

Fornix

Anterior commissure

Great cerebral vein

3rd ventricle

Straight sinus

Posterior and anterior intercavernous sinuses

Tentorium cerebelli (cut)

Hypophysis

Confluence of sinuses (cut)

Sphenoidal sinus

Basilar artery

Occipital sinus in falx cerebelli

Basilar plexus

Cerebellum

4th ventricle

Central canal of medulla oblongata and spinal cord

Cervical spinal cord

Pons

Medulla oblongata

A

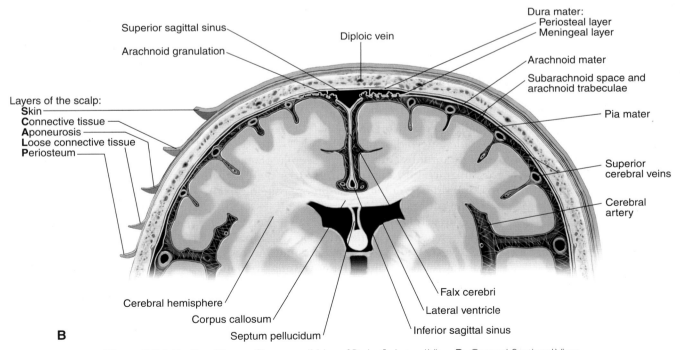

Superior sagittal sinus

Diploic vein

Dura mater:
  Periosteal layer
  Meningeal layer

Arachnoid granulation

Arachnoid mater

Subarachnoid space and arachnoid trabeculae

Layers of the scalp:
Skin
Connective tissue
Aponeurosis
Loose connective tissue
Periosteum

Pia mater

Superior cerebral veins

Cerebral artery

Cerebral hemisphere

Corpus callosum

Septum pellucidum

Falx cerebri

Lateral ventricle

Inferior sagittal sinus

B

Figure 3.2A,B. Dural Venous Sinuses and Veins of Brain. **A.** Lateral View **B.** Coronal Sectional View.

9. **Cavernous sinus**
   a. Paired; lie on each side of body of sphenoid bone
   b. Receive superior ophthalmic and middle cerebral veins and sphenoparietal sinus
   c. Drains 2 directions: superior petrosal and inferior petrosal sinus
   d. Communicates with superior ophthalmic vein and pterygoid venous plexus, and with transverse sinus via superior petrosal sinus, and internal jugular vein via inferior petrosal sinus
   e. CNs III, IV, V_1, and V_2 lie within its lateral wall made of meningeal dura, while internal carotid artery and CN VI lie within sinus
10. Intercavernous sinuses: anterior and posterior, connecting cavernous sinuses, anterior and posterior to pituitary
11. **Superior petrosal sinus**
    a. Paired; along superior border of petrous temporal bone within attached margin of tentorium; each drains part of blood from cavernous sinus
    b. Unites with transverse sinus to form sigmoid sinus
    c. Receives inferior cerebral, superior cerebellar, and tympanic veins
12. **Inferior petrosal sinus**
    a. Paired; along suture between basilar portion of occipital and petrous temporal bones; each drains part of blood from cavernous sinus
    b. Drains to superior bulb of internal jugular vein with sigmoid sinus
    c. Receives labyrinthine vein, inferior cerebellar veins, and veins from medulla
    d. Penetrated by abducent nerve (CN VI), which passes forward into cavernous sinus
13. Basilar sinuses
    a. Network on basilar portion of occipital bone; interconnects inferior petrosal sinuses
    b. Communicates with anterior vertebral plexus

II. Diploic Veins

A. Endothelial-lined channels between inner and outer tables of the calvaria; have no valves
B. Communicate with meningeal veins and dural sinuses internally, veins of the scalp externally
C. Found in frontal, temporal, and occipital regions

III. Emissary Veins

A. Direct connections between dural sinuses and veins outside skull
B. Major ones pass through foramen ovale, mastoid and parietal foramina, hypoglossal and condyloid canals

IV. Venous Drainage of Brain (Fig. 3.2F,G)

A. **Superficial (external) cerebral veins**
   1. Thin-walled, devoid of valves
   2. Arise in brain substance and first seen in pia mater
   3. Cross subarachnoid and subdural spaces; pierce arachnoid and meningeal dura to drain into dural sinuses; enter sinuses in opposite direction to that of blood flow in sinuses
   4. Major veins of brain
      a. **Superior cerebral veins**: empty into venous lacunae on either side of superior sagittal sinus (lacunae are penetrated by arachnoid villi or granulations, which appear at age 7 years and increase in size and number until adult life and which serve as a pathway for CSF fluid to enter venous circulation)
      b. **Middle cerebral veins**: drain to cavernous and sphenoparietal sinuses
      c. **Inferior cerebral veins**: drain inferior aspect of hemispheres to transverse and superior petrosal sinuses
      d. **Cerebellar veins**: drain to transverse, sigmoid, and superior and inferior petrosal sinuses
B. Deep veins of brain
   1. Drain into **great cerebral vein** (of Galen), which originates under splenium of corpus callosum from union of 2 internal cerebral veins
   2. Great cerebral vein joins inferior sagittal sinus to form straight sinus
   3. Great cerebral vein receives basal veins, posterior pericallosal, internal occipital, posterior mesencephalic, precentral, superior vermian, and superior cerebellar veins

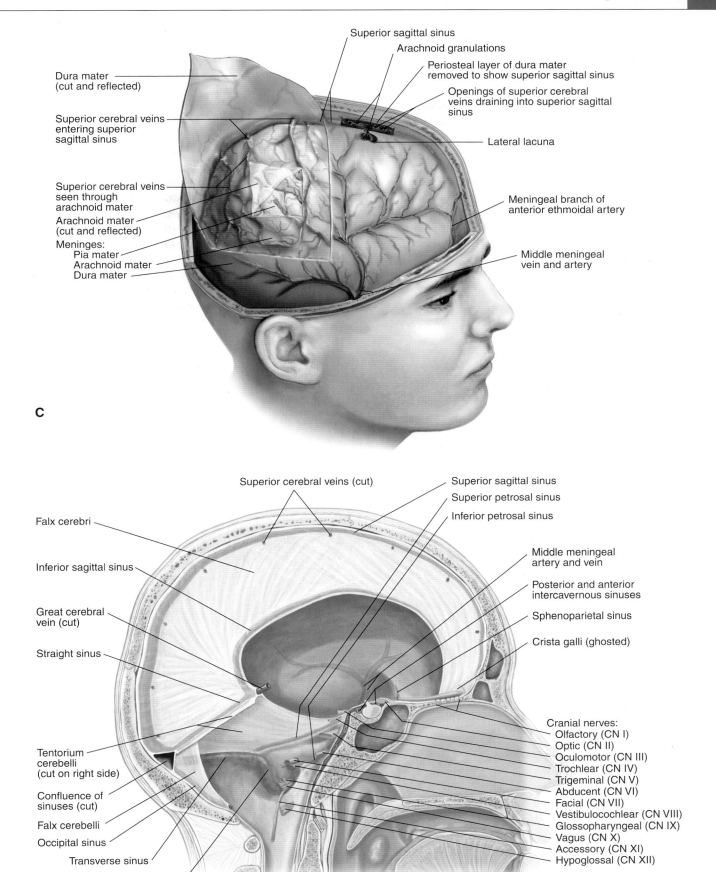

C

Superior sagittal sinus

Arachnoid granulations

Periosteal layer of dura mater removed to show superior sagittal sinus

Openings of superior cerebral veins draining into superior sagittal sinus

Dura mater (cut and reflected)

Superior cerebral veins entering superior sagittal sinus

Lateral lacuna

Superior cerebral veins seen through arachnoid mater

Arachnoid mater (cut and reflected)

Meninges:
Pia mater
Arachnoid mater
Dura mater

Meningeal branch of anterior ethmoidal artery

Middle meningeal vein and artery

D

Superior cerebral veins (cut)

Superior sagittal sinus

Superior petrosal sinus

Inferior petrosal sinus

Falx cerebri

Inferior sagittal sinus

Great cerebral vein (cut)

Straight sinus

Tentorium cerebelli (cut on right side)

Confluence of sinuses (cut)

Falx cerebelli

Occipital sinus

Transverse sinus

Sigmoid sinus

Middle meningeal artery and vein

Posterior and anterior intercavernous sinuses

Sphenoparietal sinus

Crista galli (ghosted)

Cranial nerves:
Olfactory (CN I)
Optic (CN II)
Oculomotor (CN III)
Trochlear (CN IV)
Trigeminal (CN V)
Abducent (CN VI)
Facial (CN VII)
Vestibulocochlear (CN VIII)
Glossopharyngeal (CN IX)
Vagus (CN X)
Accessory (CN XI)
Hypoglossal (CN XII)

Figure 3.2C,D.   C. Superior Sagittal Sinus, Oblique Lateral View. **D.** Dural Venous Sinuses, Lateral View.

V. Clinical Considerations

A. Dural venous sinuses present surgical hazard because they cannot be clamped if opened inadvertently; also, sinuses are related to key structures (i.e., superior petrosal sinus is located immediately superior to sensory root of CN V and sigmoid sinus lies posterosuperior to mastoid air cells)

B. Subdural hematoma (bleed)

1. Usually due to torn cerebral vein near its entry into dural sinus, especially superior sagittal sinus
2. Blood enters potential space between dura and arachnoid

C. Great cerebral vein (of Galen) attaches to straight sinus, which is fairly rigidly positioned, and is therefore liable to injury at childbirth, which can be fatal

D. Tumor cell metastasis to dural venous sinuses

1. Compression of thorax, abdomen, or pelvis (as in severe coughing and straining) may force venous blood from these body regions into internal vertebral venous plexus and from there into dural venous sinuses (because internal vertebral plexus communicates through foramen magnum with basilar plexus and occipital sinuses)
2. Thus, tumor cells or pus in abscesses can further spread into vertebrae and brain

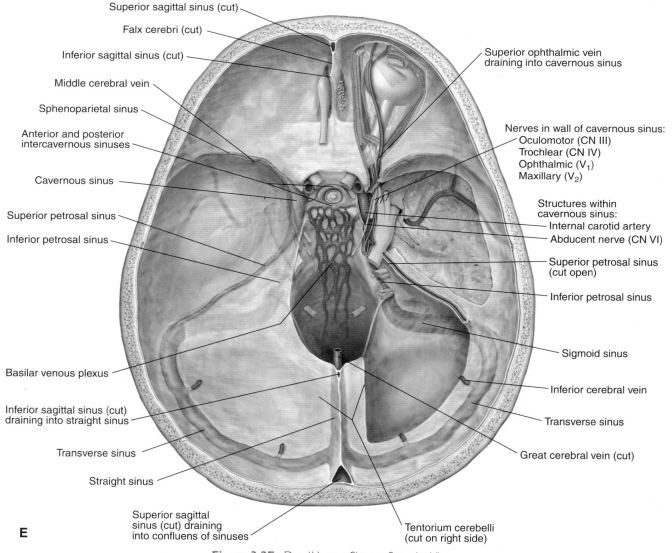

E

Figure 3.2E. Dural Venous Sinuses, Superior View.

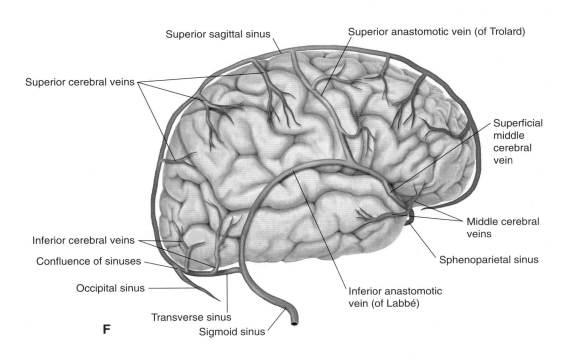

Superior sagittal sinus

Superior anastomotic vein (of Trolard)

Superior cerebral veins

Superficial middle cerebral vein

Middle cerebral veins

Sphenoparietal sinus

Inferior cerebral veins

Confluence of sinuses

Occipital sinus

Inferior anastomotic vein (of Labbé)

Transverse sinus

Sigmoid sinus

F

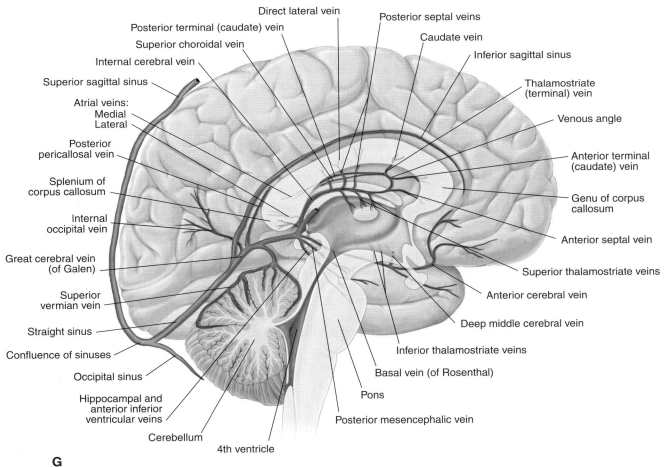

Direct lateral vein

Posterior terminal (caudate) vein

Posterior septal veins

Superior choroidal vein

Caudate vein

Internal cerebral vein

Inferior sagittal sinus

Superior sagittal sinus

Thalamostriate (terminal) vein

Atrial veins:
Medial
Lateral

Venous angle

Posterior pericallosal vein

Anterior terminal (caudate) vein

Splenium of corpus callosum

Genu of corpus callosum

Internal occipital vein

Anterior septal vein

Great cerebral vein (of Galen)

Superior thalamostriate veins

Superior vermian vein

Anterior cerebral vein

Straight sinus

Deep middle cerebral vein

Confluence of sinuses

Inferior thalamostriate veins

Occipital sinus

Basal vein (of Rosenthal)

Hippocampal and anterior inferior ventricular veins

Pons

Cerebellum

Posterior mesencephalic vein

4th ventricle

G

Figure 3.2F,G. F. Superficial Veins of the Brain, Lateral View. **G.** Deep Veins of the Brain, Sagittal View.

Cavernous Sinus

I. Location and General Features of Cavernous Sinus

A. Anteriorly: superior orbital fissure (Fig. 3.3A)

B. Posteriorly: petrous temporal bone

C. Medially: side of sella turcica and body of sphenoid bone (and anteriormost attachment of tentorium cerebelli)

D. Laterally: meningeal layer of dura with CNs III, IV, V_1, and V_2 embedded

E. Represents slit-like venous channel on each side of sphenoid body

F. Commonly made up of 1 or more venous channels (in newborn, venous plexus), lying in osseodural compartment

II. Venous Communications of Cavernous Sinus

A. Superior ophthalmic vein via superior orbital fissure; inferior ophthalmic and facial vein communicate through superior ophthalmic vein

B. Middle cerebral veins, which run in the lateral fissure of cerebral hemisphere

C. Central vein of retina usually opens into sinus directly, but it can enter superior ophthalmic vein

D. Sphenoparietal sinus, which lies along edge of lesser wing of sphenoid bone

E. Each other via intercavernous sinuses that pass anterior and posterior to hypophyseal stalk (infundibulum)

F. Pterygoid plexus of veins via inferior ophthalmic vein and emissary veins at base of skull that pass through carotid canal, foramen ovale, and sphenoidal emissary foramina

G. Drain posteriorly and inferiorly via 2 routes: superior and inferior petrosal sinuses
  1. Superior petrosal sinus: passes posterolaterally along petrous ridge within attachment of tentorium cerebelli to join transverse sinus where they curve to form sigmoid sinus
  2. Inferior petrosal sinus: passes posteroinferiorly and laterally in groove between basal portion of occipital bone and tip of petrous temporal bone to join internal jugular vein just below jugular foramen

III. Contents and Relations of Cavernous Sinuses (Fig. 3.3B)

A. Internal carotid artery and its internal carotid (sympathetic) plexus

B. Abducent nerve (CN VI), which enters inferior petrosal sinus by penetrating its meningeal dura roof; passes forward lateral to internal carotid artery within cavernous sinus

C. Within lateral wall of sinus, superior to inferior
  1. Oculomotor nerve (CN III): enters meningeal dura from above at anterior attachment of tentorium cerebelli anterior to posterior clinoid process
  2. Trochlear nerve (CN IV): enters meningeal dura beneath anterior attachment of tentorium cerebelli posterolateral to posterior clinoid process
  3. Ophthalmic division of trigeminal nerve (CN V_1): enters meningeal dura from anterior aspect of trigeminal ganglion
  4. Maxillary division of trigeminal nerve (CN V_2): enters meningeal dura from anterior aspect of trigeminal ganglion

D. Like all dural sinuses, cavernous sinus is lined by endothelium, as are internal carotid artery and abducent nerve

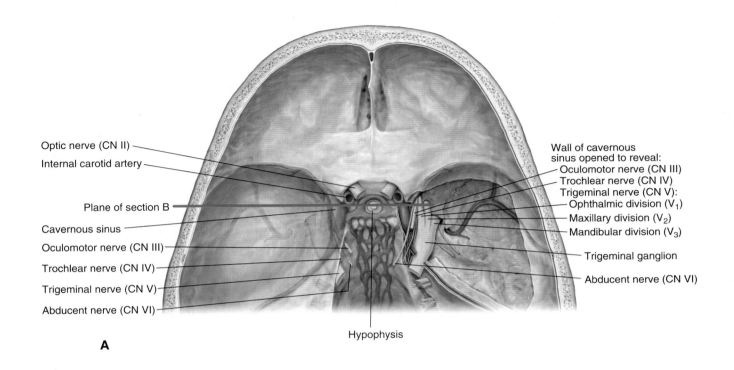

Optic nerve (CN II)

Internal carotid artery

Plane of section B

Cavernous sinus

Oculomotor nerve (CN III)

Trochlear nerve (CN IV)

Trigeminal nerve (CN V)

Abducent nerve (CN VI)

Wall of cavernous
sinus opened to reveal:
Oculomotor nerve (CN III)
Trochlear nerve (CN IV)
Trigeminal nerve (CN V):
Ophthalmic division (V$_1$)
Maxillary division (V$_2$)
Mandibular division (V$_3$)

Trigeminal ganglion

Abducent nerve (CN VI)

Hypophysis

A

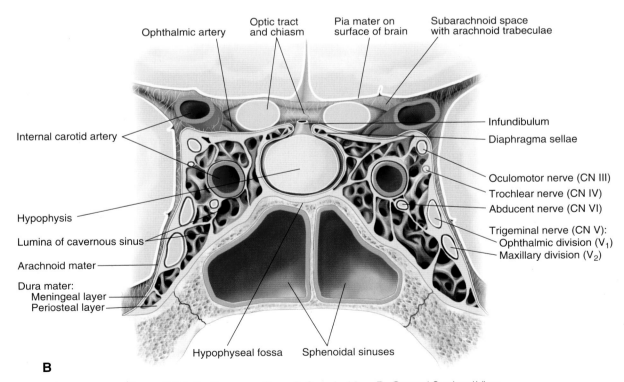

Ophthalmic artery

Optic tract
and chiasm

Pia mater on
surface of brain

Subarachnoid space
with arachnoid trabeculae

Internal carotid artery

Infundibulum

Diaphragma sellae

Oculomotor nerve (CN III)

Trochlear nerve (CN IV)

Abducent nerve (CN VI)

Hypophysis

Lumina of cavernous sinus

Trigeminal nerve (CN V):
Ophthalmic division (V$_1$)
Maxillary division (V$_2$)

Arachnoid mater

Dura mater:
Meningeal layer
Periosteal layer

Hypophyseal fossa

Sphenoidal sinuses

B

Figure 3.3A,B. Cavernous Sinus. **A.** Superior View. **B.** Coronal Sectional View.

IV. Clinical Considerations

A. Connections of facial veins are important because they communicate with ophthalmic veins and can carry infections from face (fairly frequent) to sinuses; thus, thrombophlebitis of facial vein can spread to intracranial venous system (including cortical veins of brain) because facial veins have no valves

B. Infection can spread from 1 cavernous sinus to the other via intercavernous sinuses

C. Thrombosis
  1. Results from infections in orbit, nasal sinuses, and superior part of face (**danger triangle**) because facial vein makes clinically important connections with cavernous sinus
  2. Infection often involves only 1 sinus initially, but may spread to opposite side via intercavernous sinuses
  3. Infection can also extend from cavernous sinus along central retinal vein and produce thrombosis of retinal vein branches

D. Suppuration in upper nasal cavities and in paranasal sinuses can lead to thrombophlebitis of cavernous sinus and subsequent meningitis

E. Thrombophlebitis of sinuses themselves can result in poor drainage of blood posteriorly into petrosal sinuses, resulting in swelling of cavernous sinuses with inflammatory edema of their walls
  1. Involves CNs III, IV, V_1, V_2, and VI, resulting in ocular signs
  2. Septic thrombosis of cavernous sinus frequently leads to acute meningitis

F. Poor ophthalmic venous drainage from orbit as result of pressure on veins as they enter cavernous sinus due to inflammatory edema may lead to blood stagnation, resulting in exophthalmos and edema of eyelids and conjunctivae

G. Infections of maxillary teeth can lead to thrombophlebitis of cavernous sinus

Brain: General Features

I. Principal Parts of Brain (Fig. 3.4A)

A. 3 major anatomical parts: cerebrum, cerebellum, and brainstem

B. 3 major developmental parts: forebrain, midbrain, and hindbrain

  1. Forebrain (prosencephalon)

    a. Largest portion, anterosuperiorly located

    b. 2 parts

      i. Telencephalon: anterior part of prosencephalon, consisting of cerebral hemispheres, lateral ventricles and part of 3rd ventricle, olfactory tracts, and basal nuclei (ganglia)

      ii. Diencephalon: includes epithalamus (with pineal), thalamus, subthalamus, metathalamus, and hypothalamus; optic nerve is outgrowth from brain closely associated with diencephalon

  2. Midbrain (mesencephalon)

    a. Shortest part of brain and brainstem; also known as **mesencephalon**

    b. Uppermost part of brainstem; connects forebrain with hindbrain

    c. Includes cerebral aqueduct, cerebral peduncles, corpora quadrigemina (superior and inferior colliculi), nuclei of CNs III, IV, and part of V

  3. Hindbrain (rhombencephalon)

    a. 2 parts

      i. Metencephalon: 2 parts, along with part of 4th ventricle

        a) **Pons**: consisting of transverse and longitudinal fiber tracts and nuclei of CNs V, VI, VII, and VIII

        b) **Cerebellum**: connected to midbrain, pons, and medulla

      ii. **Medulla oblongata** (myelencephalon)

        a) Lowest portion of brainstem; continues through foramen magnum as spinal cord

        b) Includes nuclei of CNs IX, X, XI, and XII and bulbar part of 4th ventricle; CN XI also arises from upper cervical spinal cord

    b. **Brainstem**: pons and medulla, together with midbrain

II. Cerebral Hemispheres (Fig. 3.4B)

A. Surface markings of hemispheres

  1. Elevations (**gyri**) and valleys (**sulci**) between gyri separate hemispheres into lobes

  2. Longitudinal fissure: a pronounced sagittally oriented valley, which separates and defines right and left cerebral hemispheres

B. Lobes of cerebrum

  1. Regions of brain roughly underlie parts of skull

  2. Central sulcus: roughly vertical sulcus divides frontal lobe from parietal lobe

    a. **Precentral gyrus**

      i. Lies anterior to central sulcus

      ii. Primary motor area of brain

    b. **Postcentral gyrus**

      i. Lies posterior to central sulcus

      ii. Primary somatic sensory area

  3. 5 cerebral lobes

    a. **Frontal lobe**: motor functions, emotions, and memory; located anterior to central sulcus; occupies anterior cranial fossa

    b. **Parietal lobe**: sensations and interpretation of sensations on basis of past experience

    c. **Occipital lobe**: mainly concerned with vision; posterior portion of cerebrum

    d. **Temporal lobe**: primarily involved with hearing and speech; occupies middle cranial fossa

    e. **Insular lobe** (**insula or island of Reil**): cerebral cortex in depth of lateral sulcus (fissure of Sylvius); involved with body awareness

C. Cerebral cortex
   1. External mantle of tissue on surface of telencephalon comprising a complex series of raised elongated strips of gray matter
   2. **Brodmann areas**: about 100 distinct functional areas, which are defined by their position, gross anatomic appearance, and histological characteristics; clinically important because even small injuries to them may result in serious motor or sensory deficits
   3. Key areas are listed below (for greater details, see textbooks of neuroscience)
      a. Areas 1, 2, and 3: primary sensory cortex; posterior to central sulcus; receives afferent axons for general sensation of touch, pressure, pain, etc.
      b. Areas 4 and 6: primary motor cortex; anterior to central sulcus; origin for axons regulating voluntary movements
      c. Area 44: motor speech area; small circular area anterior to base of central sulcus; important for voluntary expressive language (speech)
      d. Area 17: primary visual area; on medial surface of occipital lobe, deep in longitudinal fissure; receives axons excited by visual stimuli and necessary for perception of vision
      e. Areas 41 and 44: primary auditory area; on anterolateral surface of temporal lobe, just inferior to lateral fissure; receives axons excited by auditory stimuli
      f. Areas 39 and 40: receptive speech area; at posterior end of lateral fissure; necessary for comprehension of speech or other language-based input
      g. Areas 23 and 24: cingulate gyrus; on medial brain, just above corpus callosum; important role in unconscious autonomic regulation

D. Deep structures of forebrain
   1. Several masses of gray matter deep within forebrain
   2. **Basal nuclei** (formerly called **basal ganglia**) and **thalamus**: axons passing between spinal cord and cerebral cortex frequently synapse in thalamus and basal nuclei
      a. Function as reflex centers concerned particularly with voluntary muscle
      b. Injury to them may result in changes in muscle tone and in appearance of unwanted repetitive movements that interfere with carrying out desired movements
   3. **Hypothalamus**: receives neural input from many regions of brain but directs most of its output to pituitary gland

E. Midbrain
   1. Small region in which important parts of visual, auditory, and motor systems are found
   2. **Cerebral peduncles**: serve as pathways to and from cerebrum

F. Pons
   1. Small region of brainstem that has many connections with cerebellum
   2. Serves to bring cerebellar control into motor activities

G. Medulla oblongata: connects brain with spinal cord

H. Cerebellum
   1. Lies posterior to pons and medulla in posterior cranial fossa, inferior to tentorium cerebelli and occipital lobes
   2. Consists of 2 lateral lobes united by **vermis**
   3. Important in bringing coordination to motor activities, influencing muscle tonus, and maintaining balance and equilibrium

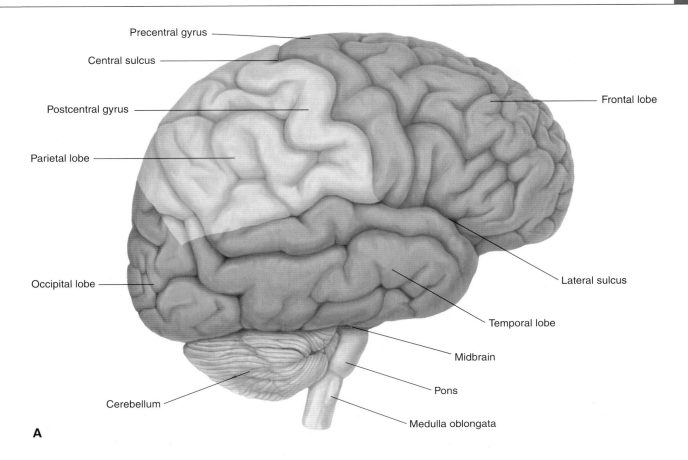

Precentral gyrus

Central sulcus

Postcentral gyrus

Parietal lobe

Occipital lobe

Frontal lobe

Lateral sulcus

Temporal lobe

Midbrain

Pons

Cerebellum

Medulla oblongata

A

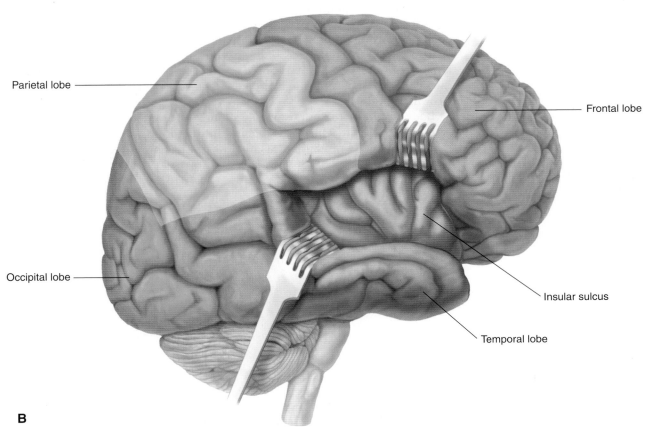

Parietal lobe

Occipital lobe

Frontal lobe

Insular sulcus

Temporal lobe

B

Figure 3.4A,B. Brain. **A.** General Features. **B.** General Features, Insula Exposed.

III. Clinical Considerations

A. Stroke: injury to brain region produced by insufficiency of blood supply to that region; may lead to blockage of artery supplying an area, producing ischemia or to hemorrhage, preventing adequate blood flow beyond hemorrhage

1. Ischemic stroke: sudden development of local neurological deficits that are usually related to impaired cerebral blood flow and generally caused by embolism on major cerebral artery; most common neurological disorder affecting U.S. adults and tend to be more disabling than fatal

2. Spontaneous cerebrovascular accidents: most common cause of stroke; includes cerebral thrombosis, cerebral embolism, cerebral hemorrhage, and subarachnoid hemorrhage

3. Symptoms
    a. Sudden weakness or numbness of face and limbs usually on 1 side of body
    b. Loss of speech or trouble talking or understanding speech
    c. Dimness or loss of vision, particularly in only 1 eye
    d. Unexplained dizziness, unsteadiness or falls
    e. Sudden severe headache

4. Treatment usually involves hospitalization for drug therapy and possible surgery and physical therapy

B. Intracranial hematomas: hemorrhages inside skull can lead to accumulation of blood in subdural or subarachnoid spaces, thereby producing pressure on underlying brain tissue; often require surgical intervention

C. White matter pathology: pathology more common in white matter than in gray matter; examples are multiple sclerosis (MS) and amyotrophic lateral sclerosis (ALS), which cause progressive deterioration of myelin and eventually lead to disturbances of normal conduction between neurons and muscle

D. Knowledge of functional localizations in the cerebral cortex can be used to determine the location of brain injury

E. Knowledge of proximity of certain structures within cranial cavity can explain combinations of symptoms; thus, a small tumor in area of optic chiasma can lead to partial or complete blindness (pressure on optic nerves), hormonal imbalance (effect on pituitary gland), and electrolyte disorders from injury to the nearby basal parts of the hypothalamus)

F. Growth of brain
1. Body weight increases postnatally about 20×, brain weight about 6.5×
2. Brain weight after birth lags behind in rate of growth, however, the brain has achieved about 80% of its final weight by end of year 2 and by year 6, brain growth has almost stopped

Brain: Basal View

I. Cerebral Hemispheres (Telencephalon) (Fig. 3.5A)

A. Frontal lobe: occupies anterior cranial fossa
   1. Frontal pole
   2. Orbital gyri
B. Temporal lobe: occupies middle cranial fossa
   1. Temporal pole
   2. Temporal gyri
C. Rhinencephalon: olfactory brain
   1. Olfactory bulb
   2. Olfactory tract
   3. Anterior perforated substance

II. Diencephalon (Fig. 3.5B)

A. Tuber cinereum
B. Mammillary bodies
C. Hypophysis
D. Optic chiasma
E. Optic tract

III. Midbrain (mesencephalon)

A. Cerebral peduncles (basis pedunculi); interpeduncular fossa
B. Posterior perforated substance

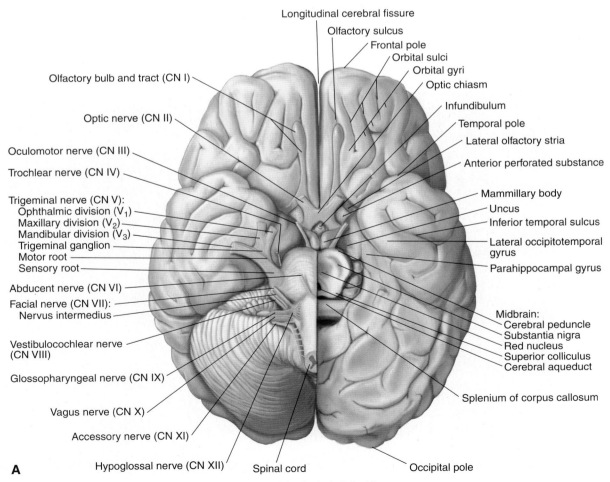

Figure 3.5A. Brain, Inferior View.

IV. Hindbrain (rhombencephalon)

A. **Metencephalon**
   1. **Pons**
      a. Basilar sulcus: for basilar artery
      b. Middle cerebellar peduncle (brachium pontis)
   2. Cerebellar hemispheres and flocculus
B. **Medulla oblongata** (**myelencephalon**): continuous with spinal cord through foramen magnum
   1. Sulci: anteromedian and anterolateral
   2. Pyramids
      a. Decussation of pyramids
      b. Inferior olive

V. Nerves

A. Olfactory nerves (CN I): lie in olfactory epithelium and penetrate cribriform plate to synapse within olfactory bulb, then extend to brain as olfactory tract
B. Optic nerve (CN II) and optic chiasm: anterior to infundibulum or stalk of hypophysis
C. Oculomotor nerve (CN III): emerge from interpeduncular fossa between posterior cerebral and superior cerebellar arteries
D. Trochlear nerve (CN IV): appear lateral to the cerebral peduncles after arising from posterior surface of midbrain
E. Trigeminal nerve (CN V): emerge from lateral side of pons
F. Abducent nerve (CN VI): emerge from groove between pons and medulla
G. Facial nerve (CN VII) and vestibulocochlear nerve (CN VIII): emerge from brainstem at the cerebellopontine angle
H. Glossopharyngeal nerve (CN IX) and vagus nerve (CN X): emerge from lateral sulcus of medulla posteroinferior to facial nerve
I. Accessory nerve (CN XI)
   1. Bulbar part joins vagus nerve (CN X)
   2. Spinal part extends upward along the side of medulla
J. Hypoglossal nerve (CN XII): emerges from sulcus between inferior olive and pyramid

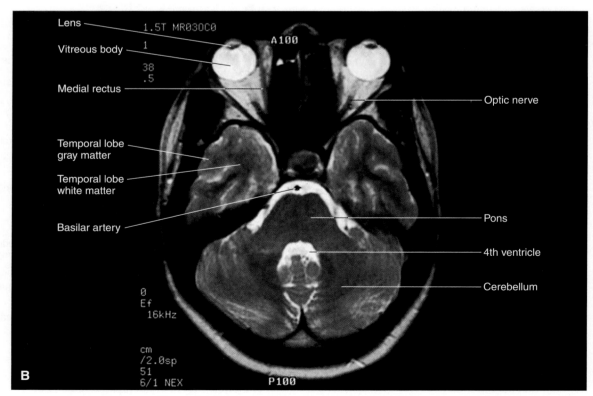

Figure 3.5B. Brain, Magnetic Resonance Image, Axial View.

Brain: Lateral View

I. Poles (Fig. 3.6A)

A. Frontal: anterior or rostral
B. Temporal: anteroinferior
C. Occipital: posterior or caudal

II. Principal Fissures or Sulci

A. **Lateral sulcus** (Sylvian): between temporal, frontal, and parietal lobes
   1. Anterior part: stem
   2. Long posterior part: posterior ramus (or limb)
   3. Near junction of stem and limb; 2 short branches, anterior horizontal and anterior ascending, extend into frontal lobe
B. **Central sulcus** (of Rolando): runs obliquely downward, from superior margin of brain, almost to lateral sulcus

III. Lobes

A. **Frontal lobe**: from frontal pole to central sulcus
   1. **Precentral sulcus**: anterior and parallel to central sulcus; superior and inferior frontal sulci run anteriorly toward frontal pole
   2. **Precentral gyrus**: between central and precentral sulci; superior frontal gyrus lies above superior frontal sulcus; middle frontal gyrus lies between superior and inferior sulci; inferior frontal gyrus lies below inferior frontal sulcus; anterior rami of lateral fissure usually divide this into triangular, opercular, and orbital portions
B. **Parietal lobe**: extends from central sulcus to parieto-occipital fissure, and a line extending from this to preoccipital notch
   1. **Postcentral sulcus**: lies parallel and posterior to central sulcus; intraparietal sulcus extends posteriorly from middle of postcentral sulcus to transverse occipital sulcus
   2. **Postcentral gyrus**: lies between central and postcentral sulci; superior and inferior parietal lobules lie above and below intraparietal sulcus
      a. In superior lobule, parieto-occipital gyrus arches over parieto-occipital sulcus
      b. In inferior lobule, supramarginal gyrus caps upper end of lateral sulcus; angular gyrus arches over superior temporal sulcus
C. **Occipital lobe**: from occipital pole to parieto-occipital fissure and its extension to preoccipital notch
D. **Temporal lobe**: from temporal pole to line extending from parieto-occipital fissure to preoccipital notch
   1. Superior and middle temporal sulci divide lobe into superior, middle, and inferior temporal gyri
   2. On upper surface of superior temporal gyrus are transverse temporal gyri
E. **Insular lobe**: at bottom of lateral sulcus, covered by opercula, from frontal, parietal, and temporal lobes (Fig. 3.6B)
   1. Encircled by circular sulcus
   2. Crossed by long and short gyri

IV. Special Features

A. **Primary motor cortex**: lies along posterior part of precentral gyrus adjoining central sulcus

B. **Primary sensory cortex**: for body sensations (pain, temperature, touch) lies in postcentral gyrus, some actually in central sulcus

C. **Primary auditory area**: lies on superior border of superior temporal gyrus in depths of lateral fissure

D. **Primary visual cortex**: as seen from lateral side, lies at occipital pole

V. Clinical Considerations

A. Cerebral concussion: abrupt, transient loss of consciousness following blow to head

   1. Results from mechanical disturbance of cerebral cells; consciousness may be lost for only a few seconds with mild injury or for hours or days following severe injury

   2. Recovery of consciousness within 6 hours usually results in excellent recovery; if "coma" lasts longer, brain tissue injury has usually occurred

B. Cerebral contusion: visible bruising of the brain due to trauma and blood leaking from small vessels

   1. Can lead to extended loss of consciousness; often results in pia being stripped from injured brain surface and can actually be torn, allowing blood to enter subarachnoid space

   2. If there is no diffuse axonal injury, brain swelling, or secondary hemorrhage, recovery is excellent

C. Chronic traumatic encephalopathy ("punchdrunk syndrome")

   1. Brain injury as result of acceleration and deceleration of head that shears or stretches axons followed by sudden stopping of head movement may result in brain hitting stationary cranium (contrecoup contusion)

   2. Characterized by weakness in lower limbs, unsteady gait, slowness of muscle movements, hand tremor, speech hesitancy, and slowness in ability to think

D. Cerebral lacerations: often associated with depressed cranial fractures (i.e., knife or gunshot wounds); result in rupture of blood vessels and bleeding into the brain and subarachnoid space, causing increased intracranial pressure and cerebral compression

E. Cerebral compression: may be result of intracranial collection of blood, excess CSF, intracranial tumors or abscesses, or brain swelling due to brain edema (due to increase in brain volume due to increase in water and sodium content)

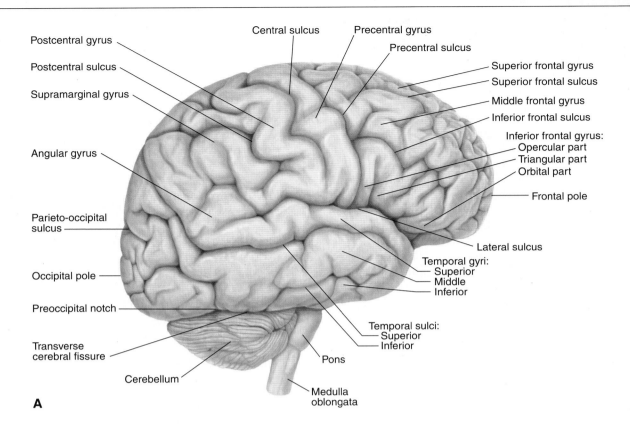

Postcentral gyrus

Postcentral sulcus

Supramarginal gyrus

Angular gyrus

Parieto-occipital sulcus

Occipital pole

Preoccipital notch

Transverse cerebral fissure

Cerebellum

Central sulcus

Precentral gyrus

Precentral sulcus

Superior frontal gyrus

Superior frontal sulcus

Middle frontal gyrus

Inferior frontal sulcus

Inferior frontal gyrus:
Opercular part
Triangular part
Orbital part

Frontal pole

Lateral sulcus

Temporal gyri:
Superior
Middle
Inferior

Temporal sulci:
Superior
Inferior

Pons

Medulla oblongata

A

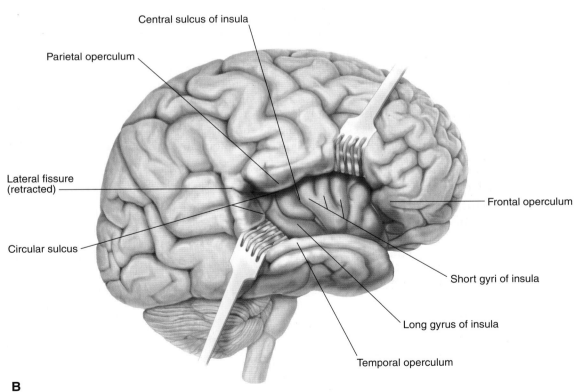

Central sulcus of insula

Parietal operculum

Lateral fissure (retracted)

Circular sulcus

Frontal operculum

Short gyri of insula

Long gyrus of insula

Temporal operculum

B

Figure 3.6A,B. Brain. **A.** Lateral View. **B.** Lateral View, Lateral Sulcus Opened.

Brain: Medial View

I. Cerebral Hemisphere (Telencephalon) (Fig. 3.7A,B)

A. Features
   1. Corpus callosum with genu, body, and splenium
   2. Fornix
   3. Septum pellucidum: stretched between corpus callosum and fornix
   4. Anterior commissure

B. Principal fissures and sulci
   1. Calcarine sulcus: starts below splenium of corpus callosum and curves upward and posteriorly toward occipital pole; primary visual cortex lies on both sides of entire length of calcarine sulcus
   2. Cingulate sulcus: curves parallel to body of corpus callosum to point posterior to central sulcus and then curves superiorly to its superior margin
   3. Parieto-occipital sulcus: begins near middle of calcarine sulcus and runs upward to its superior margin
   4. Inferior temporal sulcus: lies between fusiform and inferior temporal gyri
   5. Collateral sulcus: runs from near occipital pole, parallel to brain margin, almost to temporal pole

C. Lobes
   1. Frontal lobe: bounded posteriorly by line drawn obliquely downward and anteriorly from upper end of central sulcus to middle of corpus callosum; includes part of cingulate gyrus and paracentral lobule
   2. Parietal lobe: bounded anteriorly by posterior line of frontal lobe and posteriorly by parieto-occipital fissure
   3. Occipital lobe: bounded anteriorly by parieto-occipital fissure and line drawn inferior to preoccipital notch; posterior part of calcarine sulcus divides its medial surface into cuneus and lingual gyri
   4. Temporal lobe: bounded posteriorly by anterior boundary of occipital lobe
      a. Fusiform gyrus: lies between inferior temporal sulcus and collateral sulcus
      b. Medial to collateral sulcus are lingual gyrus and hippocampus
      c. Parahippocampal gyrus: lies medial to collateral fissure and is continuous with cingular gyrus through isthmus, which lies below splenium of corpus callosum; anteriorly, it is curved around as the uncus
      d. Hippocampal sulcus: extends from splenium of corpus callosum to medial side of uncus

II. Diencephalon

A. 3rd ventricle, thalamus, interthalamic adhesion, hypothalamus, hypothalamic sulcus, and optic recess
B. Optic chiasm and infundibulum
C. Pineal body and posterior commissure

III. Midbrain (Mesencephalon)

A. Cerebral peduncles
B. Cerebral aqueduct
C. Corpora quadrigemina (superior and inferior colliculi)

IV. Pons and Cerebellum (Metencephalon)

A. 4th ventricle
B. Superior medullary velum

V. Medulla Oblongata (Myelencephalon)

A. Inferior medullary velum
B. Central canal of medulla

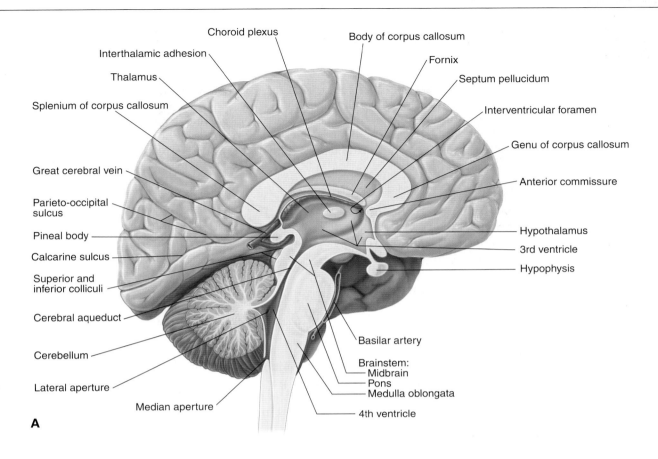

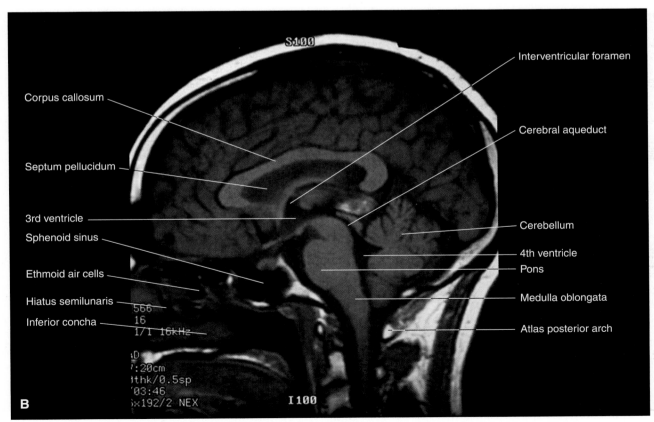

Figure 3.7A,B. Brain. **A.** Medial View. **B.** Magnetic resonance Image, Sagittal View.

Brainstem and Cerebellum

I. Forebrain (Fig. 3.8A)

A. Not part of brainstem, but closely related
B. Internal capsule: large, fan-shaped band of fibers passing to and from hemispheres; thalamus lies to medial side and lenticular nucleus on lateral side
C. Pineal body, pulvinar (large bilateral projections of dorsal thalamus), and medial geniculate bodies beneath pulvinar

II. Midbrain (Fig. 3.8B)

A. Uppermost portion of brainstem
B. Features
 1. Tectum (roof) composed of 2 pairs of swellings: **superior** and **inferior colliculi** (corpora quadrigemina)
 2. Brachium of inferior colliculus
 3. **Superior cerebellar peduncles**

III. Pons

A. Connects cerebellum with brainstem
B. Features
 1. 3 **cerebellar peduncles**: superior (conjunctivum), middle (pontis), and inferior (restiform body)
 2. Structures in floor of 4th ventricle: median fissure, sulcus limitans, medial eminence, facial colliculus, locus ceruleus, medullary stria, vestibular area

IV. Medulla Oblongata

A. Connects pons with spinal cord
B. Structures in floor of 4th ventricle: median fissure, sulcus limitans, vestibular area, hypoglossal trigone, and vagal trigone (ala cinerea)
C. Features: taenia, attachments of ventricular roof to brainstem with their horizontal part and inferiorly directed apex
D. Inferior to taenia
 1. Sulci: posterior median, intermediate, and lateral
 2. Fasciculi: gracilis, between median and intermediate sulci, ending anteriorly in swelling, the tubercle of nucleus gracilis; and cuneatus, between intermediate and lateral sulci, ending anteriorly in enlargement, the cuneate tubercle (tubercle of cuneate nucleus)

V. Nerves of Brainstem

A. Oculomotor nerve (CN III): from cerebral peduncle medially
B. Trochlear nerve (CN IV): from roof, inferior to inferior colliculus
C. Trigeminal nerve (CN V): from side of pons
D. Abducent nerve (CN VI): from pontine–medullary junction
E. Facial nerve (CN VII) and vestibulocochlear nerve (CN VIII): from pontine–cerebello–medullary junction
F. Glossopharyngeal nerve (CN IX) and vagus nerve (CN X): from upper medulla posterolateral to olive
G. Hypoglossal nerve (CN XII): from upper medulla anteromedial to olive

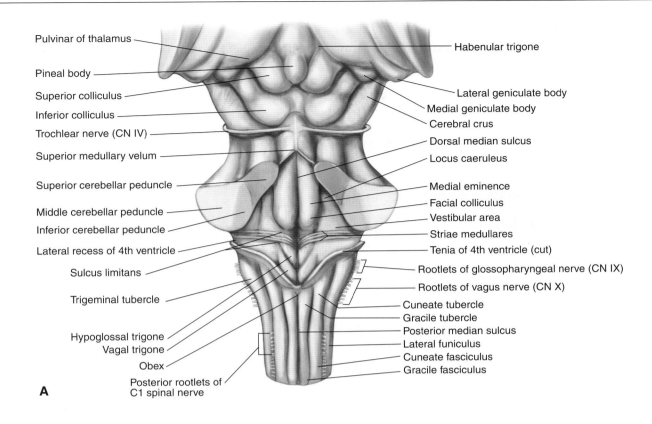

Pulvinar of thalamus

Pineal body

Superior colliculus

Inferior colliculus

Trochlear nerve (CN IV)

Superior medullary velum

Superior cerebellar peduncle

Middle cerebellar peduncle

Inferior cerebellar peduncle

Lateral recess of 4th ventricle

Sulcus limitans

Trigeminal tubercle

Hypoglossal trigone

Vagal trigone

Obex

Posterior rootlets of
C1 spinal nerve

Habenular trigone

Lateral geniculate body

Medial geniculate body

Cerebral crus

Dorsal median sulcus

Locus caeruleus

Medial eminence

Facial colliculus

Vestibular area

Striae medullares

Tenia of 4th ventricle (cut)

Rootlets of glossopharyngeal nerve (CN IX)

Rootlets of vagus nerve (CN X)

Cuneate tubercle

Gracile tubercle

Posterior median sulcus

Lateral funiculus

Cuneate fasciculus

Gracile fasciculus

A

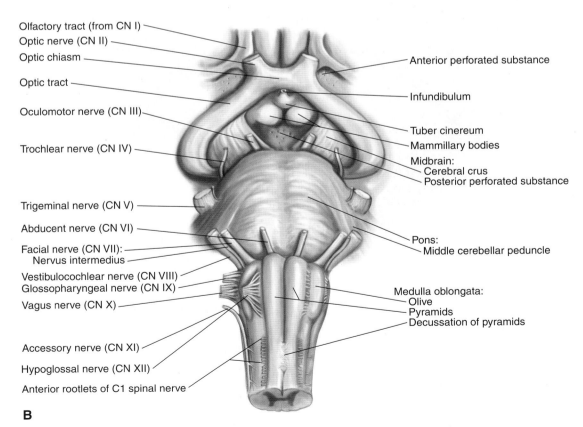

Olfactory tract (from CN I)

Optic nerve (CN II)

Optic chiasm

Optic tract

Oculomotor nerve (CN III)

Trochlear nerve (CN IV)

Trigeminal nerve (CN V)

Abducent nerve (CN VI)

Facial nerve (CN VII):
Nervus intermedius

Vestibulocochlear nerve (CN VIII)

Glossopharyngeal nerve (CN IX)

Vagus nerve (CN X)

Accessory nerve (CN XI)

Hypoglossal nerve (CN XII)

Anterior rootlets of C1 spinal nerve

Anterior perforated substance

Infundibulum

Tuber cinereum

Mammillary bodies

Midbrain:
Cerebral crus
Posterior perforated substance

Pons:
Middle cerebellar peduncle

Medulla oblongata:
Olive
Pyramids
Decussation of pyramids

B

Figure 3.8A,B. Brainstem. **A.** Posterior View. **B.** Anterior View.

VI. Cerebellum (Fig. 3.8C)

A. Location: lies within posterior cranial fossa below tentorium cerebelli and posterior portions of cerebral hemispheres
B. Major parts
    1. Cerebellar hemispheres: paired lateral parts, consisting of anterior and posterior lobe
    2. **Vermis**: smaller midline portion
    3. Cortex: with folia and fissures, that covers much larger center of white matter
    4. Cerebellar nuclei: masses of gray matter within
C. No CN is directly attached to cerebellum

VII. Clinical Considerations

A. Trauma or disease in medulla is often fatal because vital centers, such as those controlling circulation and respiration, are located here
B. A single lesion in internal capsule can result in complete unilateral motor and sensory loss
C. Damage to cerebellum may result in disturbances of voluntary movement

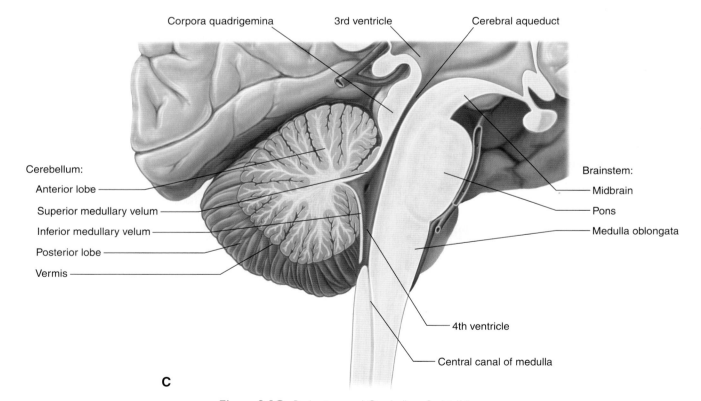

Figure 3.8C. Brain stem and Cerebellam, Sagittal View.

Pituitary Gland (Hypophysis)

I. Location, Size, and Relations (Fig. 3.9A)

A. Location: in sella turcica (hypophyseal fossa) of sphenoid bone, attached to hypothalamus by stalk (infundibulum); meningeal layer of dura stretches between clinoid processes to cover sella (diaphragma sellae) except for small hole for stalk; periosteal layer of dura lines sella

B. Size: larger in females, increases in pregnancy, and is largest in multiparous women
1. Length (anteroposterior): 1.0 cm
2. Width (transverse): 1.2–1.5 cm
3. Thickness: 0.5 cm
4. Weight: 0.5–0.6 g

C. Relations
1. Laterally: internal carotid arteries and structures in cavernous sinus and wall
2. Superior: intercavernous sinuses in diaphragma sellae and base of diencephalon
3. Anterosuperior: optic chiasm and optic tracts
4. Anteroinferior: sphenoid sinus

II. Parts (Fig. 3.8B)

A. **Adenohypophysis** (anterior lobe): largest (75%)
1. Formed from oral ectoderm
2. Developmentally, includes: pars distalis, pars infundibularis (tuberalis), and pars intermedia

B. **Neurohypophysis** (posterior lobe)
1. Formed from neural ectoderm of diencephalic floor
2. Neurohypophysis includes infundibular process (neural lobe), infundibular stem, and median eminence of hypothalamus

C. Median eminence: often classified as part of tuber cinereum; the term "infundibulum" is used for median eminence and infundibular stem; the term "hypophyseal stalk" refers to pars infundibularis and infundibulum

III. Principal Hormones and Their Effects

A. Adenohypophysis
 1. Somatotropic: promotes body growth
 2. Thyrotropic: stimulates thyroid secretion
 3. Adrenocorticotropic (ACTH): stimulates secretion of adrenal steroid hormones
 4. Gonadotropic hormones: follicle-stimulating hormone (FSH) and luteinizing hormone (LH), stimulate development of ovarian follicles and secretion of corpora lutea, respectively
 5. Prolactin: promotes secretion of mammary gland

B. Neurohypophysis
 1. Oxytocin: stimulates contraction of smooth muscle, especially of uterus
 2. Vasopressin: raises blood pressure and inhibits diuresis

IV. Blood Supply

A. Arteries
 1. **Superior hypophyseal arteries**: from internal carotid and posterior communicating arteries to stalk and adjacent anterior lobe
 2. **Inferior hypophyseal arteries**: from internal carotid artery, passing through cavernous sinus, to posterior lobe

B. Veins
 1. **Hypophyseal portal veins**: carry blood from stalk, lower hypothalamus, and pars tuberalis to most of anterior lobe
 2. **Lateral hypophyseal**: drain into cavernous and intercavernous sinuses

V. Clinical Considerations

A. Gross pituitary enlargement (tumor)
 1. Can put pressure directly on internal carotid arteries, giving symptoms of occlusion; direct pressure on optic chiasma, causing bitemporal hemianopsia
 2. Oversecretion of anterior lobe can cause gigantism, with hyperglycemia; overactivity of suprarenals, leading to Cushing's syndrome; overactivity of thyroid, which may be a factor in Graves' disease

B. Pituitary insufficiency: may lead to dwarfism, lower metabolism due to low thyroid activity, symptoms of suprarenal insufficiency, and underdevelopment of genital system

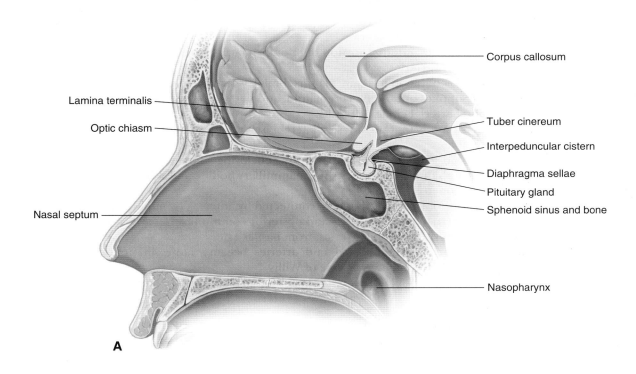

Corpus callosum

Lamina terminalis

Optic chiasm

Tuber cinereum

Interpeduncular cistern

Diaphragma sellae

Pituitary gland

Sphenoid sinus and bone

Nasal septum

Nasopharynx

A

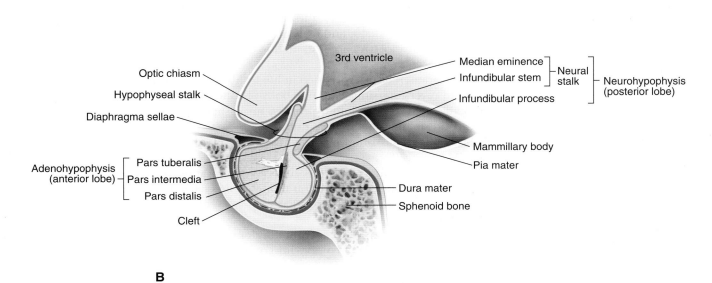

3rd ventricle

Optic chiasm

Median eminence

Infundibular stem — Neural stalk

Neurohypophysis (posterior lobe)

Hypophyseal stalk

Infundibular process

Diaphragma sellae

Mammillary body

Adenohypophysis (anterior lobe)

Pars tuberalis

Pars intermedia

Pars distalis

Pia mater

Dura mater

Sphenoid bone

Cleft

B

Figure 3.9A,B. Pituitary Gland **A.** Location. **B.** Parts.

Arteries of Brain

I. General Features of Arterial Supply of Brain (Fig. 3.10A)

A. 2 pairs of arteries
  1. Internal carotid arteries
     a. 80% of blood to brain
     b. Supplies anterior portion of brain primarily
  2. Vertebral arteries
     a. 20% of blood to brain; via vertebral–basilar system
     b. Supplies brainstem, cerebellum, and parts of temporal and occipital lobes
B. **Cerebral arterial circle** (of Willis)
  1. Anastomosis that provides collateral circulation among the 4 arteries supplying brain; variable
  2. Located beneath hypothalamus, enclosing lamina terminalis, optic chiasm, infundibulum, tuber cinereum, mammillary bodies, and posterior perforated substance
  3. Components
     a. Anterior cerebral arteries, connected by anterior communicating artery
     b. Internal carotid arteries and posterior communicating arteries
     c. Posterior cerebral arteries, from basilar artery
C. Cerebral arteries considered end arteries because large anastomoses are not found between large branches of circle of Willis
D. Capillary network of cortex is dense, and neurons rarely are more than 50 microns from a capillary

II. Internal Carotid Artery (Fig. 3.10B)

A. Course
  1. 4 parts: cervical, petrous, cavernous, and cerebral
  2. Cervical part
     a. Arises from common carotid artery at level of upper border of thyroid cartilage
     b. Ascends to base of skull; no branches in neck
  3. Petrous portion
     a. Enters petrous temporal bone through carotid canal, bends to pass roughly horizontally anteromedially, and exits near apex of petrous bone
     b. Small branch (caroticotympanic) to middle ear
  4. Cavernous part
     a. Passes over foramen lacerum (closed in life by fibrocartilage) then bends anteriorly to lie within cavernous sinus lateral to body of sphenoid bone
     b. Inferomedial to anterior clinoid process, turns superiorly in an S-shaped course, called **carotid siphon**, to penetrate dura
     c. Small branches to surrounding structures: hypophysis, trigeminal ganglion, and CNs III, IV, V, and VI
  5. Cerebral part: after leaving cavernous sinus by penetrating dura posteroinferior to optic nerve entering optic canal, gives off branches described below
B. Branches of cerebral part of internal carotid artery
  1. **Ophthalmic artery**
     a. Arises as internal carotid emerges from dura of cavernous sinus
     b. Passes anteriorly beneath optic nerve into optic canal
  2. **Posterior communicating artery**
     a. Passes posteriorly to anastomose with posterior cerebral artery
     b. Variable in size
     c. Branches supply optic tract and chiasm, hypothalamus, cerebral peduncle, thalamus, subthalamus, interpeduncular area, and hippocampal gyrus
  3. **Anterior choroidal artery**
     a. Small vessel arising 78% of time directly from internal carotid artery and remaining time from middle cerebral artery

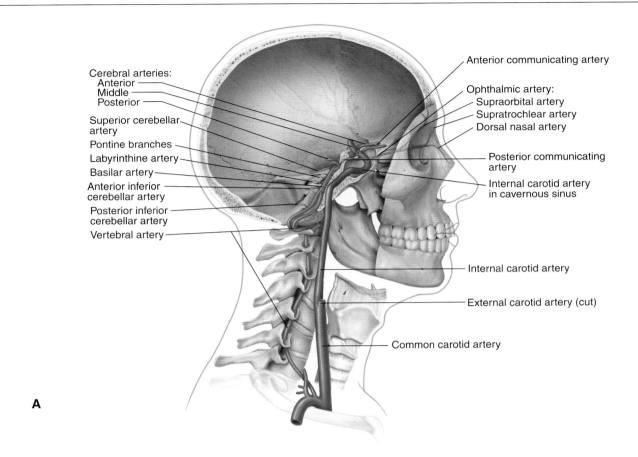

Cerebral arteries:
Anterior
Middle
Posterior

Superior cerebellar artery

Pontine branches

Labyrinthine artery

Basilar artery

Anterior inferior cerebellar artery

Posterior inferior cerebellar artery

Vertebral artery

Anterior communicating artery

Ophthalmic artery:
Supraorbital artery
Supratrochlear artery
Dorsal nasal artery

Posterior communicating artery

Internal carotid artery in cavernous sinus

Internal carotid artery

External carotid artery (cut)

Common carotid artery

A

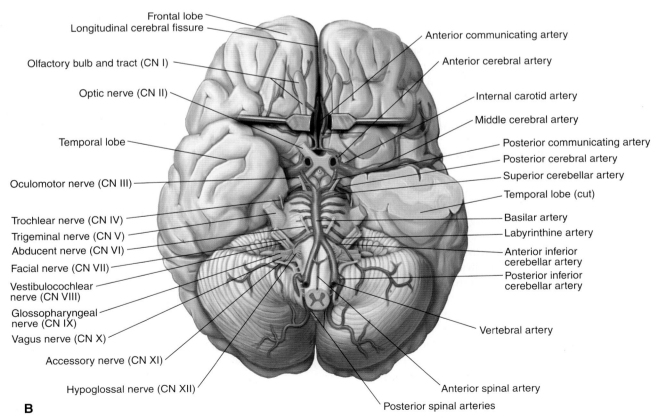

Frontal lobe
Longitudinal cerebral fissure

Olfactory bulb and tract (CN I)

Optic nerve (CN II)

Temporal lobe

Oculomotor nerve (CN III)

Trochlear nerve (CN IV)
Trigeminal nerve (CN V)
Abducent nerve (CN VI)
Facial nerve (CN VII)
Vestibulocochlear nerve (CN VIII)
Glossopharyngeal nerve (CN IX)
Vagus nerve (CN X)

Accessory nerve (CN XI)

Hypoglossal nerve (CN XII)

Anterior communicating artery

Anterior cerebral artery

Internal carotid artery

Middle cerebral artery

Posterior communicating artery
Posterior cerebral artery
Superior cerebellar artery
Temporal lobe (cut)
Basilar artery
Labyrinthine artery
Anterior inferior cerebellar artery
Posterior inferior cerebellar artery

Vertebral artery

Anterior spinal artery
Posterior spinal arteries

B

Figure 3.10A,B. Arteries of the Brain. **A.** Lateral View. **B.** Inferior View.

       b. Passes along optic tract and around cerebral peduncle to enter temporal horn of lateral ventricle to end in choroid plexus of ventricle

       c. Branches supply choroid plexus of lateral and 3rd ventricles and optic tract, tail of caudate, globus pallidus, posterior crus of internal capsule, tuber cinereum, hypothalamus, substantia nigra, red nucleus, and amygdaloid body

    4. Anterior cerebral artery (Fig. 3.10C)

       a. Smaller of 2 terminal branches of internal carotid artery

       b. Runs horizontal and anteromedial between optic nerve and anterior perforated substance to enter longitudinal fissure at midline

       c. Anterior communicating artery: short anastomotic channel between both anterior cerebral arteries

       d. Turns superiorly to arch over corpus callosum

       e. Major branches

          i. Prior to anterior communicating artery: inferior branches to optic nerve and chiasm; superior branches (via anterior perforating substance) to basal nuclei, internal capsule, and anterior hypothalamus; largest branch is medial striate artery (recurrent artery of Huebner) to head of caudate nucleus and anterior limb of internal capsule

          ii. Beyond anterior communicating artery (interhemispheric): medial orbitofrontal artery to orbital gyrus and olfactory tract and bulb; frontopolar artery to undersurface of frontal lobe and midline structures; divides into callosomarginal artery (runs in cingulate sulcus) and pericallosal artery (runs above corpus callosum), which supply medial and superior surfaces of frontal and parietal lobes, including medial part of motor and somatosensory cortex

    5. Middle cerebral artery (see Fig. 3.10C)

       a. Largest branch; passes into lateral (Sylvian) fissure

       b. Cortical branches: supply insula and claustrum and nearly all of lateral side of cerebral hemispheres (parts of frontal, parietal, and temporal lobes) except for about 1 cm–wide strip around periphery, which are supplied by branches of the anterior and posterior cerebral arteries

       c. Central branches: penetrate anterior perforated substance and comprise 2 sets, medial striate and lateral striate arteries

          i. Medial striate arteries: supply anterior parts of lenticular and caudate nuclei and of internal capsule

          ii. Lateral striate arteries: supply basal nuclei of brain (most of putamen, part of head and body of caudate, and lateral part of globus pallidus) and its internal capsule

       d. Collectively, striate arteries are known as artery of cerebral hemorrhage

III. Vertebral Artery (Fig. 3.10D)

  A. Course

    1. Arises as 1st branch of subclavian artery on each side

    2. Passes superiorly to enter transverse foramen of 6th cervical vertebra, then continues through transverse foramina to base of skull

    3. Passes behind lateral mass of atlas and between atlas and occipital bone, penetrates atlanto-occipital membrane and dura and enters skull through foramen magnum

    4. Vertebral arteries merge at pontine–medullary junction (left vertebral is usually larger than right) to form **basilar artery**

    5. Basilar artery: passes anterosuperiorly in midline anterior sulcus of pons to end at top of pons just posterior to posterior clinoid process by bifurcating into posterior cerebral arteries

    6. Supplies posterior cerebrum, brainstem, and cerebellum

  B. Branches of vertebral artery

    1. Posterior spinal arteries

       a. Multiple small branches arising directly from vertebral artery or posterior inferior cerebellar artery

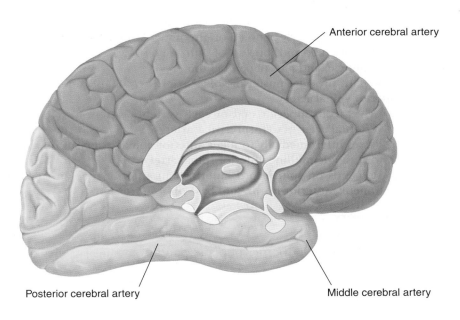

Anterior cerebral artery

Posterior cerebral artery

Middle cerebral artery

C

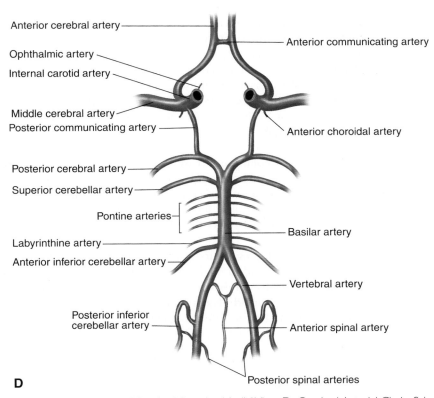

Anterior cerebral artery

Ophthalmic artery

Internal carotid artery

Middle cerebral artery

Posterior communicating artery

Posterior cerebral artery

Superior cerebellar artery

Pontine arteries

Labyrinthine artery

Anterior inferior cerebellar artery

Posterior inferior cerebellar artery

Anterior communicating artery

Anterior choroidal artery

Basilar artery

Vertebral artery

Anterior spinal artery

Posterior spinal arteries

D

Figure 3.10C,D. C. Distribution of Cerebral Arteries, Medial View. **D.** Cerebral Arterial Circle, Schematic View.

      b. Descend on cord posteriorly, associated with posterior nerve roots, and supply posterior funiculi and posterior horns

  2. Posterior inferior cerebellar artery

      a. Arises immediately superior to foramen magnum

      b. Passes posteriorly between origin of vagus and accessory nerves

      c. Supplies choroid plexus of 4th ventricle, lateral medulla, inferior cerebellar peduncle, and part of cerebellum

      d. Usually provides **posterior spinal arteries** that descend through foramen magnum

  3. Anterior spinal artery

      a. Arises from superior end of each vertebral artery near point of union of paired vertebral arteries to form basilar artery

      b. Passes inferomedially to meet anterior spinal artery of opposite side and unite to form single midline anterior spinal artery

      c. Descends on spinal cord anteriorly in anterior median sulcus to supply anterior funiculi, anterior horns, and base of posterior horns

IV. Basilar Artery

A. Origin and course

  1. Formed near lower border of pons (pontine–medullary junction) by union of paired vertebral arteries

  2. Passes anterosuperiorly in anterior sulcus of pons

  3. Terminates at upper border of pons by bifurcating into 2 posterior cerebral arteries

B. Branches

  1. **Pontine arteries**: numerous, small, penetrating to pons and anterolateral cerebellar cortex and inferior part of midbrain

  2. **Labyrinthine artery**: passes with CNs VII and VIII into internal acoustic meatus and supplies dura of canal, cochlea, labyrinth, and facial nerve; often branches from anterior inferior cerebellar artery

  3. **Anterior inferior cerebellar artery**: to brainstem and superior and middle cerebellar peduncles and anterior part of undersurface of cerebellar hemisphere

  4. **Superior cerebellar artery**: medial branches to mesencephalon, pons, medial cerebellum, and deep cerebellar nuclei; lateral branches to anterolateral part of superior 1/2 of cerebellar cortex, superior and middle cerebellar peduncles, dentate nucleus, and roof nuclei; also, the more medial superior vermian branch (anastomosis with inferior vermian branch of posterior inferior cerebellar) supplies inferior colliculi, superior cerebellar peduncles, and dentate nucleus

  5. **Posterior cerebral artery** (Fig. 3.10E,F)

      a. Passes superior to oculomotor nerve and around cerebral peduncle of midbrain in cisterna ambiens, then through tentorial notch, along medial surface of temporal and occipital lobes to end in calcarine fissure to supply visual cortex

      b. Joined by posterior communicating artery from internal carotid artery to complete cerebral arterial circle (of Willis)

      c. Branches

         i. Posteromedial ganglionic branches: posterior hypothalamus, parts of thalamus and midbrain, and medial choroidal artery to choroid plexus of 3rd ventricle

        ii. Posterior choroidal branches: to posterior thalamus, subthalamus, internal capsule and choroid plexus of 3rd ventricle, and body of lateral ventricle

        iii. Cortical branches: to inferior surface of temporal and occipital lobes

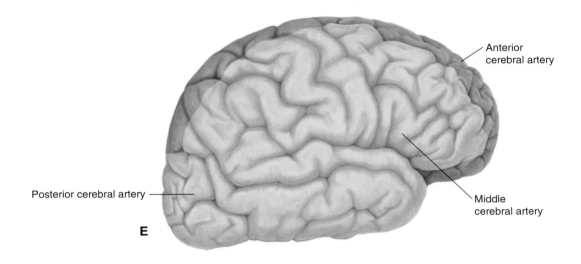

E

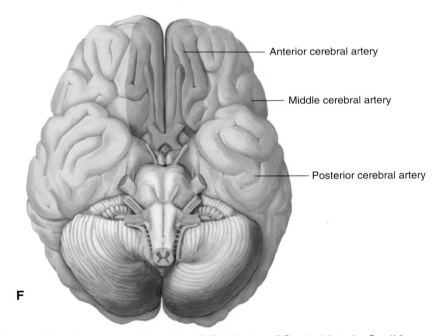

F

Figure 3.10E,F. **E.** Distribution of Cerebral Arteries, Lateral View. **F.** Distribution of Cerebral Arteries, Basal View.

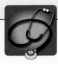

V. Clinical Considerations

A. Collateral circulation of brain

1. Although cerebral arterial circle (of Willis) appears to be effective anastomotic circuit, its efficiency in protecting against brain ischemia is only fair; in many individuals, 1 or more parts of circle are very small or even incompletely formed

2. **Autoregulation of blood flow** into cranial cavity: autonomic nerves monitor and correct for great increases and decreases in blood volume and pressure due to gravity, head position changes, etc.; sensors in carotid sinus and other parts of cerebral arterial tree enables central nervous system (CNS) to influence heart rate and muscle tone in vascular tree to maintain consistent flow and pressure of blood to brain, which is highly dependent on its blood supply for oxygen and glucose

3. On brain surface, arterial anastomoses are numerous; in substance of CNS they are rare, and those present are small; thus, occlusion or rupture of a vessel can lead to widespread and permanent destruction of nervous tissue because nerve cells do not reproduce

4. Occlusion of 1 of 3 major cerebral arteries

   a. May be caused by cerebral embolism (blood clot), which can lead to cerebral ischemia and infarction if embolus lodges where branches of the 3 cerebral arteries anastomose with each other, resulting in area of brain necrosis and severe neurologic symptoms or even death

   b. Remaining vessels must take over circulation, but supply by anastomotic vessels is usually inadequate because there is little exchange of blood between cerebral arteries via communicating arteries

   c. Infarcts usually develop, leading to vascular insufficiency; with cardiac arrest, the entire brain is affected, and unconsciousness is seen in 10 seconds

   d. Nervous tissue is extremely sensitive to lack of oxygen; with vascular insufficiency, irreversible neurologic damage can occur in 5 minutes

B. Blood–brain barrier

1. Selective anatomic and physiologic complex that controls movement of substances from general extracellular fluid of body to extracellular fluid of brain

2. Includes the arachnoid barrier layer and blood–CSF barrier and a true blood–brain barrier of rows of tight junctions between adjacent endothelial cells of cerebral capillaries

C. Cerebral angiography: femorocerebral angiography
  1. Transcutaneous technique for arterial catheterization
  2. Common method for evaluating brachiocephalic vessels
  3. Using fluoroscopic X-ray control and television monitoring of image, a preshaped, semirigid catheter is passed through cannula in femoral artery and guided up iliac vessels and aorta to aortic arch
      a. Catheter can then be selectively maneuvered into brachiocephalic, left common carotid, or left subclavian artery and then into vertebral or internal carotid artery
      b. With catheter in place, iodinated, water-soluble contrast medium is injected; rapid serial X-rays (over 8–10 sec) are taken in frontal and lateral projections, revealing, in sequence, morphologic and physiologic status of arterial, capillary, and venous phases of cerebral circulation

D. Stenosis or occlusion of vertebral artery: may lead to dizziness, fainting, spots before eyes, and transient diplopia; brainstem must then depend on other vertebral artery

E. **Transient ischemic attacks** (**TIAs**): refer to neurologic symptoms resulting from ischemia; most last only a few minutes, but some may persist for up to 1 hour; if larger vessels are affected, TIAs tend to last longer and may cause distal closure of intracranial vessels
  1. TIA symptoms may be ambiguous, cause staggering, dizziness, light-headedness, fainting, and paresthesias
  2. Patients with TIAs are at risk for ischemic stroke and myocardial infarction

F. **Subclavian steal syndrome**: rare; caused by narrowing of subclavian artery (usually left) near its origin
  1. To compensate for reduction in blood flow to limb, blood flows from right vertebral artery into left vertebral artery and into left subclavian artery
  2. Results in reduction in blood flow to brain, causing "giddiness," fainting attacks, and problems with ischemia of left upper limb

Occlusion of Major Arteries of Brain (Fig. 3.11)

Artery and Finding	Area Involved in Lesion
I. Anterior Cerebral Artery	
A. Contralateral monoplegia (leg)	Paracentral lobule
B. Contralateral sensory loss	Thalamocortical radiations
C. On dominant side	
1. Mental confusion	Frontal lobe
2. Apraxia, aphasia	Corpus callosum, cortical speech area
II. Anterior Choroidal Artery	
A. Homonymous hemianopsia	Geniculocalcarine tract (optic radiation)
B. Contralateral	
1. Hemiplegia	Corticospinal fibers of internal capsule
2. Hemianesthesia	Posterior limb of internal capsule
III. Middle Cerebral Artery	
A. Homonymous hemianopsia	Optic tract
B. Contralateral	
1. Hemiplegia	Anterior and posterior limbs of internal capsule
2. Hemianesthesia	
C. On dominant side: global aphasia	Motor and sensory speech areas
IV. Posterior Cerebral Artery	
A. Homonymous hemianopsia	Optic radiations
B. Contralateral	
1. Hemiplegia, ataxia	Internal capsule, spinocerebellar tract
2. Impaired sensation	Posterolateral ventral nucleus of thalamus
3. Burning pain	Dorsal nucleus of thalamus
4. Choreoathetoid movements	Red nucleus
V. Superior Cerebellar Artery	
A. Ipsilateral	
1. Cerebellar ataxia	Spinocerebellar tract
2. Choreiform movements	Red nucleus
3. Horner's syndrome	Reticular formation
B. Contralateral	
1. Loss of pain and temperature, face and body	Spinal nucleus of V and lemniscus system
2. Central facial weakness	Corticobulbar fibers to nucleus of VII
3. Partial deafness	Lateral lemniscus
VI. Anterior Inferior Cerebellar Artery	
A. Ipsilateral	
1. Cerebellar ataxia, deafness	Spinocerebellar tract, cochlear nuclei
2. Loss of sensation, face	Spinal tract and nucleus of V
B. Contralateral: loss of pain and temperature, body	Lemniscus system (spinothalamics)
VII. Posterior Inferior Cerebellar Artery	
A. Ipsilateral	
1. Cerebellar ataxia, nystagmus	Spinocerebellar tract
2. Horner's syndrome	Reticular formation
3. Loss of sensation, face	Spinal tract and nucleus of V
4. Dysphagia and dysphonia	Nucleus ambiguus, to IX and to X
B. Contralateral: loss of pain and temperature, body	Lateral spinothalamic tract

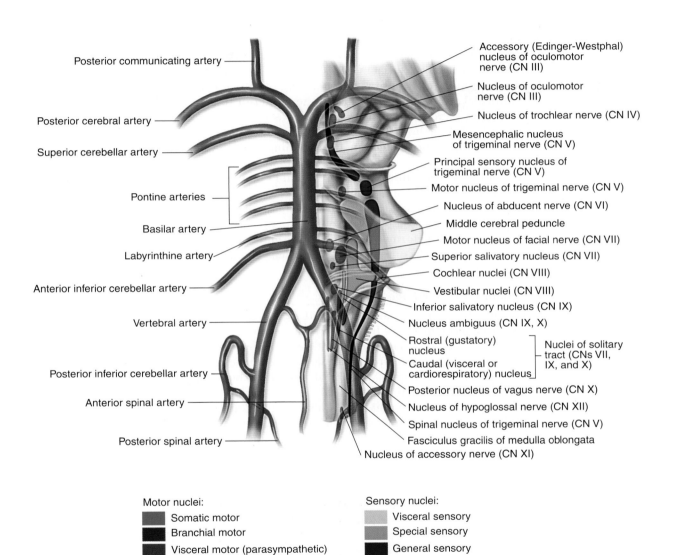

Posterior communicating artery

Posterior cerebral artery

Superior cerebellar artery

Pontine arteries

Basilar artery

Labyrinthine artery

Anterior inferior cerebellar artery

Vertebral artery

Posterior inferior cerebellar artery

Anterior spinal artery

Posterior spinal artery

Accessory (Edinger-Westphal) nucleus of oculomotor nerve (CN III)

Nucleus of oculomotor nerve (CN III)

Nucleus of trochlear nerve (CN IV)

Mesencephalic nucleus of trigeminal nerve (CN V)

Principal sensory nucleus of trigeminal nerve (CN V)

Motor nucleus of trigeminal nerve (CN V)

Nucleus of abducent nerve (CN VI)

Middle cerebral peduncle

Motor nucleus of facial nerve (CN VII)

Superior salivatory nucleus (CN VII)

Cochlear nuclei (CN VIII)

Vestibular nuclei (CN VIII)

Inferior salivatory nucleus (CN IX)

Nucleus ambiguus (CN IX, X)

Rostral (gustatory) nucleus

Caudal (visceral or cardiorespiratory) nucleus

Nuclei of solitary tract (CNs VII, IX, and X)

Posterior nucleus of vagus nerve (CN X)

Nucleus of hypoglossal nerve (CN XII)

Spinal nucleus of trigeminal nerve (CN V)

Fasciculus gracilis of medulla oblongata

Nucleus of accessory nerve (CN XI)

Motor nuclei:
Somatic motor
Branchial motor
Visceral motor (parasympathetic)

Sensory nuclei:
Visceral sensory
Special sensory
General sensory

Figure 3.11. Schematic of Blood Supply to Cranial Nerve Nuclei.

Head Injuries and Intracranial Hemorrhage

I. Introduction

A. Injuries to head are often associated with intracranial bleeding

B. Intracranial injuries occur with or without skull fracture

C. ~25% of fatal head injuries occur without skull fracture

D. Failure of respiration is usual cause of death when vital brain areas are damaged

II. Epidural (Extradural) Hemorrhage (Fig. 3.12A)

A. About 30% mortality

B. Usually due to fracture, and bleeding occurs between meningeal and periosteal dura; bleeding is usually arterial in 90% of cases and needs immediate surgical treatment

C. Most common fracture site is greater wing of sphenoid, where anterior branch of middle meningeal artery courses through bone; posterior branch is also source of bleeding

D. Classically, patient is knocked unconscious (brief concussion) at injury, may have lucid interval (of some hours) but may not, then becomes comatose as hemorrhage increases

E. A few cases are due to bleeding from meningeal or dural venous sinuses or emissary veins; onset of symptoms is often delayed for 1–3 weeks with venous bleeding

F. As fluid mass (hematoma) increases, brain compression occurs, requiring evacuation of blood and occlusion of bleeding vessel(s)

G. Commonly, 3rd nerve palsy and ipsilateral dilated, fixed pupil due to pressure on oculomotor nerve as it passes through superior orbital fissure

H. Due to hematoma formation above tentorium cerebelli resulting in rise in supratentorial pressure, herniation of temporal lobe (usually uncus) through tentorial notch near CN III origin can occur

III. Subdural Hemorrhage (Fig. 3.12B)

A. Bleeding between dura and arachnoid

B. Seen in almost all severe head injuries as result of stretching and/or tearing of dura and arachnoid; small tears in arteries and veins lead to varying degrees of bleeding

C. Most commonly results from tearing of cerebral veins where they enter superior sagittal sinus (so-called "bridging" veins); thus, is venous bleeding

D. May be acute or chronic, the latter being end result of unrecognized acute bleeding

E. May initially be widespread, but localizes in time, most often under parietal tuber

F. Bleeding is rarely of clinical significance, being overshadowed by cerebral damage

G. Subdural bleeding is common in alcoholics due to their proneness to head injuries from falls, arachnoid edema, and hemorrhagic tendency due to secondary liver damage

H. Clinical symptoms are seen 3–6 weeks after injury when clot is organized: headache, confusion, somnolence, and coma

I. CSF is under pressure and is clear or xanthochromic

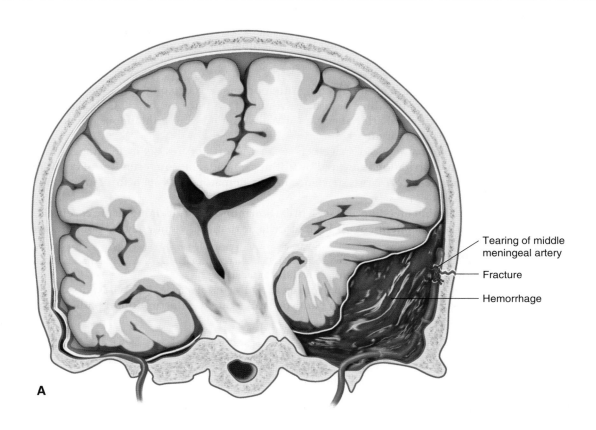

Tearing of middle meningeal artery

Fracture

Hemorrhage

A

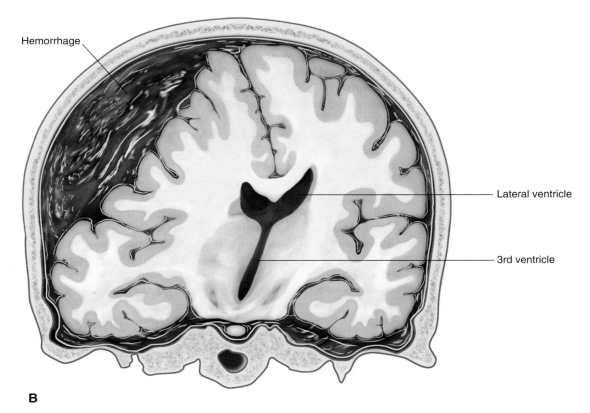

Hemorrhage

Lateral ventricle

3rd ventricle

B

Figure 3.12A,B. **A.** Epidural Hematoma. **B.** Subdural Hematoma.

IV. Subarachnoid Hemorrhage

A. Most common type of intracranial bleeding due to trauma and usually associated with cerebral or cerebellar contusion or laceration with bleeding into subarachnoid space causing bloody CSF

B. Traumatic subarachnoid bleeding often occurs over occipital lobes and cerebellum

C. Nontraumatic bleeding is usually result of rupture of berry (saccular) aneurysm of branch of cerebral arterial circle (of Willis) but may be spontaneous due to rupture of an apparently normal subarachnoid vessel

D. Blood in subarachnoid space acts as an irritant and results in meningeal inflammatory reaction or irritation indicated by stiff neck, headache, and even loss of consciousness

E. Does not result in large space-occupying hematomas as seen in epidural and subdural hematoma

F. Subarachnoid bleeding also seen in carbon monoxide poisoning, acute cerebral congestion due to status epilepticus, or in hemorrhagic diathesis (tendency to spontaneously bleed)

V. Intracerebral Hemorrhage (Fig. 3.12CD)

A. Bleeding into brain substance (usually arterial)

B. Arteries involved are often from cerebral arterial circle (of Willis) to basal nuclei or internal capsule, resulting in paralytic stroke due to interruption of pathways from cortex to brainstem and spinal cord

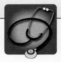

VI. Clinical Considerations

A. Aneurysms of cerebral arteries (Fig. 3.12E)

1. Often occur at division points in arteries at base of brain; many vessels of cerebral arterial circle (of Willis) intersect with each other at sharp angles, which predisposes to aneurysm formation at those sites of intersection; ruptured aneurysms in circle are common cause of death in young and middle-aged individuals

2. Classified as saccular, fusiform, or tubular

3. "Congenital" (berry or miliary) aneurysms: saccular, most common, arise from cerebral arterial circle (of Willis) and medium-size arteries at base of brain, especially anterior communicating artery, anterior or middle cerebral arteries, or basilar artery, usually at or near a point of bifurcation
   a. Vary from 10-50 mm
   b. Media of vessel is normally defective, and internal elastic membrane is deficient
   c. 20% of cases are multiple
   d. Rupture found in approximately 75% of cases
   e. May expand and rupture into subarachnoid space (subarachnoid hemorrhage) or into brain substance (intracerebral hemorrhage) or into subdural space (subdural hemorrhage)

4. Unruptured aneurysms: usually asymptomatic, but intermittent enlargements can cause throbbing headaches (due to meningeal stretching or subarachnoid bleeding) and neurologic signs: 3rd nerve palsy if associated with posterior communicating artery; anosmia (CN I compression); or unilateral hemianopia (CN II involvement)

5. Sudden rupture produces marked dizziness and unbearable, sudden, severe headache due to gross bleeding into subarachnoid space with increased intracranial pressure, meningeal irritation, and bloody CSF (under pressure); coma may follow severe hemorrhage

(Continued)

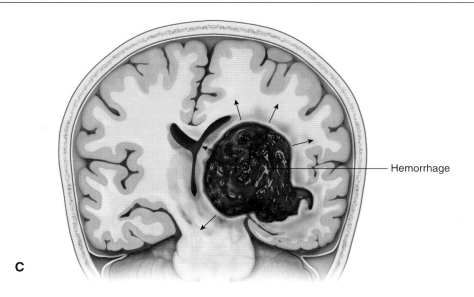

C

Hemorrhage

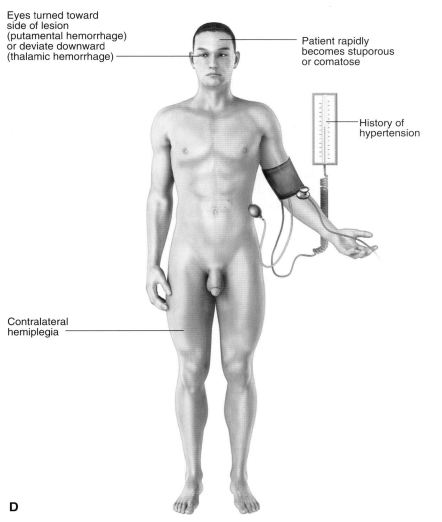

Eyes turned toward
side of lesion
(putamental hemorrhage)
or deviate downward
(thalamic hemorrhage)

Patient rapidly
becomes stuporous
or comatose

History of
hypertension

Contralateral
hemiplegia

D

Figure 3.12C,D. C. Intracerebral Hematoma. **D.** Clinical Presentation of Intracerebral Hemorrhage.

6. Atherosclerotic aneurysm: at site of atheroma in any cerebral artery; fusiform; most common in vertebral–basilar and internal carotid–cerebral axes

7. Arteriovenous aneurysm: complex tortuous network of vessels due to congenital defect in capillary bed; convulsions and/or motor and speech disturbances depend on location

8. Mycotic aneurysm: due to septic embolism (usually to middle or anterior cerebral artery)

9. Cranial nerve involvement
   a. Oculomotor nerve: passes between posterior cerebral and superior cerebellar arteries of circle; thus, aneurysm of these arteries can compress CN III
   b. CN II (optic nerve): lies just anteromedial to internal carotid artery as it enters cerebral arterial circle of Willis and may be involved if there is an aneurysm of artery

B. **Cerebrovascular accident** (CVA, or stroke)
   1. From either sudden hemorrhage into brain or interruption of blood supply leading to infarction and tissue death in area of brain supplied
      a. Clinical picture relates to size and location of infarct or bleeding
      b. "Soft" emboli that break up and pass through a vessel may produce neurologic deficits and temporary strokes
   2. Hemorrhagic type: usually due to rupture of an atherosclerotic artery or aneurysm
      a. Vary from tiny petechiae to massive hematomata; in the latter, brain bulges on affected side, gyri flatten, blood dissects through brain tissue and may rupture into ventricles
      b. Common site is lenticulostriate branch of middle cerebral artery with hemorrhage into basal nuclei and capsule
   3. Thrombotic type results from thrombosis in artery to brain or embolus that is carried from distant site via vascular system; emboli may be blood clots (usually from heart), atheromatous material (from ulcerated atheroma in medium arteries), platelet aggregates (from walls of medium arteries), or gas bubbles (from large veins opened traumatically or surgically)
   4. Striate arteries are commonly involved in CVAs

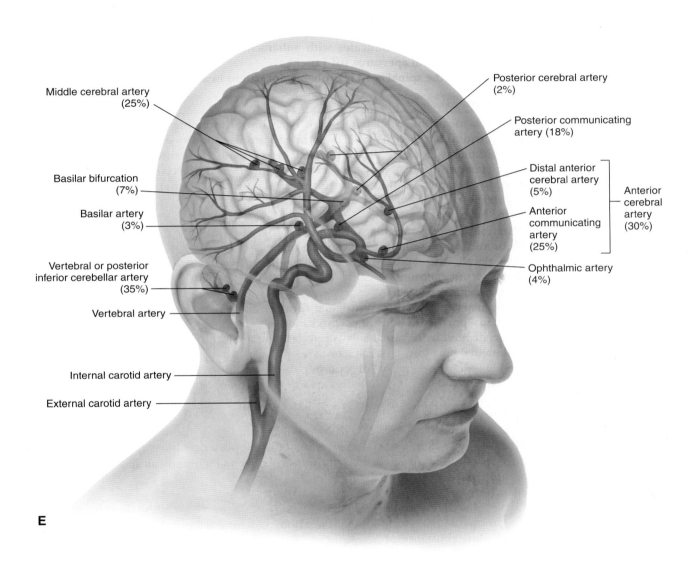

Figure 3.12E. Distribution of Aneurysms of the Brain.

Ventricles of Brain

I. General Features of Ventricles (Fig. 3.13A,B)

A. Development: core of embryonic neural tube forms continuous fluid-filled system, the ventricles, which are ependymal lined and found in cerebral hemispheres and brainstem

B. Variable in size and contain about 35 mL of CSF; comprise paired lateral ventricles and midline 3rd and 4th ventricles

C. Each lateral ventricle contains about 7–10 mL of fluid with remainder in 3rd and 4th ventricles

D. Ventricular system communicates with subarachnoid space via **median aperture** (**of Magendie**) and **lateral apertures** (**of Luschka**)

E. **Central canal of the spinal cord** is probably not patent in adults

II. Lateral Ventricles (Fig. 3.13C–E)

A. C-shaped cavities within each hemisphere; have "horns" radiating from center, the **collateral trigone** (atrium) of ventricle, which lies under parieto–temporo–occipital junction; glomus of choroid plexus lies here; from trigone, horns radiate to an anterior (frontal) horn, an inferior (temporal) horn, and a posterior (occipital) horn; interventricular foramina (of Monro) are at junction of anterior horns and bodies and connect lateral ventricles with 3rd ventricle

B. Anterior horn
1. Anterior to interventricular foramen (of Monro)
2. Floor and lateral wall: head of caudate nucleus
3. Medial wall: rostral part of septum pellucidum
4. Roof: corpus callosum

C. Body (par centralis)
1. Runs posterior from interventricular foramen to level of splenium of corpus callosum
2. Roof: midportion of body of corpus callosum
3. Floor: divided by terminal sulcus into lateral part formed by body of caudate nucleus and medial part formed by thalamus
4. Medial wall: posterior part of septum pellucidum above and fornix below

D. Collateral trigone (atrium): junction area of body and occipital and temporal horns

E. Posterior horn
1. Extends into occipital lobe
2. Roof and lateral wall: tapetum of corpus callosum
3. Medial wall: 2 longitudinal elevations, bulb of posterior horn formed by occipital portion of radiation of corpus callosum (forceps major), and calcar avis produced by anterior part of calcarine fissure

F. Inferior horn
1. Curves anteriorly into temporal lobe
2. Lies in the medial part of lobe but not quite reaching temporal pole
3. Roof: white substance of hemisphere; along its medial border are stria terminalis and tail of caudate nucleus
4. Amygdaloid nucleus bulges into terminal end of horn
5. Floor and medial wall: from within out, by fimbria, hippocampus, and collateral eminence
6. Choroid plexus is superimposed on fimbria and hippocampus

G. **Interventricular foramina** (**of Monro**): from lateral ventricles to 3rd ventricle

III. Third Ventricle

A. Small, narrow, midline vertical cleft of diencephalon

B. Bridged by interthalamic adhesion of thalamus

C. Lateral wall: thalamus and hypothalamus

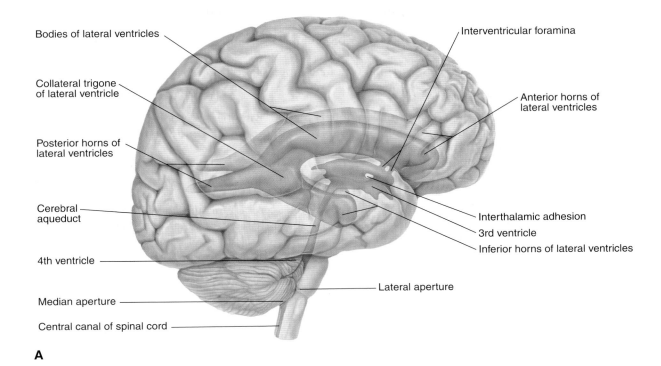

Bodies of lateral ventricles

Collateral trigone of lateral ventricle

Posterior horns of lateral ventricles

Cerebral aqueduct

4th ventricle

Median aperture

Central canal of spinal cord

Interventricular foramina

Anterior horns of lateral ventricles

Interthalamic adhesion

3rd ventricle

Inferior horns of lateral ventricles

Lateral aperture

A

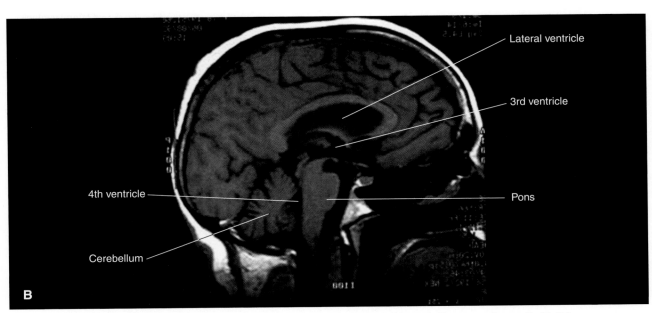

Lateral ventricle

3rd ventricle

4th ventricle

Pons

Cerebellum

B

Figure 3.13A,B. A. Ventricles of the Brain, Lateral View. **B.** Brain, Magnetic Resonance Image, Sagittal View.

D. Roof: choroid tela and choroid plexus
   1. At posterior end of roof is suprapineal recess
   2. Below this, in posterior wall, is habenular commissure
   3. Pineal body is attached below the latter; beneath pineal body is posterior commissure
E. Floor: contains optic chiasm, infundibulum, tuber cinereum, mammillary bodies, and subthalamus
F. Anterior wall: contains anterior commissure, anterior pillars of fornix, and lamina terminalis
J. Openings: 2 interventricular foramina superolaterally, cerebral aqueduct posteroinferiorly

IV. Fourth Ventricle

A. Lozenge-shaped cavity of rhombencephalon, lying between pons and medulla oblongata anteriorly and cerebellum posteriorly; continuous with central canal of closed portion of medulla posteroinferiorly
B. Floor (rhomboid fossa): posterior surfaces of pons and open part of medulla
C. Lateral boundaries of floor: superior and inferior cerebellar peduncles, cuneate tubercles, and clavae
D. Roof: superior and inferior medullary vela, cerebellum, and choroid tela
E. Openings: cerebral aqueduct anterosuperiorly; central canal of closed part of medulla posteroinferiorly; median aperture (of Magendie) at level of obex; lateral apertures (of Luschka) at lateral angles at level of CN VIII; median and lateral apertures open into subarachnoid space

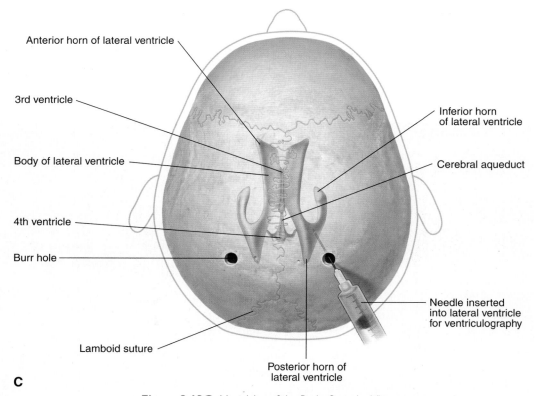

Anterior horn of lateral ventricle

3rd ventricle

Body of lateral ventricle

4th ventricle

Burr hole

Inferior horn of lateral ventricle

Cerebral aqueduct

Needle inserted into lateral ventricle for ventriculography

Lamboid suture

Posterior horn of lateral ventricle

C

Figure 3.13C. Ventricles of the Brain, Superior View.

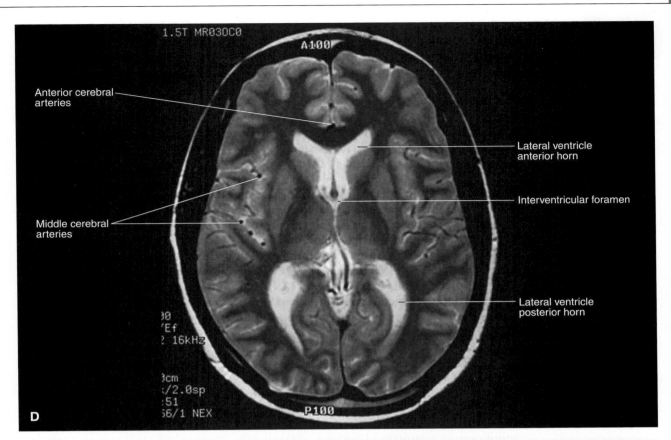

Anterior cerebral arteries

Middle cerebral arteries

Lateral ventricle anterior horn

Interventricular foramen

Lateral ventricle posterior horn

D

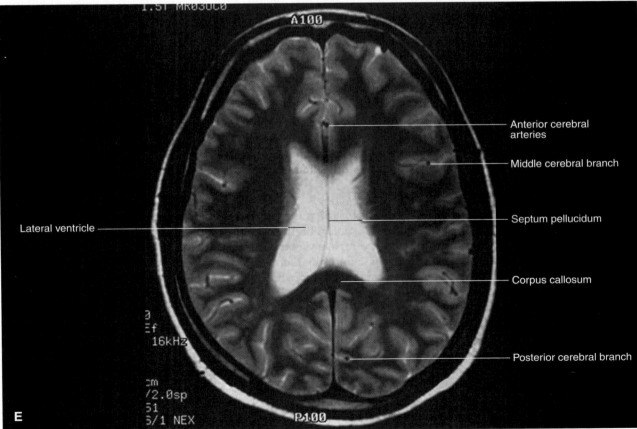

Lateral ventricle

Anterior cerebral arteries

Middle cerebral branch

Septum pellucidum

Corpus callosum

Posterior cerebral branch

E

Figure 3.13D,E. Brain, Magnetic Resonance Images, Axial Views.

Circulation of Cerebrospinal Fluid

I. Choroid Plexus (Fig. 3.14A)

A. Definition
   1. Ventricles are covered by ependymal epithelium and pia mater (tela choroidea); in some areas, a rich capillary plexus called choroid plexus develops and invaginates ependymal layer into ventricular system
   2. Line of attachment of plexus is called **taenia**

B. Locations
   1. Floor of bodies and inferior horns of lateral ventricles and roof of 3rd and 4th ventricles
   2. None is seen in frontal or occipital horns of lateral ventricles
   3. Plexus in lateral ventricles is largest and most important and is continuous with that of 3rd ventricle via interventricular foramina
   4. Lateral apertures of 4th ventricle (foramina of Luschka) also contain choroid plexus, which protrudes through them and secretes CSF into subarachnoid space
   5. Choroid plexus is enlarged in region of collateral trigone (triangular prominence of floor of lateral ventricle at transition between occipital and temporal horn; caused by penetration of collateral sulcus of temporal lobe), and here it is called the **glomus** (Latin, *glomus* = ball of thread)

II. Cerebrospinal Fluid

A. Composition
   1. Colorless, crystal clear; contains Na^+ (148 mEq/L), K^+ (2.88 mEq/L), Cl^- (120–130 mEq/L), glucose (50–75 mg/100 mL), HCO_3^- (22.9 mEq/L), and has a pH of 7.3
   2. Differs from blood in having virtually no cells (0–5 white blood cells per mm^3; usually lymphocytes) or protein (15–45 mg/100 mL; 80% albumin, 6%–10% gamma globulin)
   3. After secretion, it is further modified by choroid plexuses and pia during its circulation
   4. Because it does not resemble an ultrafiltrate of blood, suggests active secretion and absorption of ions rather than it being a simple diffusion across membranes

B. Formation
   1. At choroid plexuses and perhaps by vessels in subarachnoid space
   2. Formed at rate of 0.3–0.4 mL/min, with total volume being replaced about every 6 hours
   3. Formation is independent of ventricular, subarachnoid, or systemic blood pressures (rate does decrease at high back pressures)
   4. Each lateral ventricle has approximately 7 mL of fluid; entire ventricular system has approximately 35 mL; and subarachnoid space and spinal spaces approximately 100–125 mL of CSF

C. Drainage of CSF
   1. CSF passes from lateral to 3rd ventricle via interventricular foramina (of Monro) as result of hydrostatic pressure in highly convoluted choroid plexuses
   2. Passes from 3rd to 4th ventricle via **cerebral aqueduct** (**of Sylvius**)
   3. Passes from 4th ventricle into subarachnoid cisterns (cerebellomedullary and pontine) of posterior cranial fossa through median aperture (of Magendie) and lateral apertures (of Luschka)
   4. From cisterns, some CSF passes inferiorly around spinal cord and posterosuperiorly over cerebellum, whereas most flows up through tentorial notch in subarachnoid space around midbrain (interpeduncular cistern, right and left cisterna ambiens, and superior cistern)
   5. From these, CSF spreads up through sulci and fissures on median and superolateral surfaces of cerebral hemispheres (probably aided by cerebral arterial pulsations); also passes into extensions of subarachnoid spaces around CNs

D. Absorption
   1. Rate directly related to CSF pressure

2. Major sites of absorption are into venous blood, especially superior sagittal sinus and its lateral lacunae, via protrusion of arachnoid into dural sinus (arachnoid or Pacchionian granulations) with granulations acting as 1-way "valves"

3. Also absorbed by ventricular ependymal lining, in spinal subarachnoid space, through capillary walls in the pia, and into lymphatics adjacent to subarachnoid space around cranial and spinal nerves

E. Function

1. Protects brain by cushioning blows to head and vibration; brain floats in water bath, reducing effect of gravity on its weight; buoyancy prevents weight of brain from compressing CN roots and blood vessels against inside of cranium

2. Separates brain from bones of cranial cavity and vertebral canal

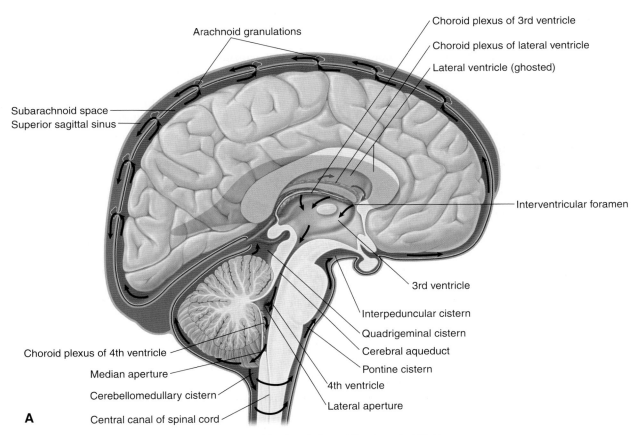

Figure 3.14A. Circulation of Cerebrospinal Fluid.

III. Subarachnoid Space

A. Between arachnoid and pia; receives CSF from 4th ventricle via median and lateral apertures (of Magendie and Luschka); subpial space does not exist

B. Above layer of pial cells, meshwork of arachnoid cells makes filmy membrane with depth of up to a few millimeters

C. CSF contained between arachnoid trabeculations of this meshwork

D. Blood vessels of brain enter and leave brain through this space

E. Removal of this membrane will disrupt vessels, producing bloody CSF

IV. Subarachnoid Cisterns

A. Definition: in some areas at base of brain, subarachnoid space is larger than over hemisphere and forms fluid spaces, or cisterns, which appear to function in supporting brain or cushioning base of brain against bony ledges of fossae of base of skull

B. Major cisterns and their contents

1. Posterior cisterns

a. **Superior (cerebellar)**: under tentorium and over upper surface of cerebellum

b. **Pericallosal**: above corpus callosum and between and below cingulate gyri

c. **Quadrigeminal** (cistern of great cerebral vein)

i. Location: under splenium of corpus callosum and over quadrigeminal plate; in front of tentorial notch

ii. Contents: pineal gland, great cerebral vein, terminal parts of basal veins, and posterior cerebral artery

d. P**osterior cerebellomedullary cistern** (**cisterna magna**): largest space found below cerebellum on posterior side of medulla; can be punctured between cerebellum and posterior margin of foramen magnum

i. Location: beneath cerebellar tonsils above and behind foramen magnum (between undersurface of cerebellum and dorsum of medulla)

ii. Contents: posterior inferior cerebellar arteries

2. Anterior cisterns

a. **Medullary**

i. Location: between medulla and lower clivus of skull

ii. Contents: CNs IX, X, XI, and XII and vertebral and posterior inferior cerebellar arteries

b. **Interpeduncular**

i. Location: on anterior aspect of brainstem between cerebral peduncles

ii. Contents: CN III and internal carotid, middle cerebral, anterior choroidal, posterior communicating, posterior cerebral, superior cerebellar, and basilar arteries

c. **Cistern of lateral cerebral fossa**: lies in lateral sulcus of cerebrum between frontal, temporal, and parietal lobes

d. **Pontine**

i. Location: beside pons and between it and upper clivus of skull

ii. Contents: CNs V and VI and basilar and anterior inferior cerebellar arteries

e. **Cerebellopontine**

i. Location: in front of cerebellar hemisphere and cerebellar peduncle; behind petrous ridges

ii. Contents: CNs VII, VIII, X, and XI and anterior inferior cerebellar artery

f. **Chiasmatic**

i. Location: extension of interpeduncular cistern anterosuperior to optic chiasm

ii. Contents: anterior cerebral arteries

g. **Crural**

i. Location: around cerebral peduncles

ii. Contents: posterior cerebral and anterior choroidal arteries

3. Intercommunicating cisterns

a. **Basal**: consists of combination of chiasmatic cistern and interpeduncular cistern

b. **Ambient**

      i. Location: lateral extensions of quadrigeminal cistern, continuous with interpeduncular and pontine cisterns; free edge of tentorial notch is lateral; between corpus callosum and thalamus

      ii. Contents: CN IV; posterior cerebral, superior cerebellar, and choroidal arteries; and basal and internal cerebral veins

c. **Of lamina terminalis**

      i. Location: in front of lamina terminalis; free edge of falx is anterior and corpus callosum forms its roof

      ii. Contents: anterior cerebral and frontopolar arteries

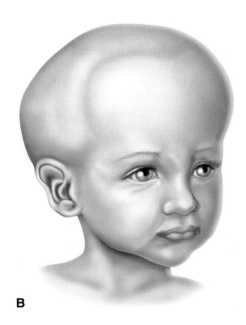

B

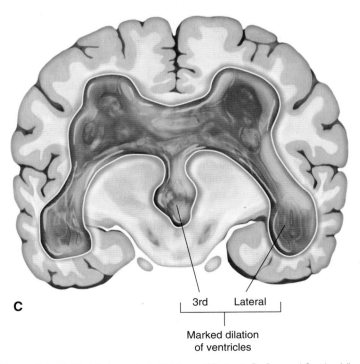

C

3rd   Lateral

Marked dilation
of ventricles

Figure 3.14B,C. Hydrocephaly. **B.** View of Patient. **C.** Coronal Section View.

V. Clinical Considerations (Fig. 3.14B,C)

A. **Meningitis** (inflammation of the meninges)

 1. Disease processes that cause inflammation of the arachnoid membrane (meningitis) or produce elevations of pressure within venous system (congestive heart failure) which tend to retard normal flow of CSF

 2. May produce "pus" in subarachnoid spaces of brain and spinal cord and in cisterns

B. **Hydrocephalus**

 1. Overproduction of CSF or blockage of normal drainage of ventricular system leads to dilation of ventricles (hydrocephalus) and subsequent destruction of surrounding brain tissue

   a. In a small child, condition can force separation of unossified skull sutures and increase infant's head size

   b. Chronic hydrocephalus may be treated by placing ventriculoperitoneal shunt, where a catheter is placed into lateral ventricle and drains CSF downward into abdominal cavity or into superior vena cava

 2. **Obstructive hydrocephalus** (internal or noncommunicating)

   a. Obstruction of flow of CSF within ventricles (at interventricular foramen or cerebral aqueduct) or at their exit apertures

   b. Aqueduct stenosis: blockage most commonly occurs at cerebral aqueduct (of Sylvius); may be result of nearby tumor in midbrain or by cellular debris following intraventricular hemorrhage or bacterial and fungal infection of CNS

   c. Dye placed in lateral ventricle does not appear in lumbar cistern

 3. **Communicating (external) hydrocephalus**

   a. Blockage of reabsorption of CSF at arachnoid granulations, often as result of meningitis; involves blockage to flow, which does not involve ventricles or passages between them

   b. Dye appears in lumbar cistern after being injected into lateral ventricle

 4. Hydrocephalus is more common in infants than in adults and, in most cases, no definitive cause can be found (of communicating type)

 5. Adult type of hydrocephalus is generally due to some mechanical obstruction of CSF circulation

 6. **Posthemorrhagic hydrocephalus**: seen in infants following intracranial hemorrhage that distends ventricles and obstructs normal pathways for CSF

 7. **Ototic hydrocephalus:** caused by spread of inflammation of otitis media to cranial cavity

 8. Normal pressure occult hydrocephalus: causes dementia, ataxia, and urinary incontinence with enlarged ventricles associated with inadequacy of subarachnoid spaces but with normal CSF pressure

C. When subarachnoid space is opened, CSF leaks out because fluid is normally under pressure; after surgical procedure, it is not possible to close subarachnoid space by suturing arachnoid because it is flimsy and transparent; leakage of CSF is prevented by carefully suturing dura mater

D. CSF leakage: can be distinguished from mucus by testing its glucose level which reflects that of blood; CSF leakage from nose and ear may indicate cranial base fracture; infection can spread to meninges resulting in meningitis

 1. Fractures in floor of middle cranial fossa: can lead to leakage of CSF from external acoustic meatus (CSF otorrhea) if meninges superior to middle ear are torn and tympanic membrane is ruptured

 2. Fractures in floor of anterior cranial fossa: can involve cribriform plate of ethmoid, resulting in CSF leakage through nose (CSF rhinorrhea)

E. Imaging ventricular system and related structures: ventriculography and encephalography are means to replace fluid in subarachnoid space and ventricular system with contrast medium of differing density to X-rays; air injected into spaces outlines and fills them and, being less opaque on X-ray film, cavities appear more intensely exposed and darker on radiographs; sometimes radiopaque oil is injected

1. **Fractional pneumoencephalography** (**PEG**): Approximately 35 cc of air, in 10- to 15-cc increments, is slowly injected into the lumbar cistern with patient sitting upright
   a. CSF pressure monitored carefully, and only if not abnormally high is air injected and CSF removed alternately in small amounts
   b. Patient's head is flexed and extended such as to fill different parts of subarachnoid cisterns and ventricular system sequentially
   c. Air bubble can be kept in different parts of ventricular system by maneuvering head; thus, system can be outlined

2. **Ventriculography**: if intracranial pressure is elevated, it is safer to inject air (or positive contrast medium) into lateral ventricle, following trephination (perforating skull with surgical instrument) in posterior part of frontal bone or in parietal bone; air is exchanged for ventricular fluid; of value in diagnosing size of ventricular system and possible obstructions or encroachments on ventricular system

3. **Radionuclide encephalography**: injection of a radioactive isotope into the lumbar cistern and scanning the brain at intervals over 24–48 hours
   a. If CSF is normal, most of the isotope passes into the basilar cisterns and over the convexities of the hemispheres
   b. If obstruction occurs, the isotope refluxes into the ventricles
   c. Useful method for locating an atrophic or space-occupying lesion

F. **Lumbar puncture** (**spinal tap**)
   1. CSF may be removed for diagnostic purposes from any part of ventricular system or from subarachnoid space; most common site is lumbar cistern, the subarachnoid space in lower lumbar part of vertebral column below level of spinal cord (which ends at L2 vertebral level)
   2. CSF may also be removed from lateral ventricles and cisterna magna
   3. **Spinal anesthesia**: anesthetic agent can be added to CSF via lumbar puncture

Summary of Cranial Nerves

I. Table of Cranial Nerves (Fig. 3.15A,B)

Number	Nerve	Nuclei of Origin and Termination	Distribution	Function
CN I	Olfactory	Central or deep process of olfactory bulb	Nasal mucous membranes	Special sensory (smell)
CN II	Optic	Ganglionic cells of retina	Retina of eye	Special sensory (vision)
CN III	Oculomotor	Nucleus in floor of cerebral aqueduct; Edinger-Westphal	Levator palpebrae superioris, superior, inferior, and medial recti, inferior oblique, ciliary, sphincter pupillae muscles	Motor
CN IV	Trochlear	Nucleus in floor of cerebral aqueduct	Superior oblique muscle	Motor
CN V	Trigeminal	Fibers of sensory root arise from trigeminal ganglion	V_1 Ophthalmic: cornea, ciliary body, iris, lacrimal gland, conjunctiva, mucous membrane of nasal cavity, skin of forehead, eyelid, eyebrow, and nose	Sensory
			V_2 Maxillary: lower eyelid, upper lip, gums and teeth of upper jaw, mucous membranes and skin of cheek and nose, dura	Sensory
		Fibers of motor root arise from nucleus in pons	V_3 Mandibular: temple, auricle of ear, lower lip, skin over mandible, teeth and gums of mandible, mucous membrane of anterior part of tongue	Sensory
			Muscles of mastication (temporalis, masseter, medial and lateral pterygoid), and mylohyoid and anterior belly of digastric, tensor tympani and tensor veli palatini muscles	Motor
CN VI	Abducent	Nucleus beneath floor of 4th ventricle	Lateral rectus muscle	Motor
CN VII	Facial	Nucleus in lower part of pons	Muscles of facial expression, stapedius, stylohyoid and posterior belly of digastric muscles	Motor
		Geniculate ganglion	Anterior 2/3 tongue via chorda tympani	Sensory (taste)
		Lacrimal nucleus	Lacrimal gland	Secretomotor
		Superior salivatory nucleus	Submandibular and sublingual glands	Secretomotor
CN VIII	Vestibulocochlear	Cochlear from bipolar cells in spiral ganglion of cochlea	Organ of Corti	Sensory (hearing)
		Vestibular from bipolar cells in vestibular ganglion	Semicircular canals	Sensory (equilibrium)

(Continued)

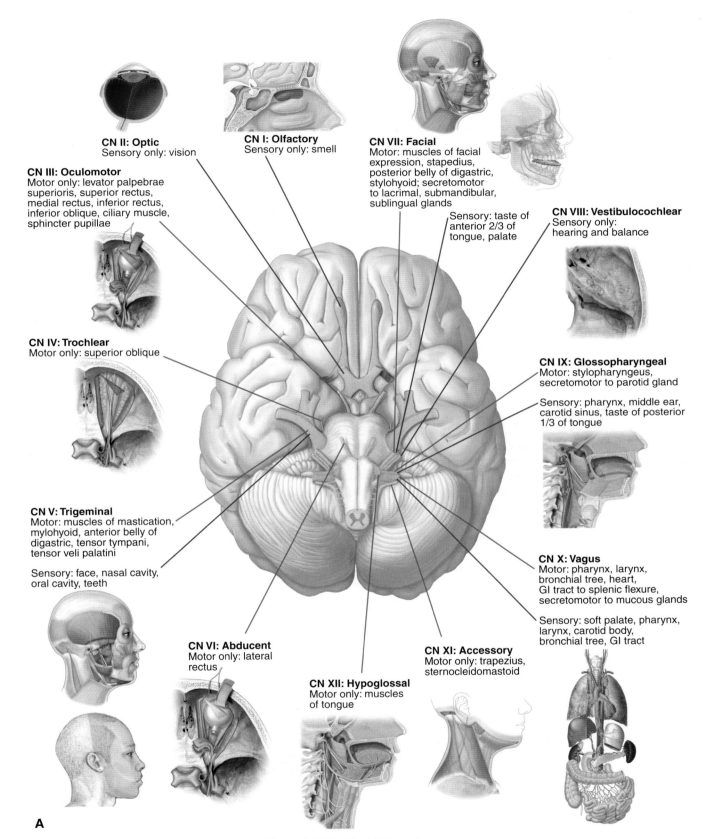

CN II: Optic
Sensory only: vision

CN I: Olfactory
Sensory only: smell

CN VII: Facial
Motor: muscles of facial
expression, stapedius,
posterior belly of digastric,
stylohyoid; secretomotor
to lacrimal, submandibular,
sublingual glands

CN III: Oculomotor
Motor only: levator palpebrae
superioris, superior rectus,
medial rectus, inferior rectus,
inferior oblique, ciliary muscle,
sphincter pupillae

Sensory: taste of
anterior 2/3 of
tongue, palate

CN VIII: Vestibulocochlear
Sensory only:
hearing and balance

CN IV: Trochlear
Motor only: superior oblique

CN IX: Glossopharyngeal
Motor: stylopharyngeus,
secretomotor to parotid gland

Sensory: pharynx, middle ear,
carotid sinus, taste of posterior
1/3 of tongue

CN V: Trigeminal
Motor: muscles of mastication,
mylohyoid, anterior belly of
digastric, tensor tympani,
tensor veli palatini

Sensory: face, nasal cavity,
oral cavity, teeth

CN X: Vagus
Motor: pharynx, larynx,
bronchial tree, heart,
GI tract to splenic flexure,
secretomotor to mucous glands

Sensory: soft palate, pharynx,
larynx, carotid body,
bronchial tree, GI tract

CN VI: Abducent
Motor only: lateral
rectus

CN XI: Accessory
Motor only: trapezius,
sternocleidomastoid

CN XII: Hypoglossal
Motor only: muscles
of tongue

A

Figure 3.15A. Cranial Nerve Summary.

Number	Nerve	Nuclei of Origin and Termination	Distribution	Function
CN IX	Glossopharyngeal	Superior and inferior ganglia	Mucous membranes of fauces, tonsils, pharynx, and posterior 3rd tongue	Sensory (taste and general sense)
		Nucleus ambiguus	Stylopharyngeus muscle	Motor
		Inferior salivatory nucleus	Parotid gland	Secretomotor
CN X	Vagus	Superior and inferior ganglion (nodose) to solitary nucleus	Mucous membranes of larynx, trachea, lungs, esophagus, stomach, intestines, and gallbladder	Sensory and secretomotor
		Dorsal motor nucleus	Smooth muscle of lower esophagus, stomach, small intestine, and part of large intestine	Motor (smooth muscle)
			Excitatory fibers to gastric and pancreatic glands	Secretomotor
			Heart	Motor (cardiac muscle)
		Nucleus ambiguus	Muscles of pharynx, larynx, soft palate, and upper esophagus	Motor
CN XI	Accessory	Spinal cord C1 to C5	SCM and trapezius muscles	Motor
CN XII	Hypoglossal	Hypoglossal nucleus in medulla	Muscles of tongue	Motor

II. Nerve Components

A. Simplified classification of components
   1. Somatic motor: CNs III, IV, VI, VII, IX, X, XI, and XII
   2. Visceral or autonomic motor: CNs III, VII, IX, and X
   3. Somatic sensory: CNs II, V, VII, VIII, IX, and X
   4. Visceral sensory: CNs I, VII, IX, and X

B. Traditional classification of components: 7 types of fibers
   1. **General somatic efferent** (**GSE**): motor supply to skeletal muscle of myotomal origin (CNs III, IV, VI, XII)
      a. CN III: oculomotor nucleus to orbital muscles (except lateral rectus and superior oblique)
      b. CN IV: to superior oblique muscle
      c. CN VI: to lateral rectus muscle
      d. CN XII: to extrinsic and intrinsic muscles of tongue
      e. Spinal nerves to body musculature
   2. **Special visceral efferent** (**SVE**): motor to skeletal muscle of branchial arch origin (CNs V, VII, IX, and X)
      a. CN V: from motor nucleus of trigeminal to muscles of mastication, mylohyoid, anterior belly of digastric, tensor veli palatini, and tensor tympani muscles
      b. CN VII: from facial motor nucleus to muscles of facial expression and stylohyoid, posterior belly of digastric, and stapedius
      c. CN IX: from nucleus ambiguus to stylopharygeus muscle
      d. CN X: from nucleus ambiguus to muscles of palate, pharynx, esophagus, and larynx
      e. CN XI: from spinal cord to sternocleidomastoid (SCM) and trapezius muscles

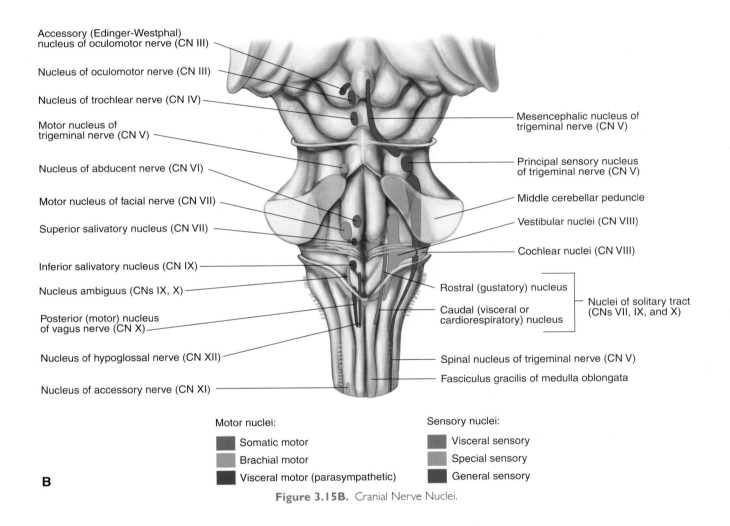

Accessory (Edinger-Westphal) nucleus of oculomotor nerve (CN III)

Nucleus of oculomotor nerve (CN III)

Nucleus of trochlear nerve (CN IV)

Motor nucleus of trigeminal nerve (CN V)

Nucleus of abducent nerve (CN VI)

Motor nucleus of facial nerve (CN VII)

Superior salivatory nucleus (CN VII)

Inferior salivatory nucleus (CN IX)

Nucleus ambiguus (CNs IX, X)

Posterior (motor) nucleus of vagus nerve (CN X)

Nucleus of hypoglossal nerve (CN XII)

Nucleus of accessory nerve (CN XI)

Mesencephalic nucleus of trigeminal nerve (CN V)

Principal sensory nucleus of trigeminal nerve (CN V)

Middle cerebellar peduncle

Vestibular nuclei (CN VIII)

Cochlear nuclei (CN VIII)

Rostral (gustatory) nucleus

Caudal (visceral or cardiorespiratory) nucleus

Nuclei of solitary tract (CNs VII, IX, and X)

Spinal nucleus of trigeminal nerve (CN V)

Fasciculus gracilis of medulla oblongata

Motor nuclei:
- Somatic motor
- Brachial motor
- Visceral motor (parasympathetic)

Sensory nuclei:
- Visceral sensory
- Special sensory
- General sensory

B

Figure 3.15B. Cranial Nerve Nuclei.

3. **General visceral efferent** (**GVE**): motor supply, including secretomotor to visceral structures such as gut, glands, etc. (CNs III, VII, IX, and X)
   a. CN III: from Edinger-Westphal nucleus to ciliary ganglion to ciliary and pupillary constrictor muscles
   b. CN VII: from superior salivatory nucleus via nervus intermedius to pterygopalatine ganglion to lacrimal gland and glands of nasal and oral mucosae and palate; from same nucleus, via chorda tympani, to submandibular ganglion to submandibular and sublingual glands
   c. CN IX: from inferior salivatory nucleus to tympanic plexus to lesser petrosal nerve to otic ganglion to parotid gland (via auriculotemporal nerve)
   d. CN X: from dorsal motor nucleus to trachea and thoracic and abdominal viscera with synapse in intrinsic organ ganglia
4. **General somatic afferent** (**GSA**): general sensations such as touch, pain, temperature, and proprioception (sense of position of joints and amount of contraction of muscles) (CNs V, VII, IX, and X)
   a. CN V: trigeminal ganglion
      i. Ophthalmic nerve (CN V_1): from forehead, upper lid, cornea, conjunctivae, meninges, sinuses, nasal septum and anterior lateral nasal wall, dorsum of nose, lacrimal caruncle, and sac
      ii. Maxillary (CN V_2): from cheeks, lower lid, orbital periosteum, upper teeth and gums, upper lip, palate, maxillary sinus, and nasal cavity
      iii. Mandibular (CN V_3): from lower teeth and gums, lower lip, chin, lower face, external ear and scalp over temporal region, anterior tongue and mouth, and (temporomandibular joint) TMJ
      iv. From muscles of mastication and external ocular muscles for proprioception with central fibers passing to mesencephalic nucleus
      v. CN VII: geniculate ganglion to external acoustic meatus and small area of skin behind ear
   b. CN IX: superior ganglion to posterior 3rd of tongue, palatine tonsil, oropharynx, and auditory tube
   c. CN X: superior ganglion to external acoustic meatus, small area of skin behind ear, and dura of posterior cranial fossa
5. **General visceral afferent** (**GVA**): sensations from visceral structures such as gut, glands, etc. (CNs VII, IX, and X)
   a. CN VII: from sensory receptors of palatine tonsils, soft palate and middle ear to cell bodies in geniculate ganglion; central fibers pass to inferior solitary nucleus and tract (tractus solitarius) for general sensation
   b. CN IX: from sensory receptors of posterior 3rd of tongue, soft palate, palatine tonsil, oropharynx, auditory tube, middle ear, and carotid body and sinus with cell bodies in petrosal ganglion and central fibers to solitary nucleus and tract in brainstem
   c. CN X: from sensory receptors on posterior surface of epiglottis, larynx, pharynx, trachea, respiratory bronchi, and digestive (esophagus, stomach, small intestine, ascending and transverse colons) system and circulatory system (heart; aortic arch; and, possibly, carotid body), and aortic bodies; cell bodies in nodose ganglion with central fibers to solitary nucleus of brainstem
   d. Spinal nerves: from viscera and organs
6. **Special somatic afferent** (**SSA**): special sensations of vision and equilibrium (CNs II and VIII)
   a. CN II: from rods and cones of retina to ganglion cells of retina and then via optic nerves to lateral geniculate bodies of brain and then to visual cortex, for vision
   b. CN VIII
      i. From hair cells of organ of Corti via bipolar cells of spiral ganglia to dorsal and ventral cochlear nuclei of brainstem, for hearing
      ii. From hair cells of cristae and maculae of ampullae of semicircular canals and from utricle and saccule to vestibular ganglion and then to vestibular nuclei of brainstem

7. **Special visceral afferent** (**SVA**): special sensations of smell and taste from visceral structures related to gut (CNs I, VII, IX, and X)
    a. CN I: from hair cells of superior nasal concha and upper 3rd of nasal septum mucosa to bipolar cell of olfactory bulbs and then to brain via olfactory tracts for olfaction
    b. CN VII: for taste from anterior 2/3 of tongue and soft palate via chorda tympani with cell bodies in geniculate ganglion and then centrally to solitary tract nucleus
    c. CN IX: for taste from posterior 3rd of tongue to cell bodies in petrosal ganglion and then centrally to solitary tract nucleus
    d. CN X: for taste from epiglottis to cell bodies in nodose ganglion and then centrally to solitary tract nucleus
8. **General proprioception**: receptors for cranial musculature are same as those found in limbs and trunk

C. Summary of cranial nerve components
    1. Olfactory (CN I): sensory (SVA)
    2. Optic (CN II): sensory (SSA)
    3. Oculomotor (CN III): somatic and visceral motor (GSE, GVE, and proprioception)
    4. Trochlear (CN IV): somatic motor (GSE and proprioception)
    5. Trigeminal (CN V): sensory and somatic motor (SVE, GSA, and proprioception)
    6. Abducent (CN VI): somatic motor (GSE and proprioception)
    7. Facial (CN VII): sensory and somatic and visceral motor (SVE, GVE, GVA, SVA, GSA, and proprioception)
    8. Vestibulocochlear (CN VIII): sensory (SSA)
    9. Glossopharyngeal (CN IX): sensory and somatic and visceral motor (SVE, GVE, GVA, SVA, GSA, and proprioception)
    10. Vagus (CN X): sensory and somatic and visceral motor (SVE, GVE, GVA, SVA, and GSA)
    11. Accessory (CN XI): somatic motor (SVE)
    12. Hypoglossal (CN XII): somatic motor (GSE and proprioception)

Cranial Nerve I: Olfactory Nerve

I. General features of Olfactory Nerve (CN I)

A. Approximately 20 in number
B. Sensory only; nerve of smell

II. Origin, Course, and Branches (Fig. 3.16A–C)

A. From olfactory mucosa: sensory cell bodies in olfactory epithelium of walls of upper nasal cavity pass upward through cribriform plate to synapse in olfactory bulb where 1st-order neurons end and 2nd-order neurons of olfactory tract begin
B. Nerves pass in **olfactory tracts** to brain
C. No branches

III. Clinical Considerations

A. Testing CN I: patient is asked to close eyes and inhale, with 1 nostril occluded, test substances brought close to open nostril; substance must be non-irritating volatile oil solutions or oil of cloves or lemon, vanilla, tobacco, freshly ground coffee, etc.; each nostril is thus tested separately

B. **Anosmia**: lack of sense of smell
  1. Unilateral anosmia suggests compression of olfactory bulb or tract by frontal lobe abscess or glioma, olfactory groove meningioma, sphenoid ridge meningioma, or pituitary or parasellar tumors
  2. Central lesions in hemispheres do not produce anosmia, due to decussation of olfactory fibers in anterior commissure
  3. A tumor may extend posterolaterally and involve ipsilateral optic nerve causing optic atrophy or increased intracranial pressure with papilledema of opposite optic nerve; combination of unilateral anosmia, ipsilateral optic atrophy and contralateral papilledema is called **Foster-Kennedy syndrome**
  4. Consistent loss of sense of smell on 1 side is more significant than bilateral loss, unless patient's chief complaint is acute sudden loss

C. Olfactory hallucinations: false perception of smell; may accompany lesions in temporal lobe

D. Lesion irritating lateral olfactory area (deep to uncus) may result in temporal lobe epilepsy or "uncinate" fits, which are characterized by imaginary disagreeable odors and involuntary lip and tongue movements

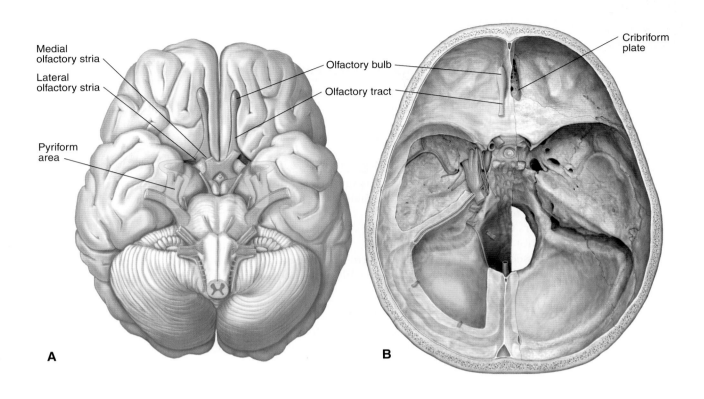

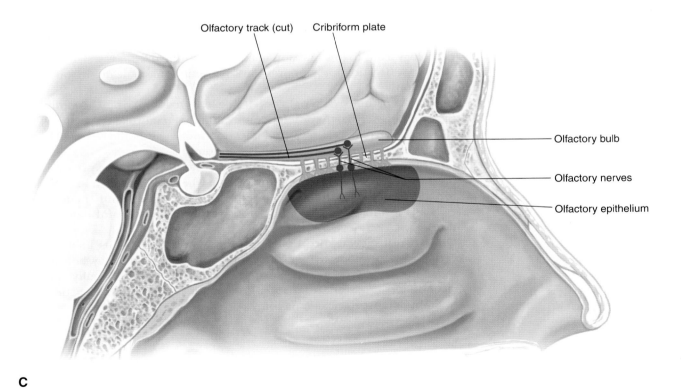

Figure 3.16A–C. Olfactory Nerve. **A.** Origin from Brain. **B.** Exit from Skull. **C.** Distribution, Sagittal View.

Cranial Nerve II: Optic Nerve

I. General Features of Optic Nerve (CN II)

A. Forward projecting tract (rather than a nerve) of diencephalon

B. 4-mm thick and consists of axons of the 3rd-order neurons from ganglion cells of retina in visual pathway

C. Sensory only

II. Origin, Course, and Branches (Fig. 3.17A–C)

A. From retina, passes above ophthalmic artery and through optic canal into cranial cavity

B. In front of sella turcica, in prechiasmatic groove of sphenoid bone, nerves of both sides unite to form **optic chiasm**

C. Fibers from medial or nasal halves of retinae cross in chiasm; those from temporal retina do not cross

D. Crossed and uncrossed fibers form **optic tracts**, which pass directly behind pulvinar and around cerebral peduncles to the 4th-order neurons in lateral geniculate bodies

III. Clinical Considerations

A. Testing of the visual system: involves testing the following

1. Visual acuity: evaluation of near and distant vision

2. Ophthalmoscopic examination: examining cornea for abrasions or opacities; aqueous humor; iris; lens; vitreous body; and retina (optic nerve head or disk for papilledema, optic atrophy, retrobulbar neuritis; and fovea centralis)

3. Examination (plotting) of visual fields: each side and in binocular vision; looking for scotoma (area of depressed vision in visual field surrounded by normal or less depressed area)

B. Pathology in optic nerve leads to ipsilateral (monocular) blindness; optic tract pathology leads to loss of vision in contralateral field

C. Pathology (section or compression) of optic chiasm leads to bitemporal hemianopsia

D. Optic tract pathology: on right or left side leads to loss of vision in contralateral field, respectively (right or left homonymous hemianopsia, respectively)

E. Close relation of these nerves and tracts to hypophysis should be noted because tumors of gland often induce visual symptoms

F. Optic nerves and demyelinating diseases: because optic nerves are CNS tracts, myelin sheaths around sensory fibers from where fibers penetrate sclerae are formed by glial cells (oligodendrocytes) instead of Schwann (neurolemma) cells as in other CNs; thus, they are susceptible to effects of demyelinating diseases of CNS (e.g., MS)

G. **Optic neuritis**: related to lesions of optic nerve that results in decrease in visual acuity without changes in peripheral visual fields; may be caused by inflammatory demyelination or some toxic disorders (i.e., methyl and ethyl alcohol, tobacco, lead, or mercury); nerve looks pale and smaller than usual on ophthalmoscopic examination

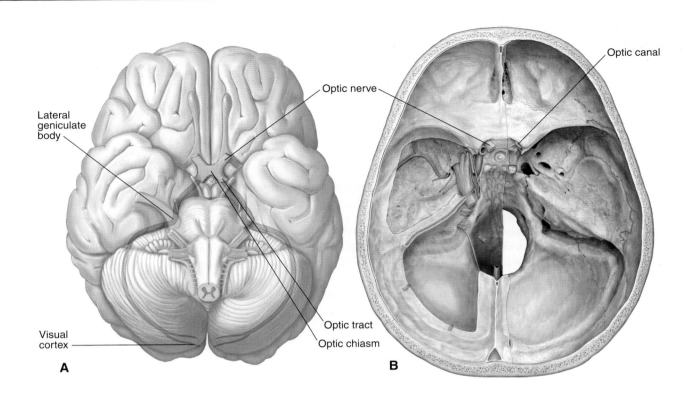

Lateral
geniculate
body

Optic nerve

Optic canal

Visual
cortex

Optic tract

Optic chiasm

A

B

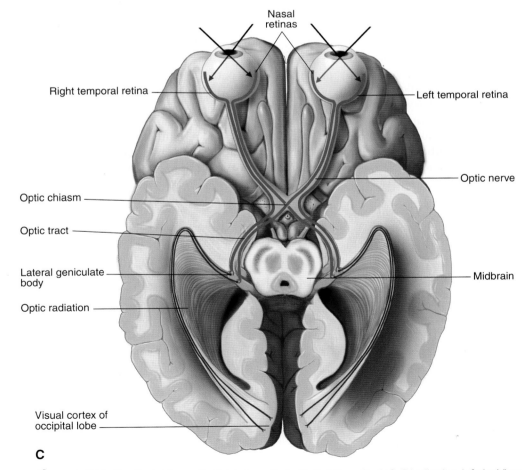

Nasal
retinas

Right temporal retina

Left temporal retina

Optic nerve

Optic chiasm

Optic tract

Lateral geniculate
body

Midbrain

Optic radiation

Visual cortex of
occipital lobe

C

Figure 3.17A–C. Optic Nerve. **A.** Origin from Brain. **B.** Exit from Skull. **C.** Distribution, Inferior View.

Cranial Nerve III: Oculomotor Nerve

I. General Features of Oculomotor Nerve (CN III)

A. Innervates most muscles of orbit
B. Carries somatic motor fibers (general somatic efferent) for 5 voluntary muscles controlling eye movements and eyelid and parasympathetic motor (general visceral efferent) to 2 smooth muscles of eyeball

II. Origin, Course, and Branches (Fig. 3.18A,B)

A. Leaves midbrain on medial side of cerebral peduncles
B. Passes between posterior cerebral and superior cerebellar arteries (near termination of basilar artery) and leaves posterior cranial fossa to penetrate dura of cavernous sinus and pass forward in its lateral wall
C. Enters medial angle of superior orbital fissure within common ring tendon to enter orbit
D. Can be injured against sharp edge of tentorium cerebelli (tentorial notch)
E. Branches (Fig. 3.18C)
   1. Superior division: supplies levator palpebrae superioris and superior rectus (supplying both from below)
   2. Inferior division: supplies medial rectus, inferior rectus, and inferior oblique muscles and presynaptic parasympathetic motor root to ciliary ganglion
F. **Ciliary ganglion** (Fig. 3.18D)
   1. Approximately 2-mm diameter and lies in orbital fat, lateral to optic nerve and medial to lateral rectus muscle, near apex of orbit
   2. Contains cell bodies of postsynaptic parasympathetic nerve fibers for ciliary muscle (for accomodation) and sphincter pupillae muscle (for pupil constriction)
   3. Connections of ganglion
      a. Parasympathetic motor root: presynaptic fibers from Edinger-Westphal nucleus pass in oculomotor nerve to ganglion
      b. Sympathetic root: postsynaptic sympathetic fibers originating in superior cervical ganglion and traveling in internal carotid plexus, from which fibers pass through ciliary ganglion without synapsing
      c. Sensory root: sensory fibers from eye to nasociliary nerve (CN V_1)
      d. **Short ciliary nerves**: 10–20 neurons, which contain postsynaptic parasympathetic fibers from ciliary ganglion, postsynaptic sympathetic fibers from sympathetic root, and sensory nerve fibers from sensory root to nasociliary nerve

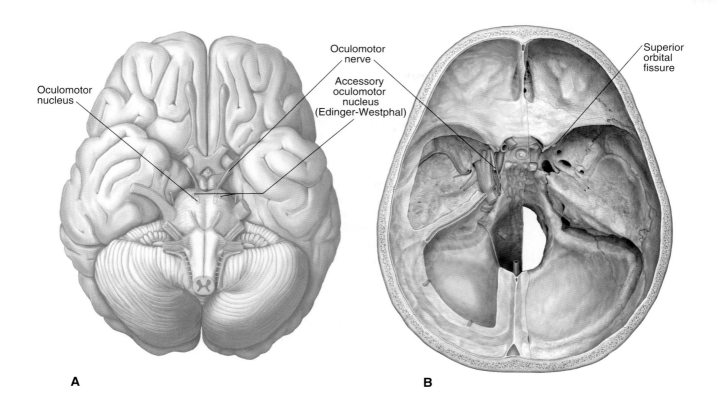

A

Oculomotor nucleus

Oculomotor nerve

Accessory oculomotor nucleus (Edinger-Westphal)

Superior orbital fissure

B

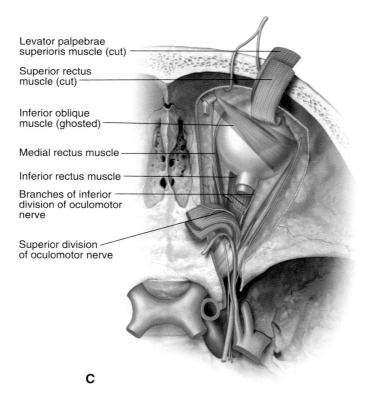

Levator palpebrae superioris muscle (cut)

Superior rectus muscle (cut)

Inferior oblique muscle (ghosted)

Medial rectus muscle

Inferior rectus muscle

Branches of inferior division of oculomotor nerve

Superior division of oculomotor nerve

C

Figure 3.18A–C. Oculomotor Nerve. **A.** Origin from Brain. **B.** Exit from Skull. **C.** Distribution, Superior View.

III. Clinical Considerations

A. Eyeball reflexes

1. **Light reflex**: light shined into eye is picked up by the retina and impulses are carried by optic nerve to brain centers

   a. There are direct connections between these centers and Edinger-Westphal nucleus of CN III

   b. Presynaptic parasympathetic cells are stimulated and impulses pass via CN III to ciliary ganglion where they synapse

   c. Postsynaptic fibers travel to sphincter pupillae muscle to constrict pupil and complete reflex

2. **Accommodation reflex**: involves convergence of eyes, which is effected by voluntary action of contracting the 3 muscles used to move eye medially (medial rectus, superior rectus, and inferior oblique); increase in thickness of the lens (accomplished by the circularly and radially arranged ciliary muscles); and constriction of pupil (by action of sphincter pupillae)

3. **Reflex dilation**: includes inhibition of Edinger-Westphal nucleus through hypothalamic connections via reticular activating system and activation of sympathetic fibers

4. **Argyl Robertson pupils**: due to lesion of fibers that pass from pretectal area of midbrain to Edinger-Westphal nucleus; however, only the anteriorly placed fibers subserving the light reflex are involved, whereas posterior fibers responsible for near-vision reflex are unaffected

   a. Thus, retina is sensitive to light (patient can see), but pupils do not constrict in response to light stimuli

   b. Accommodation is intact because this pathway does not utilize pretectal area but involves visual stimulation of cortical areas and an undefined pathway from cortex to Edinger-Westphal nucleus of oculomotor complex

   c. Effect is almost always bilateral

5. Lesions of ciliary ganglion (**tonic pupil**; **Holmes-Adie**, or **Adie syndrome**): pupil tends to be large and fails to contract or shows very slow, delayed constriction to light; similar response seen with near vision in which pupil slowly contracts and remains small for some time before returning to normal size

B. Lesion of oculomotor nerve

1. Eye moves inferiorly and laterally (down and out), leading to double vision (lateral rectus and superior oblique muscles are only extraocular muscles innervated)

2. Severe ptosis (loss of levator palpebrae superioris muscle)

3. Dilated pupil and inability to accommodate for near vision (loss of parasympathetic fibers to sphincter pupillae and ciliary muscles

4. Slight prominence of eye (loss of tone of orbital muscles)

5. Pupillary reflex on side of lesion is lost

6. Symptoms will vary in degrees depending on how much of nerve has been traumatized

7. In any pathology of CN III, expect vascular pathology in area of cavernous sinus or posterior cerebral or superior cerebellar arteries to be involved

8. Oculomotor nerve compression: rapidly rising intracranial pressure (i.e., due to an extradural hematoma) commonly compresses CN III against crest of petrous temporal bone

   a. Because parasympathetic fibers in CN III are superficial, they are affected 1st

   b. Results in pupil on injured side dilating progressively, and there is ipsilateral slowness of pupillary response to light

9. Aneurysm of posterior cerebral or superior cerebellar artery may exert pressure on CN III as it passes between vessels; clinical findings depend on degree of pressure

10. Because CN III is located in lateral wall of cavernous sinus, injuries or infections of sinus also affect nerve

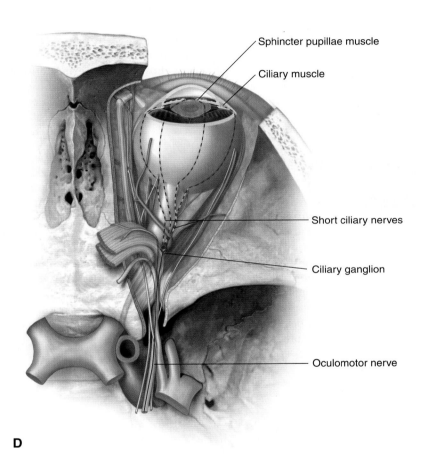

Sphincter pupillae muscle

Ciliary muscle

Short ciliary nerves

Ciliary ganglion

Oculomotor nerve

D

Figure 3.18D. Oculomotor Nerve, Parasympathetic Distribution, Superior View.

Cranial Nerve IV: Trochlear Nerve

I. General Features of Trochlear Nerve (CN IV)

A. Smallest CN

B. Only CN to arise from posterior surface of brainstem

C. Carries somatic motor fibers (general somatic efferent) for 1 voluntary muscle controlling eye movement, superior oblique muscle

II. Origin, Course, and Branches (Fig. 3.19A–C)

A. Arises from posterior surface of midbrain behind quadrigeminal plate and passes anteriorly around sides of cerebral peduncles of midbrain, inferior and parallel to tentorium cerebelli (behind CN III)

B. Penetrates undersurface of tentorium cerebelli posterolateral to its attachment to posterior clinoid process to enter upper lateral wall of cavernous sinus

C. Passes through superior orbital fissure above common ring tendon, crosses medially over origin of levator palpebrae superioris to supply 1 voluntary muscle (no smooth muscle) in orbit, the superior oblique, which it enters from above and laterally

D. Branches: none

III. Clinical Considerations

A. If interrupted, patient cannot move eye laterally and inferiorly
   1. Eye moves in opposite direction when movement in above direction is attempted, resulting in diplopia (double vision)
   2. Patient may hold head in such a position as to prevent diplopia

B. Proximity of nerve to posterior cerebral and superior cerebellar arteries and to cavernous sinus should be considered as possible source of any pathology

C. Superior oblique muscle is primary muscle producing intorsion of eyeball; primary muscle producing extorsion is inferior oblique; if superior oblique is unopposed, direction of gaze and rotation of eyeball about its anteroposterior axis becomes different for the 2 eyes when attempt is made to look down and medially

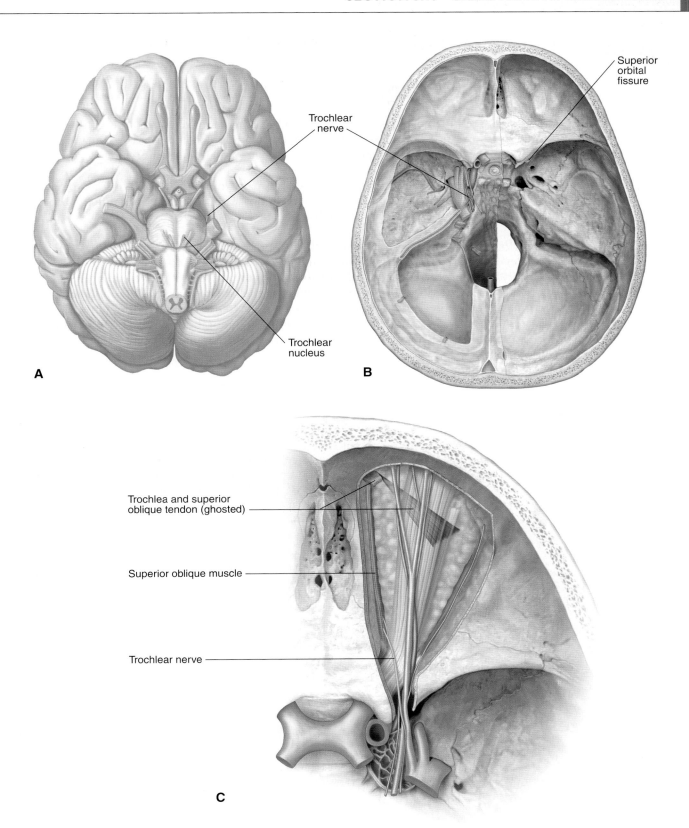

Figure 3.19A–C. Trochlear Nerve. **A.** Origin from Brain. **B.** Exit from Skull. **C.** Distribution, Superior View.

Cranial Nerve V: Trigeminal Nerve

I. General Features of Trigeminal Nerve (CN V)

A. Largest CN

B. 3 divisions: ophthalmic, maxillary, and mandibular nerves or divisions

C. All 3 divisions carry somatic sensory fibers; only mandibular nerve carries somatic motor fibers for 8 voluntary muscles controlling jaw movements or embryologically related structures

D. All 3 divisions have at least 1 branch that carries parasympathetic fibers to some target in head; however, these parasympathetic fibers do not arise within trigeminal nerve but are delivered to its branches from other CNs (namely CN VII or IX)

II. Origin, Course, and Branches (Fig. 3.20A,B)

A. Nuclei of origin: 4 trigeminal nuclei; 1 motor (motor nucleus of trigeminal nerve) and 3 sensory (mesencephalic, principal sensory, and spinal nucleus of trigeminal nerve)

B. Arises from lateral side of pons (near middle cerebellar peduncle) by 50 root filaments

C. Forms 2 roots: large sensory root (portio major); small motor root (portio minor)

D. Passes anteriorly over anteromedial tip of petrous temporal bone and under attachment of tentorium cerebelli to petrous ridge to reach trigeminal ganglion (semilunar, or Gasserian)

E. Trigeminal ganglion

   1. Largest sensory ganglion in body

   2. Lies under meningeal dura in trigeminal impression (cavum trigeminale) on apex of petrous temporal bone in middle cranial fossa

F. Branches (Fig. 3.20C,D)

   1. 3 divisions arise from trigeminal ganglion

   2. Ophthalmic and maxillary nerves (CNs V_1 and V_2) pass anteriorly in lateral wall of cavernous sinus; mandibular nerve (CN V_3) passes inferiorly through foramen ovale

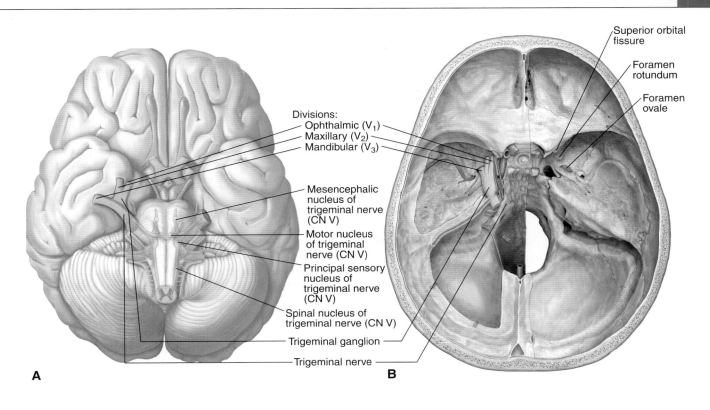

Divisions:
Ophthalmic (V₁)
Maxillary (V₂)
Mandibular (V₃)

Mesencephalic nucleus of trigeminal nerve (CN V)

Motor nucleus of trigeminal nerve (CN V)

Principal sensory nucleus of trigeminal nerve (CN V)

Spinal nucleus of trigeminal nerve (CN V)

Trigeminal ganglion

Trigeminal nerve

A

Superior orbital fissure

Foramen rotundum

Foramen ovale

B

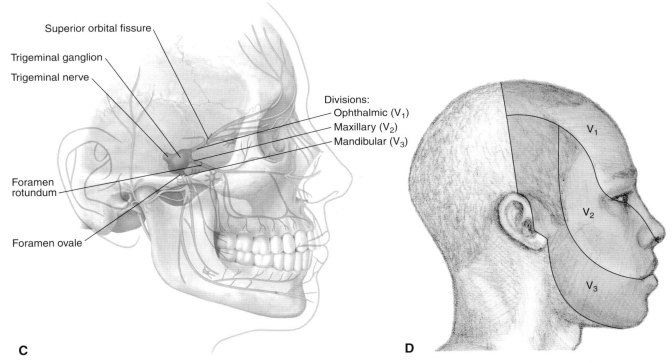

Superior orbital fissure

Trigeminal ganglion

Trigeminal nerve

Divisions:
Ophthalmic (V₁)
Maxillary (V₂)
Mandibular (V₃)

Foramen rotundum

Foramen ovale

C

V₁

V₂

V₃

D

Figure 3.20A–D. Trigeminal Nerve. **A.** Origin from Brain. **B.** Exit from Skull. **C.** Sensory Distribution, Lateral View. **D.** Dermatome Distribution, Lateral View.

III. Divisions of Trigeminal Nerve

A. Ophthalmic nerve (CN V$_1$) (Fig. 3.20E,F)

   1. Carries somatic sensory fibers only (although it has branch that may carry parasympathetic secretomotor fibers briefly)

   2. In contrast to other 2 CN V divisions, it does not supply derivatives of a branchial arch, but supplies structures derived from paraxial mesoderm of embryonic frontonasal process

   3. Passes anteriorly from trigeminal ganglion within lateral wall of cavernous sinus and branches into 3 nerves before passing into orbit through superior orbital fissure (small meningeal branch supplies tentorium cerebelli, falx cerebri, and adjacent dura)

   4. Branches

     a. **Frontal nerve**

       i. Largest branch of ophthalmic nerve

       ii. Enters orbit through superior orbital fissure above common ring tendon; runs anteriorly beneath periorbita as most superior structure in orbit

       iii. Divides into supraorbital and supratrochlear nerves

         a) **Supraorbital nerve**: larger and lateral, passes through supraorbital notch or foramen and supplies skin of forehead as far superiorly as vertex and skin and conjunctiva of upper eyelid

         b) **Supratrochlear nerve**: smaller and medial; runs anteriorly in position above trochlea of superior oblique muscle; leaves orbit to supply medial side of upper eyelid and conjunctiva and root of nose and skin of medial part of forehead

     b. **Lacrimal nerve** (Fig. 3.20G)

       i. Enters orbit by passing through superior orbital fissure above common ring tendon

       ii. Passes anterolaterally within orbit above lateral rectus muscle and into region of lacrimal gland to reach skin of upper eyelid and conjunctiva laterally

       iii. Near or adjacent to lacrimal gland, it often receives communicating branch from zygomaticotemporal nerve carrying postsynaptic parasympathetic fibers from pterygopalatine ganglion and postsynaptic sympathetic fibers from internal carotid plexus to lacrimal gland

     c. **Nasociliary nerve**

       i. Enters orbit via superior orbital fissure within common ring tendon between 2 divisions of CN III

       ii. Passes anteromedially between superior rectus muscle and optic nerve to end as anterior ethmoidal and infratrochlear nerves

       iii. Branches

         a) Sensory root to ciliary ganglion: for conjunctiva of eyeball

         b) **Long ciliary nerves**: pass forward parallel and superomedial to optic nerve to enter back of eyeball; run forward within eyeball to be sensory to conjunctiva

         c) **Posterior ethmoidal nerve**: passes medially between superior oblique and medial rectus muscles to leave orbit via posterior ethmoidal foramen and enter ethmoidal air cells; sensory to posterior ethmoid air cells and sphenoid sinus

         d) **Anterior ethmoidal nerve**: 1 of terminal branches of nasociliary nerve; passes medially between superior oblique and medial rectus muscles to leave orbit via anterior ethmoidal foramen and enter anterior cranial fossa on cribriform plate; passes anteriorly over plate, gives off a meningeal branch, and leaves cranial fossa to enter nasal cavity, where it gives off branches to septum and lateral wall and then continues anteriorly and inferiorly to emerge between nasal bone and nasal cartilage and finally terminates as **external nasal branch** supplying skin on lower half of nose

         e) **Infratrochlear nerve**: 1 of terminal branches of nasociliary; continues anteriorly and leaves orbit at point above medial angle of eye; supplies upper half of nose, upper medial eyelid, lacrimal sac, and lacrimal caruncle

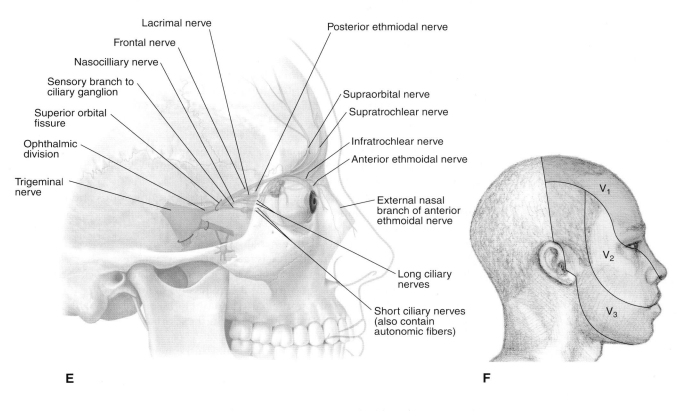

Lacrimal nerve

Frontal nerve

Nasocilliary nerve

Sensory branch to
ciliary ganglion

Superior orbital
fissure

Ophthalmic
division

Trigeminal
nerve

Posterior ethmiodal nerve

Supraorbital nerve

Supratrochlear nerve

Infratrochlear nerve

Anterior ethmoidal nerve

External nasal
branch of anterior
ethmoidal nerve

Long ciliary
nerves

Short ciliary nerves
(also contain
autonomic fibers)

E

V_1

V_2

V_3

F

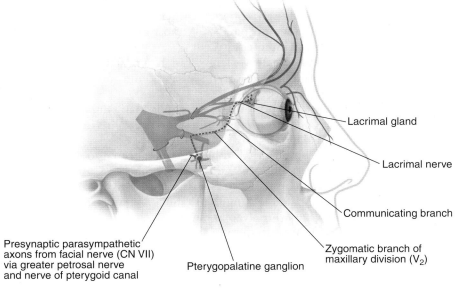

Presynaptic parasympathetic
axons from facial nerve (CN VII)
via greater petrosal nerve
and nerve of pterygoid canal

Pterygopalatine ganglion

Lacrimal gland

Lacrimal nerve

Communicating branch

Zygomatic branch of
maxillary division (V_2)

G

Figure 3.20E–G. Ophthalmic Nerve. **E.** Sensory Distribution. **F.** Dermatome Distribution. **G.** Associated
Parasympathetic Fibers.

B. Maxillary nerve (CN V$_2$) **(Fig. 3.20H,I)**
  1. Carries sensory fibers only; although many branches carry postsynaptic parasympathetic secretomotor fibers from pterygopalatine ganglion to mucous glands of nasal and oral cavities and to lacrimal gland
     a. Carries taste fibers from palate via palatine nerves to nerve of pterygoid canal and greater petrosal nerve to geniculate ganglion of facial nerve
     b. Innervates derivatives of maxillary prominence of 1st pharyngeal arch
  2. Arises from anterior margin of trigeminal ganglion to pass forward within lateral wall of cavernous sinus inferior to ophthalmic nerve; leaves middle cranial fossa by passing through foramen rotundum to enter pterygopalatine fossa, where it ends by branching (small meningeal branch is given off within middle cranial fossa to adjacent dura)
  3. Branches
     a. **Pterygopalatine nerves** **(Fig. 3.20J)**
        i. Connect maxillary nerve with pterygopalatine ganglion below it
        ii. Carry sensory fibers to pterygopalatine ganglion and postsynaptic parasympathetic fibers back to maxillary nerve
        iii. Small orbital branches pass forward into orbit and sphenoid sinus and posterior ethmoid air cells to innervate mucous glands
     b. **Greater palatine nerve**
        i. Descends within greater palatine canal to reach greater palatine foramen and distribute to mucosa of hard palate as far anteriorly as incisor teeth
        ii. Branches: posterior inferior lateral nasal branches distribute to mucosa of lateral nasal wall over middle and inferior nasal concha and meatuses
        iii. Carries sensory and postsynaptic parasympathetic secretomotor fibers from pterygopalatine ganglion to mucous glands in these areas
     c. **Lesser palatine nerve**
        i. Passes inferiorly within greater palatine canal and emerges from lesser palatine foramina to distribute to mucosa of soft palate and palatine tonsil
        ii. Carries sensory (somatic and taste) and postsynaptic parasympathetic secretomotor fibers from pterygopalatine ganglion to mucous glands in these areas
     d. **Posterior superior lateral nasal nerve**
        i. Passes through sphenopalatine foramen to distribute to mucosa of upper posterior lateral nasal wall, most of nasal septum, and small portion of hard palate behind incisor teeth
        ii. **Nasopalatine nerve:** large branch of posterior superior lateral nasal nerve, which passes anteroinferiorly on nasal septum and through incisive canal to reach hard palate
        iii. Carries sensory and postsynaptic parasympathetic secretomotor fibers from pterygopalatine ganglion to mucous glands in these areas
     e. **Pharyngeal nerve**
        i. Passes posteriorly within pharyngeal canal to distribute to mucosa of sphenoid sinus, nasopharynx, and auditory tube
        ii. Carries sensory and postsynaptic parasympathetic secretomotor fibers from pterygopalatine ganglion to mucous glands in these areas
     f. **Posterior superior alveolar nerve**
        i. Passes inferolaterally through pterygomaxillary fissure to enter posterior alveolar canal on back of maxilla
        ii. Carries sensory fibers to upper molar teeth and gingivae and mucosa of posterior maxillary sinus and postsynaptic parasympathetic secretomotor fibers to mucosa in these areas

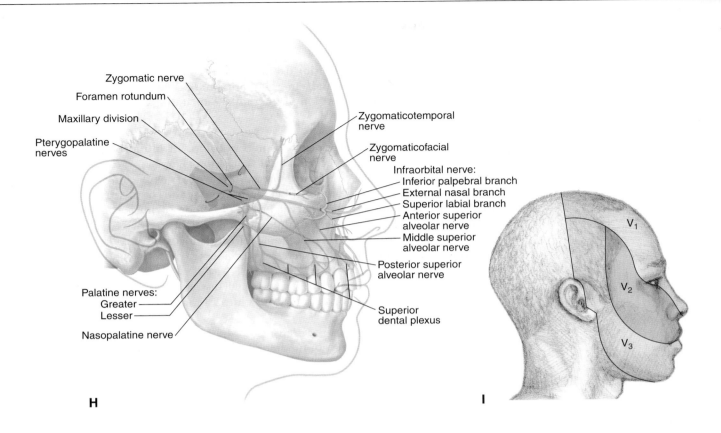

Zygomatic nerve
Foramen rotundum
Maxillary division
Pterygopalatine nerves

Zygomaticotemporal nerve
Zygomaticofacial nerve
Infraorbital nerve:
  Inferior palpebral branch
  External nasal branch
  Superior labial branch
  Anterior superior alveolar nerve
  Middle superior alveolar nerve
Posterior superior alveolar nerve

Palatine nerves:
  Greater
  Lesser
Nasopalatine nerve

Superior dental plexus

V_1
V_2
V_3

H

I

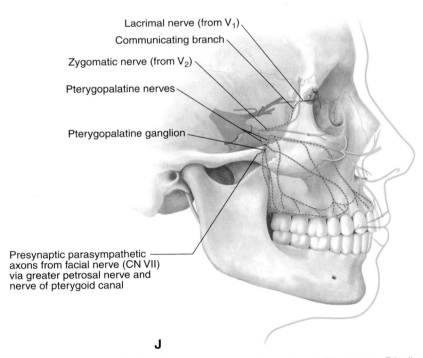

Lacrimal nerve (from V_1)
Communicating branch
Zygomatic nerve (from V_2)
Pterygopalatine nerves
Pterygopalatine ganglion

Presynaptic parasympathetic axons from facial nerve (CN VII) via greater petrosal nerve and nerve of pterygoid canal

J

Figure 3.20H–J. Maxillary Nerve. **H.** Sensory Distribution. **I.** Dermatome Distribution. **J.** Associated Parasympathetic Fibers.

g. **Infraorbital nerve**
   i. Largest branch of maxillary nerve and largest cutaneous branch of trigeminal nerve
   ii. Passes anteriorly through inferior orbital fissure to enter floor of orbit and lie in infraorbital groove and canal, emerging onto midface at infraorbital foramen to supply sensory fibers from skin of the midface including lower eyelid, lateral nose, and upper lip
   iii. Branches
      a) **Middle superior alveolar nerve**: penetrates floor of infraorbital groove to descend along inner aspect of lateral wall of maxillary sinus; carries sensory fibers from premolar teeth and mucosa of maxillary sinus and postsynaptic parasympathetic secretomotor fibers to mucous glands of this area
      b) **Anterior superior alveolar nerve**: penetrates floor of infraorbital canal to descend along inner aspect of anterolateral wall of maxillary sinus; carries sensory fibers from incisor and canine teeth and mucosa of maxillary sinus and postsynaptic parasympathetic secretomotor fibers to mucous glands of this area

h. **Zygomatic nerve**
   i. Passes anterolaterally through inferior orbital fissure to reach floor of orbit, passes onto lateral wall of orbit and divides into 2 branches
   ii. Branches
      a) **Zygomaticofacial nerve**: penetrates zygomatic bone to emerge at zygomaticofacial foramen onto cheek to supply sensory fibers from skin of this area
      b) **Zygomaticotemporal nerve**: gives off communicating branch to lacrimal gland before penetrating lateral margin of orbit to emerge at sphenozygomatic suture or zygomaticoorbital foramen; carries sensory fibers from skin over lateral orbital margin
      c) Communicating branch to lacrimal gland: usually given off by zygomaticotemporal nerve; passes superiorly to reach lacrimal gland, sometimes joining lacrimal nerve adjacent to gland; carries postsynaptic parasympathetic secretomotor fibers from pterygopalatine ganglion and postsynaptic sympathetic fibers from internal carotid plexus to lacrimal gland

i. **Pterygopalatine ganglion**
   i. Hangs below maxillary nerve within pterygopalatine fossa, suspended from it by pterygopalatine nerves
   ii. Receives presynaptic parasympathetic fibers and postsynaptic sympathetic fibers from nerve of pterygoid canal which joins it from posterior; nerve of pterygoid canal represents union of greater petrosal nerve from facial nerve (carrying presynaptic parasympathetic fibers) and deep petrosal nerve from internal carotid plexus (carrying postsynaptic sympathetic fibers)
   iii. Supplies postsynaptic autonomic fibers to all branches of maxillary nerve to supply mucous glands and lacrimal gland (parasympathetic) and vascular smooth muscle, sweat glands, and arrector pili muscles (sympathetic) of nasal and upper oral cavities and skin of midface

C. Mandibular nerve (CN V$_3$) **(Fig. 3.20K,L)**
   1. Largest division of trigeminal nerve; innervates derivatives of mandibular prominence of 1st pharyngeal arch
   2. Carries motor root of trigeminal nerve; only division of trigeminal to carry both sensory and motor fibers
   3. Supplies 8 muscles associated with movements of the jaw or embryonic development of jaw
   4. Passes inferiorly from trigeminal ganglion through foramen ovale to enter infratemporal fossa and end as its branches; divides into anterior and posterior divisions
      a. Anterior division is primarily motor with 1 sensory branch
      b. Posterior division is primarily sensory with 1 motor branch

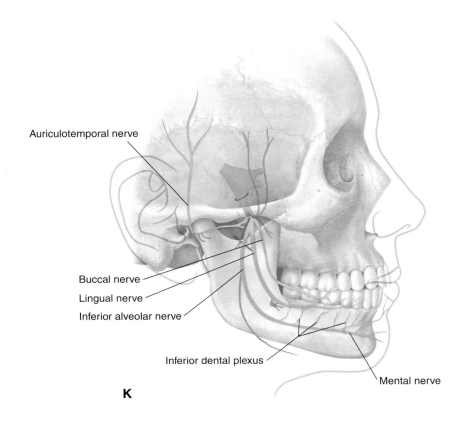

Auriculotemporal nerve

Buccal nerve

Lingual nerve

Inferior alveolar nerve

Inferior dental plexus

Mental nerve

K

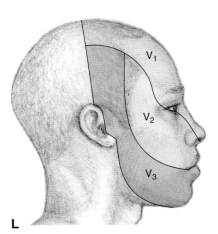

V_1

V_2

V_3

L

Figure 3.20K,L. Mandibular Nerve. **K.** Sensory Distribution. **L.** Dermatome Distribution.

5. Branches (Fig. 3.20M,N)
   a. Meningeal branch: from main trunk; passes superiorly through foramen ovale to carry sensory fibers to dura in middle cranial fossa
   b. **Nerve to medial pterygoid muscle**: from main trunk; passes anteromedially into medial pterygoid muscle to supply it; gives off branches to tensor veli palatini and tensor tympani muscles
   c. **Masseteric nerve**: from anterior division; passes laterally over mandibular notch to innervate masseter muscle
   d. **Deep temporal nerves**: anterior and posterior; from anterior division; pass laterally to turn superiorly at infratemporal crest and run deep to and innervate temporalis muscle
   e. **Nerve to lateral pterygoid muscle**: from anterior division; passes laterally to reach and innervate lateral pterygoid muscle
   f. **Buccal nerve**: from anterior division; passes anterolaterally between 2 heads of lateral pterygoid muscle, against insertion of temporalis muscle (usually passing through some of muscle), then continuing anteroinferiorly on lateral surface of buccinator muscle; some branches pass through buccinator to innervate mucosa of oral vestibule, whereas others pass to skin overlying buccal area
   g. **Auriculotemporal nerve**: from posterior division via 2 roots (sensory and parasympathetic) that encircle middle meningeal artery
      i. Passes on medial surface of TMJ capsule, which it innervates, then turns laterally behind joint capsule to reach root of zygomatic arch and deliver multiple postsynaptic parasympathetic secretomotor fibers from otic ganglion to parotid gland, then turns superiorly to run with superficial temporal vessels anterior to auricle
      ii. Supplies skin of anterosuperior portion of auricle and small area of scalp anterosuperior to auricle; supplies branches to external acoustic meatus and tympanic membrane

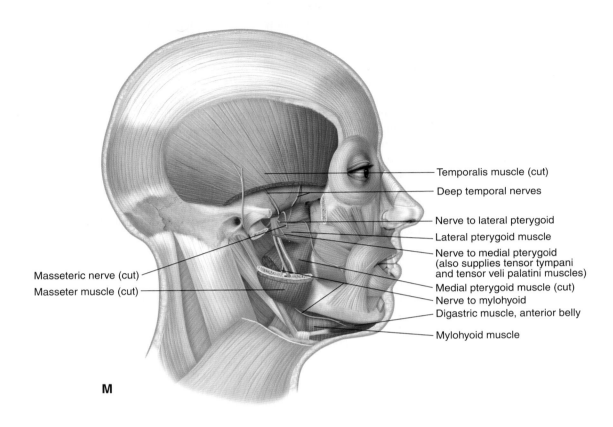

Temporalis muscle (cut)

Deep temporal nerves

Nerve to lateral pterygoid

Lateral pterygoid muscle

Nerve to medial pterygoid
(also supplies tensor tympani
and tensor veli palatini muscles)

Medial pterygoid muscle (cut)

Nerve to mylohyoid

Digastric muscle, anterior belly

Mylohyoid muscle

Masseteric nerve (cut)

Masseter muscle (cut)

M

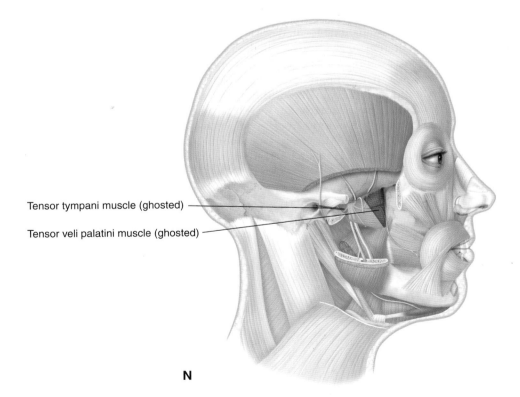

Tensor tympani muscle (ghosted)

Tensor veli palatini muscle (ghosted)

N

Figure 3.20M,N. Mandibular Nerve, Motor Distribution. **M.** Superficial. **N.** Deep.

h. **Lingual nerve**: from posterior division
  i. Passes inferoanteriorly on lateral surface of medial pterygoid muscle where it receives chorda tympani nerve from facial nerve carrying presynaptic parasympathetic fibers and taste fibers for anterior 2/3 of tongue
  ii. Passes below lower margin of superior pharyngeal constrictor muscle and enters paralingual space
  iii. Submandibular branches hang submandibular ganglion below nerve and deliver presynaptic parasympathetic fibers which synapse, some passing to submandibular gland and some rejoining lingual nerve to reach sublingual gland
  iv. Lingual nerve then crosses submandibular duct laterally then inferiorly to pass into tongue
  v. Carries sensory fibers from anterior 2/3 of tongue (and taste via chorda tympani)
i. **Inferior alveolar nerve**: from posterior division
  i. Passes inferoanteriorly lateral to sphenomandibular ligament toward mandibular foramen
  ii. Gives off slender **nerve to mylohyoid** muscle posteroinferiorly, which lies medially on mandibular ramus and inferior surface of mylohyoid muscle to reach anterior belly of digastric muscle
  iii. Inferior alveolar nerve then runs through mandibular canal, innervating all mandibular teeth and gingivae
  iii. Sends **mental nerve** through mental foramen to reach skin of chin
j. Parasympathetic ganglia associated with mandibular nerve: both concerned with innervation of salivary glands **(Fig. 3.20O)**
  i. **Otic ganglion**: lies on medial surface of mandibular nerve below foramen ovale
    a) Presynaptic fibers originate in tympanic branch of glossopharyngeal nerve, passes upward through inferior tympanic canaliculus, forms tympanic plexus on promontory of middle ear, then sends off lesser petrosal nerve which passes across middle cranial fossa, through foramen ovale to reach ganglion
    b) Postsynaptic parasympathetic secretomotor fibers travel in auriculotemporal nerve to reach parotid gland
  ii. **Submandibular ganglion**: located within posterior end of paralingual space, inferior to lingual nerve and connected to deep portion of submandibular gland via postsynaptic parasympathetic fibers
    a) Presynaptic parasympathetic fibers from facial nerve travel via chorda tympani to join lingual nerve within infratemporal fossa
    b) Postsynaptic parasympathetic secretomotor fibers reach submandibular gland (some presynaptic fibers synapse on diffuse ganglion cells within gland), while some postsynaptic parasympathetic fibers rejoin lingual nerve to travel anteriorly to reach and innervate sublingual gland

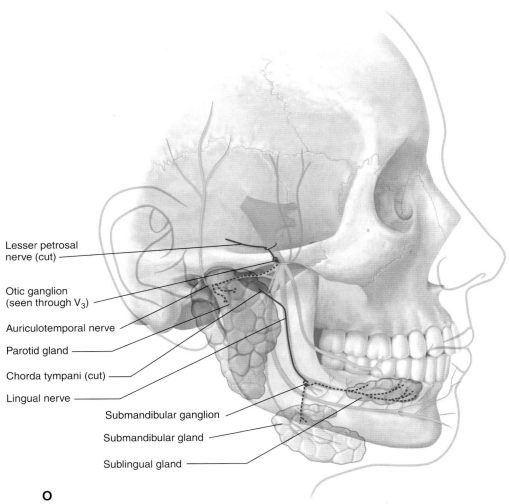

Lesser petrosal
nerve (cut)

Otic ganglion
(seen through V$_3$)

Auriculotemporal nerve

Parotid gland

Chorda tympani (cut)

Lingual nerve

Submandibular ganglion

Submandibular gland

Sublingual gland

O

Figure 3.20O. Mandibular Nerve, Associated Parasympathetic Fibers, Lateral View.

IV. Clinical Considerations

A. **Trigeminal neuralgia** (**tic douloureux**): condition of unknown cause associated with excruciating, severe, sharp, lightening-like jabs of facial pain, especially along maxillary and mandibular divisions of trigeminal nerve; can last for 15 minutes or more; may be severe enough to create psychological changes, leading to depression and even suicide; in conditions of intractable pain, may be relieved by alcohol injections either into trigeminal ganglion via foramen ovale or along root involved as it leaves skull; sometimes necessary to transect entire sensory part of nerve between ganglion and pons; motor division must be preserved, if possible, to avoid paralysis of muscles of mastication; fibers of ophthalmic division should also be preserved to retain corneal reflex because denervation of cornea invariably results in ulceration

   1. Paroxysms (sudden sharp pain) can be set off by touching face (special sensitive trigger zone is found around tip of nose or cheek), brushing teeth, shaving, drinking, or chewing
   2. Maxillary nerve (CN V_2) is most frequently involved
   3. Specific cause is uncertain
      a. In many cases, caused by pressure of small aberrant artery, and symptoms have disappeared with removal of vessel
      b. Suggested that it is a pathological process affecting neurons of trigeminal ganglion
      c. Cause may also be result of carious teeth, sinus disease, or irritating lesions in cranium
      d. Many treatments both medical and surgical have been used in attempt to alleviate pain
   4. Branches of trigeminal nerve on face communicate with branches of facial nerve (CN VII); thus, a lesion in the territory of trigeminal nerve may cause reflex spasm involving facial muscles and produce so-called facial "tic"

B. Entire trigeminal nerve lesion: results in widespread anesthesia to anterior half of scalp, face (except for area around angle of jaw, cornea, and conjunctivae) and mucous membranes of nose, mouth, and anterior part of tongue

   1. Paralysis of muscles of mastication of same side
   2. If only CN V_1 and V_2 are severed, loss is entirely sensory, but if CN V_3 is involved, there is sensory loss and paralysis of mastication

C. **Herpes zoster virus infection of trigeminal ganglion**: ganglion involvement seen in approximately 20% of cases and characterized by eruption of groups of vesicles, which tend to follow course of nerves

   1. Any nerve division can be involved, but most commonly ophthalmic nerve is affected
   2. Tends to involve cornea, resulting in painful corneal ulceration leading to scarring of cornea

D. Although all 4 cranial parasympathetic ganglia are located close to or on some branch of CN V, the presynaptic fibers to these ganglia actually come from other nerves: CNs III, VII, and IX; postsynaptic fibers join and are distributed with peripheral branches of trigeminal nerve (except for CN III)

E. **Testing of CN V**

   1. Includes evaluation of corneal reflex, sensation over face and scalp, motor function, and jaw jerk
   2. **Corneal reflex**: tested by light application of cotton to cornea

     a. Examiner pulls cotton head from applicator into fine, thin point, asks patient to look upward, and brings cotton toward eye from lateral position and gently touches cornea

     b. Should normally be prompt bilateral reflex closure of eyelids; response is compared on both sides, and patient asked if sensation seemed to be equal on the 2 sides

     c. Afferent loop of reflex is ophthalmic division of CN V; efferent reflex involves CN VII (to orbicularis oculi)

3. Face and scalp sensation: cotton is applied to forehead on 1 side, followed by similar application to other side, then to cheeks on both sides, and finally jaws on both sides

     a. Patient's responses are monitored, and patient also asked whether sensations appeared to be equal or otherwise on the 2 sides

     b. Test usually repeated using small, sharp pin with gentle application to ophthalmic, maxillary, and mandibular areas of both sides

4. Motor function: place fingers over temporalis muscles and ask patient to clench teeth or bite

     a. Muscle will be felt to contract on both sides

     b. Masseter muscle also thus tested

     c. Test pterygoids by having patient deviate jaw to 1 side against resistance; in unilateral lesions, jaw deviates toward side of lesion

5. **Jaw jerk**: place index finger in midline of patient's jaw and ask patient to open mouth approximately 30° and then relax

     a. Examiner then strikes index finger with reflex hammer, which should produce stretching of masseter and pterygoid muscles, followed by reflex contraction of these muscles, and jaw jerks toward closed position

     b. Reflex may be absent in normal individuals or may create minimal movement

     c. Reflex usually exaggerated in corticobulbar tract lesions above midpons

     d. Reflex is highest stretch reflex that can be tested in neurological examination (Note: normal jaw jerk with increased tendon reflexes in upper limbs suggests that lesion is located below pons, but above C5)

F. Pain referred from 1 branch of division to another of same division (i.e., infection in teeth may be referred to ear and TMJ, or pressure on tentorium cerebelli may be referred to forehead)

Cranial Nerve VI: Abducent Nerve

I. General Features of Abducent Nerve (CN VI)

A. Carries somatic motor fibers (general somatic efferent) to 1 muscle controlling movements of eyeball and lateral rectus

B. Most of its course lies beneath or within meningeal dura; has very short course through subarachnoid space

II. Origin, Course, and Branches (Fig. 3.21A–C)

A. Abducens nucleus: in pons near median plane

B. Arises at inferior border of pons just above medullary pyramids (pontine–medullary junction)

C. Passes anteriorly to pierce dura covering inferior petrosal sinus at anteromedial tip of petrous temporal bone, runs through notch below posterior clinoid processes, and enters cavernous sinus; lies lateral to internal carotid artery within sinus, then passes into orbit via superior orbital fissure within common ring tendon and buries itself into medial surface of lateral rectus muscle, which it innervates

D. Branches: none

III. Clinical Considerations

A. Testing of CN VI: have patient follow your finger with eyes, without any head movement; test both right and left eyes

    1. Any weakness in abducting (turning eye to outside) indicates some involvement of CN VI

    2. Diplopia often increases on attempted abduction and distant vision

B. Relation of nerve at its origin to anterior inferior cerebellar artery and to internal carotid artery in cavernous sinus makes it liable to vascular pathology

C. Closeness of nerve to superior edge of petrous portion of temporal bone may involve it in fractures of base of skull

D. When nerve is traumatized, patient's eye will be drawn medially due to unopposed action of CN III and medial rectus muscle, resulting in diplopia

E. Lesion of this nerve in pons produces internal strabismus at rest due to paralysis of lateral rectus muscle, diplopia at rest, and increased diplopia on attempting to gaze toward side of lesion

F. Destruction of nucleus of CN VI produces all of the above and in addition, is usually associated with CN VII paralysis on same side due to close association of CN VII to nucleus of CN VI in pons

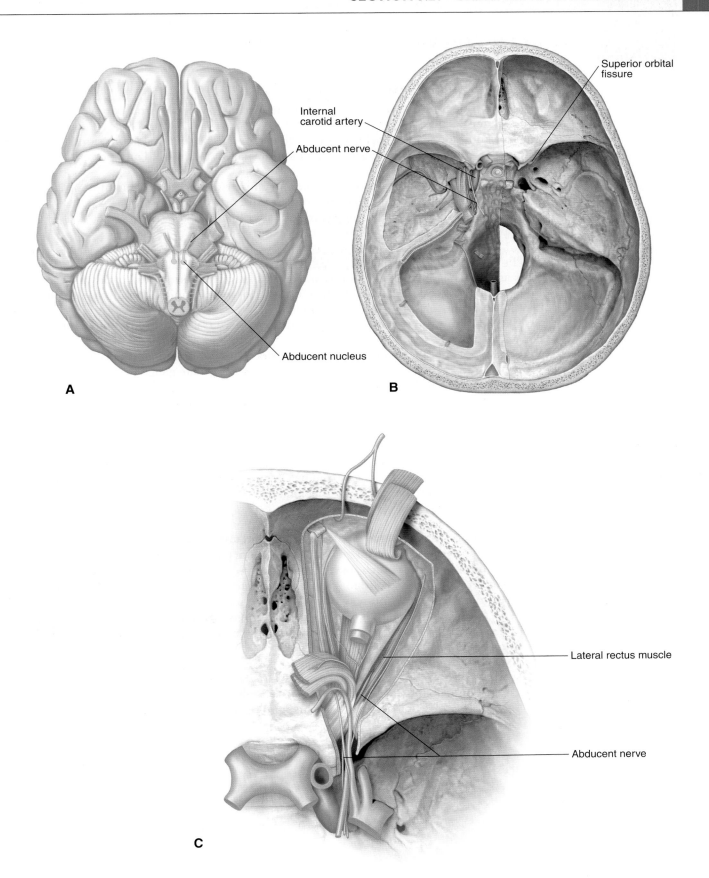

Figure 3.21A–C. Abducent Nerve. **A.** Origin from Brain. **B.** Exit from Skull. **C.** Distribution, Superior View.

Cranial Nerve VII: Facial Nerve

I. General Features of Facial Nerve (CN VII)

A. Arises by 2 roots: large voluntary motor and smaller mixed sensory and parasympathetic (**nervus intermedius**)

B. Primarily known for carrying somatic motor fibers for muscles of facial expression but also delivers these fibers to stapedius muscle in middle ear and stylohyoid and posterior belly of digastric muscle

    1. Carries presynaptic parasympathetic fibers that innervate lacrimal, submandibular, and sublingual glands and mucous glands of nasal and oral cavities

    2. Carries taste sensory fibers from palate and anterior 2/3 of tongue

    3. Supplies small area of skin of auricle near external acoustic meatus

II. Origin, Course, and Branches (Fig. 3.22A,B)

A. Arises as 2 roots: larger skeletal motor and smaller nervus intermedius (parasympathetic and taste) from lateral surface of medulla just inferior to pons and anterior to cerebellum (cerebellopontine angle) in company with CN VIII

B. Passes laterally in posterior cranial fossa and then above CN VIII as both enter internal acoustic meatus

    1. At end of meatus, bends in right angle in posterolateral direction and thus forms **genu** (bend) of CN VII (where its sensory ganglion, the **geniculate ganglion**, is located) and enters **facial canal** (lying in medial and posterior walls of tympanic cavity)

    2. Facial canal passes posterolaterally above oval window then bends inferiorly to deliver facial nerve at stylomastoid foramen

    3. Passes anteroinferiorly into parotid gland to end as branches to facial muscles

C. Geniculate ganglion

    1. Location: at bend of facial nerve as it enters facial canal

    2. Sensory ganglion: for taste fibers from palate and anterior 2/3 of tongue

    3. Greater petrosal nerve branches from geniculate ganglion

D. Branches (Fig. 3.22C–E)

    1. **Greater petrosal nerve**

        a. Carries presynaptic parasympathetic fibers and taste sensory fibers

        b. Passes anteromedially from geniculate ganglion; penetrates petrous temporal bone on floor of middle cranial fossa at hiatus for greater petrosal nerve (facial hiatus); continues anteromedially in groove for greater petrosal nerve to pass beneath trigeminal ganglion and across foramen lacerum to its anterior margin, where it enters pterygoid canal and fuses with **deep petrosal nerve** from internal carotid plexus, which carries postsynaptic sympathetic fibers, to form nerve of pterygoid canal

        c. **Nerve of pterygoid canal** (Vidian nerve) passes anteriorly to reach pterygopalatine ganglion within pterygopalatine fossa, where parasympathetic fibers synapse

        d. Postsynaptic parasympathetic fibers distribute on maxillary nerve branches to mucous glands of nasal and oral cavities and paranasal sinuses and to lacrimal gland in orbit; taste fibers reach palate

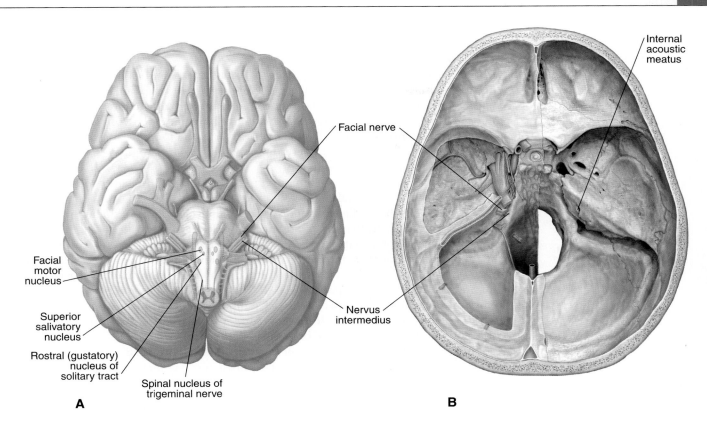

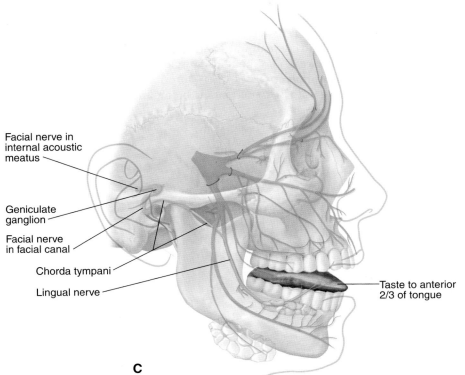

Figure 3.22A–C. Facial Nerve. **A.** Origin from Brain. **B.** Exit from Skull. **C.** Sensory Distribution, Lateral View.

2. **Nerve to stapedius muscle**: very small, leaves facial nerve in its descending part to supply muscle

3. **Chorda tympani**

   a. Leaves facial nerve in descending part of facial canal, arches superoanteriorly, enters tympanic cavity and passes across medial surface of tympanic membrane and handle of malleus, exits petrous bone through petrotympanic fissure and descends in infratemporal fossa to join posterior border of lingual nerve (from CN V_3)

   b. Carries taste sensory fibers from anterior 2/3 of tongue and presynaptic parasympathetic fibers that synapse in submandibular ganglion to innervate submandibular and sublingual glands

4. **Posterior auricular nerve**: below stylomastoid foramen; passes posteriorly to innervate posterior auricular and occipitalis muscles

5. **Nerves to posterior belly of digastric and stylohyoid muscles**: short branches near exit from stylomastoid foramen that innervate these muscles

6. Branches to muscles of facial expression: facial nerve passes anteroinferiorly into parotid gland and branches into 2 divisions, the temporofacial and cervicofacial divisions, which pass anteriorly within parotid gland lateral to retromandibular vein; 5 types of branches emerge from parotid gland

   a. **Temporal branches**: pass superiorly from temporofacial division across zygomatic arch to reach and innervate anterior and superior auricular muscles and frontalis, corrugator, and upper portion of orbicularis oculi muscles

   b. **Zygomatic branches**: pass anterosuperiorly from temporofacial division toward lateral corner of eye to innervate orbicularis oculi and zygomaticus major

   c. **Buccal branches**: pass roughly transversely anteromedially from both temporofacial and cervicofacial divisions, above and below parotid duct and usually communicating across duct; innervate facial muscles of midface, including buccinator, zygomaticus major and minor, levator labii superioris, levator anguli oris, nasalis, procerus, risorius, and upper fibers of orbicularis oris muscles

   d. **Marginal mandibular branch**: passes anteroinferiorly from cervicofacial division to cross facial vessels near premasseteric notch; roughly parallels lower border of mandible to curve upward and reach and innervate depressor anguli oris, depressor labii inferioris, and mentalis muscles

   e. **Cervical branch**: passes inferoanteriorly from cervicofacial division to lie deep to and innervate platysma muscle below angle of mandible

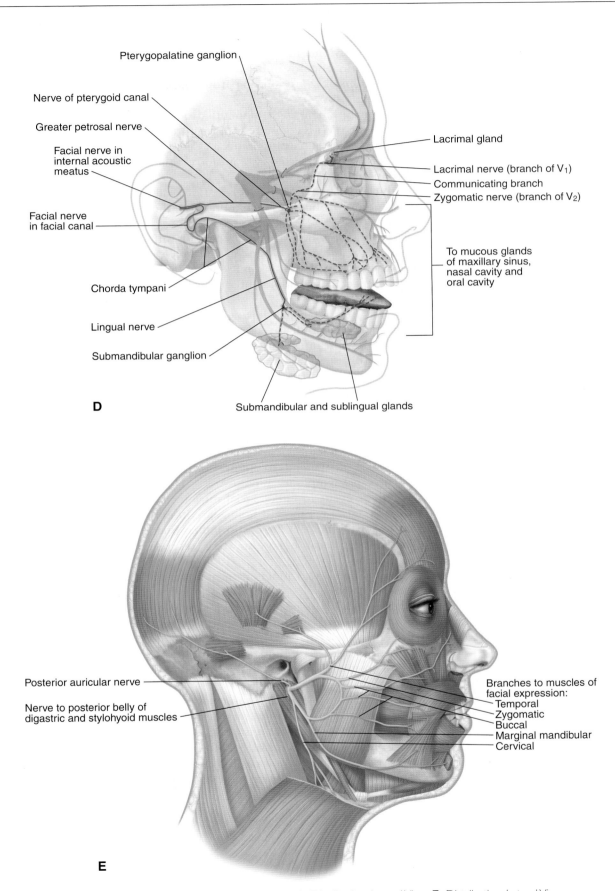

Pterygopalatine ganglion

Nerve of pterygoid canal

Greater petrosal nerve

Facial nerve in
internal acoustic
meatus

Facial nerve
in facial canal

Chorda tympani

Lingual nerve

Submandibular ganglion

Lacrimal gland

Lacrimal nerve (branch of V₁)

Communicating branch

Zygomatic nerve (branch of V₂)

To mucous glands
of maxillary sinus,
nasal cavity and
oral cavity

Submandibular and sublingual glands

D

Posterior auricular nerve

Nerve to posterior belly of
digastric and stylohyoid muscles

Branches to muscles of
facial expression:
Temporal
Zygomatic
Buccal
Marginal mandibular
Cervical

E

Figure 3.22D,E. Facial Nerve. **D.** Parasympathetic Distribution, Lateral View. **E.** Distribution, Lateral View.

III. Clinical Considerations

A. After leaving stylomastoid foramen, nerve runs forward in substance of parotid gland and is in jeopardy in parotid surgery

 1. Lacerations or contusions in parotid region may result in paralysis of facial muscles

 2. Eye remains open, angle of mouth droops, but forehead does not wrinkle

B. Damage to CN VII is common with fractures of temporal bone and is usually immediately detectable after injury

C. CN VII may also be affected by brain and cranial tumors, aneurysms, meningeal infections, and herpes viruses

D. In intracranial hematoma (stroke), forehead wrinkles because of bilateral innervation of frontalis muscle; otherwise, there is paralysis of contralateral facial muscles

E. **Bell's palsy**: symptoms exhibited by patients with lesions of facial nerve depend on whether pathology is located in supranuclear position (in fibers leading to facial nucleus), in facial nucleus itself, or infranuclear position (in facial nerve itself); even in latter case, symptoms will vary with location of lesion along nerve pathway

 1. If entire nerve is involved, patient will have dry eye (lack of lacrimal fluid), dryness of the mouth, hyperacusis due to loss of action of stapedius muscle, loss of taste on anterior 2/3 of tongue, paralysis of stylohyoid and posterior belly of digastric, and paralysis of all muscles of facial expression, leading to lowered eyebrow; distinct facial drooping; 1-sided smile; and inability to blink (conjunctiva usually becomes ulcerous), dilate nostrils, and contain food or saliva in mouth (drooling)

   a. All symptoms are ipsilateral (on side of lesion)

   b. Most lesions either occur to nerve in petrous part of temporal bone (due to fractures) or at stylomastoid foramen (classic Bell's palsy), where edema tends to put pressure on nerve (Note: most cases of Bell's palsy are temporary in nature)

 2. If lesions occur in either facial nucleus or its peripheral fibers, there is total unifacial paralysis; if lesions are in either the facial area of cerebral cortex or the descending corticobulbar fibers, only muscles below eye will be paralyzed because those above eye receive cortical fibers from both sides of brain

F. Exact distribution and function of many of the sensory fibers of the facial nerve are not known

 1. Some thought to be concerned with deep pain from face, some are apparently distributed to small part of soft palate, a few may reach middle ear cavity, a few cutaneous fibers are distributed to skin on posterior surface of the ear, along with similar fibers from CNs IX and X)

 2. Best-known sensory fibers in this nerve are those for taste on anterior 2/3 of tongue

 3. Although injuries to CN VII cause paralysis of facial muscles, sensory loss in small area of skin on posteromedial surface of auricle and around opening of external acoustic meatus is rare

 4. Hearing is not usually impaired, but ear may become more sensitive to low tones when stapedius muscle (supplied by CN VII) is paralyzed, because muscle functions to dampen stapes vibration

G. Testing of CN VII: patient asked to contract facial muscles and show teeth
   1. Contraction should be symmetric on both sides and performed simultaneously
   2. Patient then asked to close the eyes tightly, and examiner makes an effort to open the eyelids; normally this is not possible even with exertion of considerable force
   3. Then patient is asked to wrinkle forehead in an upward direction; this, too, should be symmetric on both sides
   4. Upper motor neuron lesions involving corticobulbar pathways: weakness of lower portion of face with normal function is seen when patient is asked to wrinkle forehead
   5. Involvement of facial nucleus in pons or facial nerve itself will produce total involvement of muscles of facial expression on same side, and lower facial muscles and forehead are equally involved
   6. Sense of taste: tested by placing test substance (sugar for sweet; vinegar for sour; and, possibly, quinine for bitter) on anterior part of tongue
      a. Patient asked to protrude tongue and expose 1 side; latter is dried and test substance that has been prepared in solution is gently applied with cotton applicator
      b. Patient should signal when substance is identified and can then draw tongue back into mouth and indicate what solution felt like; both sides can thus be tested independently
H. Due to divergent radiation of branches of facial nerve, surgeons prefer radial type incision for face operations because when trunk of nerve of 1 side is lost, all facial branches are affected and results in peripheral facial paralysis

Cranial Nerve VIII: Vestibulocochlear Nerve

I. General Features of Vestibulocochlear Nerve (CN VIII)

A. Consists of 2 roots: cochlear root (medial, for hearing) and vestibular root (lateral, for balance)

B. Carries sensory fibers only (special somatic afferent)

II. Origin, Course, and Branches (Fig. 3.23A–C)

A. Arises from upper lateral surface of brainstem (at cerebellopontine angle), passes laterally into internal acoustic meatus with CN VII; near lateral end of the meatus, it divides into its 2 parts, cochlear and vestibular

B. Each part of CN VIII has its own ganglion: cochlear ganglion and vestibular ganglion; the latter ganglion is further divided into 2 parts

   1. **Cochlear or spiral ganglion**: sensory fibers (special afferent fibers) come from the part connected with hearing (receptor cells of the spiral organ of Corti in the cochlea of the inner ear)

   2. **Vestibular ganglion** (both parts): sensory fibers (general somatic afferent) come from parts of the ear connected with balance (semicircular canals, saccule and utricle); nerve fibers from the receptor cells enter the ganglion in 2 parts, superior and inferior

     a. Superior part: carries fibers (utriculo-ampullar and lateral ampullar nerves) from the anterior and lateral semicircular ducts and a utricular nerve from the macula utriculi which passes with the anterior ampullary nerve

     b. Inferior part: carries fibers from the posterior semicircular duct via the posterior ampullary nerve and fibers from the macula sacculi via the saccular nerve

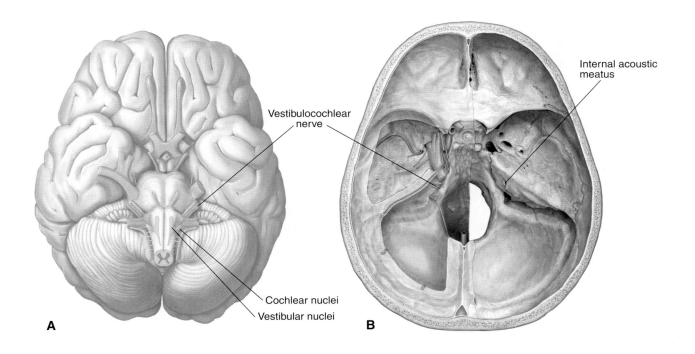

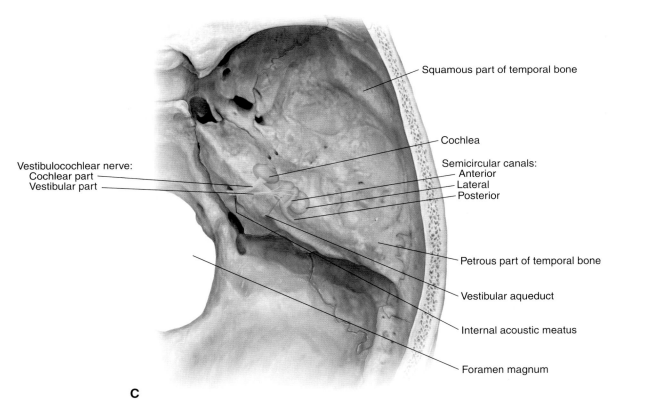

Figure 3.23A–C. Vestibulocochlear Nerve. **A.** Origin from Brain. **B.** Exit from Skull. **C.** Distribution, Superior View.

III. Clinical Considerations

A. Testing for hearing: requires audiograms and is not accurate at bedside

    1. **Conduction tests**: useful because normally, air conduction is more sensitive than bone conduction.

        a. **Rinne test**: tuning fork placed over mastoid process and patient asked to let you know when sound can no longer be heard

            i. At this point, fork placed at level of external acoustic meatus, and patient asked whether sound is audible; normally, this will be the case

            ii. Thus, a (+) test is when air conduction is more sensitive and a (−) test when reverse is true; this indicates some obstruction of sound transmission by disease that involves external acoustic meatus (i.e., foreign body or wax), eardrum malfunction, or middle ear problem

        b. **Weber test**: tuning fork placed on center of forehead, and patient asked to locate sound; it should be heard equally well in both ears or on forehead

            i. If air conduction impaired on 1 side, test lateralizes to that ear

            ii. If cochlea or cochlear nerve is involved, test will lateralize to side opposite diseased ear

    2. Diseases of cochlea or CN VIII: produce hearing impairment and both air and bone conduction are diminished, but Rinne test remains (+)

B. Vestibular function tests

    1. Vestibular system is very sensitive, and disturbances of function of system or vestibular part of CN VIII are usually accompanied by **vertigo** (sensation of movement in which objects seem to be moving in a rotating manner around subject or when subject has illusion of rotation); it is always accompanied by **nystagmus**, or involuntary rapid movement (horizontal, vertical, rotatory or mixed) of eyeball, due to connections of vestibular system with CNs III, IV, and VI via medial longitudinal fasciculus

    2. Tests usually performed

        a. **Barany test**: testing the semicircular canals by rotating the patient in a chair (10× in 20 sec) to produce stimulation of cristae in canals

            i. Eyes are closed, head is inclined forward 30° to test lateral canal or extended back 60° to test anterior canal

            ii. When chair is stopped rotating, inertia of endolymph continues to stimulate cristae, producing sensation of vertigo in opposite direction to rotation; accompanied by nystagmus, past-pointing, and eye deviation in direction of rotation

iii. Vertigo normally lasts about 35 seconds; reduced in disease of stimulated canal or vestibular nerve; increased in conditions that produce dysfunction of vestibular system

b. **Caloric testing**: tilt head of supine patient forward 30° (placing horizontal semicircular canal in horizontal position) and irrigate the external acoustic canal of 1 side with 5–10 cc of ice water or warm water for 30 seconds

   i. Effect of caloric stimulation is reduced in disease of canal, vestibular apparatus, vestibular nerve, or central connections

   ii. With ice water: normally, eyes will slowly deviate to ipsilateral side with quick correction return to midline; thus, because nystagmus is named for the fast movement, injecting in left ear leads to right nystagmus

   iii. With warm water: slow phase is to opposite side, and warm water in left ear leads to left nystagmus

   iv. With dysfunction of cerebral hemispheres, there is ipsilateral tonic deviation of eyes with cold water and contralateral tonic deviation with warm water (just the reverse of normal)

   v. With no caloric response, there is probably disruption of connections between vestibular nuclei, and CN VI nucleus is indicated

C. Lesions of CN VIII

   1. Usually result of fracture of petrous part of temporal bone (CN VII may also be involved), in which case permanent deafness can occur on affected side; or they can be inflammatory in nature, in which case, deafness may only be temporary; vertigo and nystagmus will usually occur in these cases due to involvement of vestibular part of the nerve

   2. Although vestibular and cochlear nerves are relatively independent, peripheral lesions tend to produce concurrent clinical effects due to their close relationship; thus, symptoms may result in **tinnitus** (noises in ear such as ringing or buzzing), vertigo (dizziness, loss of balance), and loss or impairment of hearing

D. **Acoustic neuroma** (tumor of the nerve): may lead to progressive unilateral hearing loss, and tinnitus

Cranial Nerve IX: Glossopharyngeal Nerve

I. General Features of Glossopharyngeal Nerve (CN IX)

A. Arises from side of medulla just above vagus nerve, by multiple small rootlets like vagus nerve

B. Carries somatic motor (branchial motor) for 1 muscle of pharynx, presynaptic parasympathetic fibers for parotid gland, taste sensory fibers for posterior 3rd of tongue, general sensory fibers for posterior 3rd of tongue, palatine tonsil, auditory tube, middle ear, and oropharynx, and special sensory fibers from carotid body and sinus

II. Origin, Course, and Branches (Fig. 3.24A,B)

A. Small nerve arising from 5 or 6 rootlets from side of medulla oblongata between inferior cerebellar peduncle and inferior olive, in line with rootlets of CN X

  1. Passes laterally in posterior cranial fossa and through jugular foramen to enter carotid sheath; just below base of skull it bears 2 ganglia close together, **superior** (**jugular**) and **inferior** (**petrosal**)

  2. Below ganglia, it passes inferolaterally to leave carotid sheath and pass obliquely posterolaterally around stylopharyngeus muscle to reach base of tongue and end as branches to tongue and oropharynx

B. Branches (Fig. 3.24C,D)

  1. Tympanic branch

    a. Carries presynaptic parasympathetic fibers for parotid gland

    b. Immediately below jugular foramen, passes up through inferior tympanic canaliculus to enter tympanic cavity and form tympanic plexus on promontory with postsynaptic sympathetic fibers from superior cervical ganglion

    c. **Lesser petrosal nerve**: arises from upper part of tympanic plexus and passes through hiatus of lesser petrosal nerve in petrous temporal bone to pass anteromedially across floor of middle cranial fossa; passes through foramen ovale to reach **otic ganglion** on medial surface of mandibular nerve (CN V_3)

    d. Postsynaptic parasympathetic fibers pass posteriorly from otic ganglion to join sensory fibers from mandibular nerve and form auriculotemporal nerve around middle meningeal artery

    e. Auriculotemporal nerve carries postsynaptic parasympathetic secretomotor fibers to parotid gland

  2. Carotid sinus nerve: passes vertically from carotid sinus and body to provide sensory feedback on blood pressure (carotid sinus) and blood gases (carotid body)

  3. Pharyngeal branches: several branches join pharyngeal plexus on pharyngeal wall; sensory from oropharynx primarily

  4. Nerve to stylopharyngeus: innervates muscle as it lies against it; only muscle innervated by IX and only muscle of pharynx not innervated by X

  5. Lingual branches: IX travels through lower portion of tonsilar fossa to reach tongue; carries general and taste sensory fibers from posterior 3rd of tongue

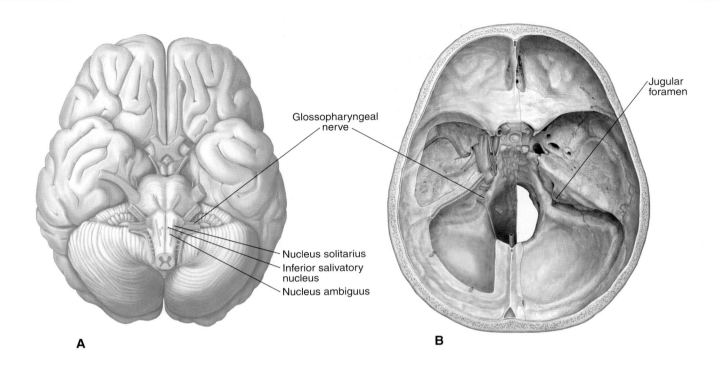

Glossopharyngeal
nerve

Nucleus solitarius

Inferior salivatory
nucleus

Nucleus ambiguus

Jugular
foramen

A

B

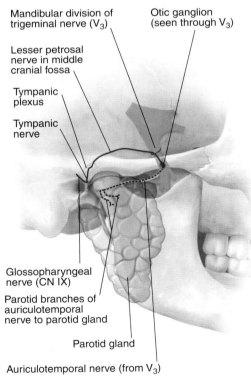

Mandibular division of
trigeminal nerve (V₃)

Otic ganglion
(seen through V₃)

Lesser petrosal
nerve in middle
cranial fossa

Tympanic
plexus

Tympanic
nerve

Glossopharyngeal
nerve (CN IX)

Parotid branches of
auriculotemporal
nerve to parotid gland

Parotid gland

Auriculotemporal nerve (from V₃)

C

Figure 3.24A–C. Glossopharyngeal Nerve. **A.** Origin from Brain. **B.** Exit from Skull. **C.** Parasympathetic
Distribution, Lateral View.

III. Clinical Considerations

A. Lesions of CN IX do not induce obvious symptoms in patients (assuming vagus is intact for contraction of pharyngeal constrictors)

B. **Jugular foramen syndrome**: injuries of CN IX are usually accompanied by signs of involvement of adjacent nerves; because CNs IX, X, and XI pass through jugular foramen, tumors there produce multiple CN palsies

C. Intactness of IX can be tested by afferent limb (CN IX) of gag reflex by stimulating pharyngeal wall (CN X forms efferent limb) or by testing for taste on posterior 3rd of tongue

D. Isolated brainstem lesion or deep laceration of neck: may result in loss of taste and sensation on posterior 3rd of tongue, changes in swallowing, absence of gag reflex on side of lesion, and deviation of palate toward unaffected side

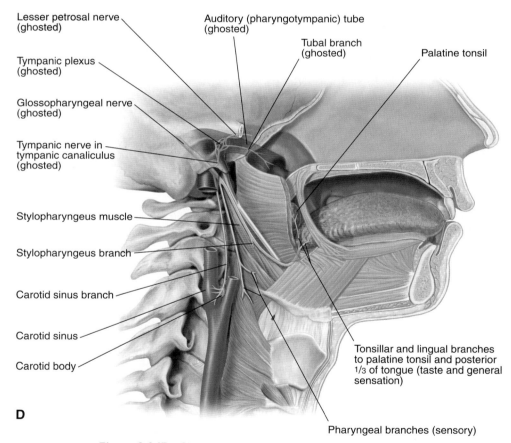

D

Figure 3.24D. Glossopharyngeal Nerve, Distribution, Lateral View.

Cranial Nerve X: Vagus Nerve

I. General Features of Vagus Nerve (CN X)

A. Longest cranial nerve: distributes to organs from neck to abdomen

B. Fiber types
   1. Somatic motor fibers to larynx, pharynx, soft palate, and upper 2/3 of esophagus
   2. Presynaptic parasympathetic fibers (visceral motor)
      a. Mucous glands in head, neck, thorax, and abdomen
      b. Glands of gastrointestinal (GI) tract and suprarenal gland
      c. Smooth muscle in GI and respiratory tracts, cardiac muscle
   3. Visceral sensory fibers from carotid body, base of tongue, pharynx, larynx, trachea, bronchi, lungs, heart, esophagus, stomach, and intestines
   4. Taste sensory fibers from epiglottis and palate
   5. Somatic sensory fibers: cutaneous sensation from small portion of external ear and external acoustic meatus and sensation from dura mater of posterior cranial fossa

II. Origin, Course, and Branches (Fig. 3.25A,B)

A. Arises by 8–10 rootlets emerging from lateral border (dorsolateral sulcus) of medulla between inferior cerebellar peduncle and inferior olive and posteroinferior to CN IX; rootlets join to form nerve as they pass through anteromedial part of jugular foramen, with CN XI just behind, in common dural sleeve

B. **Cranial accessory nerve**: fibers carry skeletal motor fibers that vagus delivers to larynx, pharynx, soft palate, and upper esophagus
   1. Traditionally, cranial portion of accessory nerve has been described as joining vagus nerve in or near jugular foramen
   2. However, current opinion assigns this cranial root as vagal fibers, without invoking any claim of accessory nerve ownership

C. 2 sensory ganglia: small superior (jugular) and large inferior sensory (nodose) ganglion located just below skull

D. Course (Fig. 3.25C)
   1. In neck: CN X passes downward in carotid sheath posteriorly between internal jugular vein and internal/common carotid artery; passes through superior thoracic opening between subclavian artery and brachiocephalic vein
   2. In chest (Fig. 3.25D)
      a. On right side, passes inferiorly on right side of trachea, then behind right main bronchus and medially posterior to esophagus, becoming plexiform with left vagus and forming esophageal plexus; passes through esophageal hiatus of diaphragm posterior and right of esophagus as posterior vagal trunk
      b. On left side, passes anterolateral to aortic arch and behind left main bronchus to course medially onto anterior surface of esophagus and become plexiform; passes through esophageal hiatus of diaphragm on anterior surface of esophagus as anterior vagal trunk
      c. Note: although most of posterior vagal trunk fibers are from right vagus and most of anterior vagal trunk is from left vagus, there is approximately 10% crossover
   3. In abdominal cavity: vagal trunks branch to distribute to stomach, liver, and gallbladder directly and join celiac and superior mesenteric plexuses to distribute perivascularly to gut structures as far distal as proximal 2/3 of transverse colon

E. **Branches**
  1. **Meningeal branch**: retrograde from its superior ganglion to dura in part of posterior cranial fossa
  2. **Auricular branch**: from superior ganglion through mastoid canaliculus to exit from tympanomastoid fissure and innervate skin that lines posterior inferior wall of external acoustic meatus and lower part of tympanic membrane
  3. **Pharyngeal nerves**: usually 2 branches from inferior (nodose) ganglion; run down between external and internal carotid arteries to side of pharynx to join pharyngeal plexus; send motor fibers to muscles of pharynx except stylopharyngeus (CN IX) and muscles of soft palate except tensor veli palatini (CN V_3)
  4. **Superior laryngeal nerve**: arises from inferior (nodose) ganglion and divides into external and internal branches
     a. **Internal branch**: mainly sensory; enters laryngopharynx by passing through thyrohyoid membrane; sensory and secretomotor to mucous membrane of upper part of larynx as far as vocal cords (origin of cough reflex), and to posterior surface of epiglottis and valleculae epiglottica
     b. **External branch**: motor to cricothyroid muscle and lower fibers of inferior pharyngeal constrictor muscle
  5. **Superior** and **inferior cervical cardiac branches**: superior branches near base of skull, inferior branches in root of neck; pass into thorax to join cardiac plexuses and innervate cardiac muscle
  6. **Recurrent laryngeal nerves**: recur around subclavian artery on right and arch of aorta and ligamentum arteriosum on left
     a. Course superiorly in tracheoesophageal groove to reach larynx; responsible for sensory and secretomotor supply to mucous membrane below vocal cords and motor supply to all muscles of larynx except for cricothyroid
     b. Branches also innervate trachea and upper esophagus, and several branches join cardiac plexuses
     c. Becomes **inferior laryngeal nerve** at lower border of cricoid cartilage
  7. **Thoracic cardiac branches**: several branches pass anteromedially to join cardiac plexuses
  8. **Pulmonary and bronchial branches**: multiple small branches form pulmonary plexus as vagus passes against posterior surface of lung root; pulmonary plexus passes through hilum to innervate mucous glands and bronchial smooth muscle of lung
  9. **Esophageal plexus**: formed by right and left vagus nerves on esophagus below level of lung roots; innervates smooth muscle and mucous glands of esophagus
  10. **Anterior vagal trunk**: formed as esophageal plexus passes through esophageal hiatus; primarily from left vagus nerve fibers
     a. **Anterior gastric branches**: spread onto anterior surface of stomach to supply smooth muscle and glands of stomach; 1 large gastric branch, anterior nerve of lesser curvature, reaches pylorus
     b. **Hepatic branches**: pass to liver and gallbladder in upper portion of hepatogastric ligament; gives pyloric branch inferiorly in hepatoduodenal ligament to pylorus
  11. **Posterior vagal trunk**: formed as esophageal plexus passes through esophageal hiatus; primarily from right vagus nerve fibers
     a. **Posterior gastric branches**: spread onto posterior surface of stomach to supply smooth muscle and glands of stomach; 1 large gastric branch, posterior nerve of lesser curvature, reaches pylorus
     b. **Celiac branches**: pass to celiac plexus on celiac trunk to become part of perivascular celiac plexus
        i. Anterior vagal trunk may also contribute celiac branches
        ii. From here, vagal fibers reach superior mesenteric and renal plexuses, innervating smooth muscle and glands of GI tract nearly to splenic flexure of transverse colon

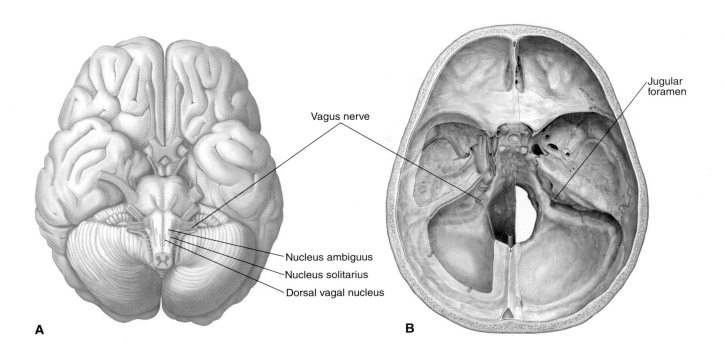

Vagus nerve

Nucleus ambiguus
Nucleus solitarius
Dorsal vagal nucleus

Jugular foramen

A

B

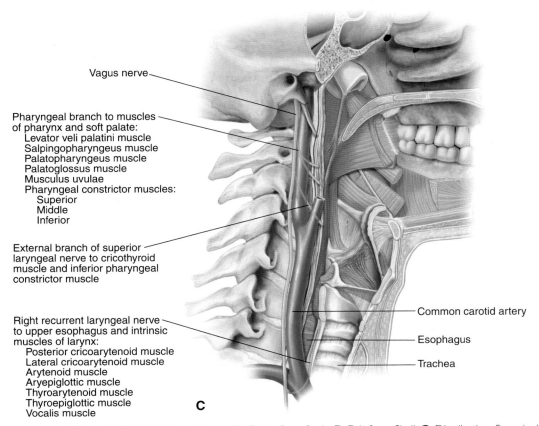

Vagus nerve

Pharyngeal branch to muscles
of pharynx and soft palate:
    Levator veli palatini muscle
    Salpingopharyngeus muscle
    Palatopharyngeus muscle
    Palatoglossus muscle
    Musculus uvulae
    Pharyngeal constrictor muscles:
        Superior
        Middle
        Inferior

External branch of superior
laryngeal nerve to cricothyroid
muscle and inferior pharyngeal
constrictor muscle

Right recurrent laryngeal nerve
to upper esophagus and intrinsic
muscles of larynx:
    Posterior cricoarytenoid muscle
    Lateral cricoarytenoid muscle
    Arytenoid muscle
    Aryepiglottic muscle
    Thyroarytenoid muscle
    Thyroepiglottic muscle
    Vocalis muscle

Common carotid artery

Esophagus

Trachea

C

Figure 3.25A–C. Vagus Nerve. **A.** Origin from Brain. **B.** Exit from Skull. **C.** Distribution, Superior View.

III. Clinical Considerations

A. Lesions of CN X

1. Not common, but do occur

2. Symptoms are usually palpitation accompanied by increased pulse rate, constant nausea, decreased rate of respiration, sensation of suffocation, and changes in speech; symptoms will vary depending on where the nerve is traumatized

   a. **Dysphonia** (difficulty in speaking): due to paralysis of larynx or vocal cords as result of lesion of recurrent laryngeal nerve

   b. **Dysarthria** (difficulty in articulation): leads to speech imperfection as result of weakness of soft palate (which gives nasal quality to the voice); voice is hoarse and volume is reduced

   c. With both nerves paralyzed, there is also **stridor** (harsh, high-pitched breath sounds) because of unrestricted action of the cricothyroid muscles and partial vocal cord paralysis, causing them to lie close together in midline

   d. Patient may complain of difficulty in swallowing (**dysphagia**)

3. Tests used to confirm lesion of CN X

   a. Efferent end of gag reflex is mediated by pharyngeal branches of vagus; test contraction of pharyngeal constrictors on touching pharyngeal wall

   b. Faulty movement of uvula: patient is asked to open the mouth and say "Ah"

      i. Normally, soft palate elevates symmetrically and uvula remains in midline

      ii. Unilateral CN X paralysis results in failure of palatal movement on 1 side; soft palate does not elevate on affected side, and uvula is drawn to opposite side by contraction and arching of palate on nonaffected side

   c. Paralyzed vocal cord on affected side as seen with laryngoscope

B. Irritations of auricular branch can be referred to larynx and commonly manifest as coughs or to gastric area, inducing nausea

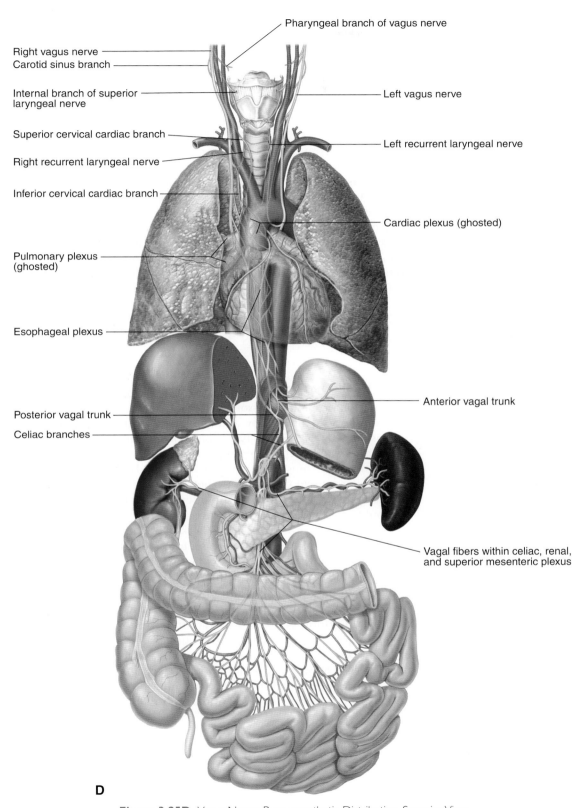

Pharyngeal branch of vagus nerve

Right vagus nerve

Carotid sinus branch

Internal branch of superior
laryngeal nerve

Left vagus nerve

Superior cervical cardiac branch

Left recurrent laryngeal nerve

Right recurrent laryngeal nerve

Inferior cervical cardiac branch

Cardiac plexus (ghosted)

Pulmonary plexus
(ghosted)

Esophageal plexus

Anterior vagal trunk

Posterior vagal trunk

Celiac branches

Vagal fibers within celiac, renal,
and superior mesenteric plexus

D

Figure 3.25D. Vagus Nerve, Parasympathetic Distribution, Superior View.

Cranial Nerve XI: Accessory Nerve

I. General Features of Accessory Nerve (CN XI)

A. Second longest cranial nerve (vagus is longest)

B. Carries somatic motor fibers to 2 muscles: SCM and trapezius muscles; does not carry proprioceptive sensory fibers from these muscles, so must rely on branches of cervical nerves C2–C4

II. Origin, Course, and Branches (Fig. 3.26A–C)

A. Traditionally said to arise from 2 sets of rootlets

B. Current opinion assigns cranial root to vagus nerve

    1. Cranial rootlets (vagal part): from nucleus ambiguus in lower medulla

       a. Exits in line with vagal rootlets in dorsolateral sulcus of medulla

       b. These join vagus nerve near brainstem and may be considered part of vagus nerve

       c. Carry somatic motor fibers for pharynx, larynx, and upper esophagus

    2. Spinal rootlets: from nucleus of accessory nerve in anterior horn of segments C1–C5 of spinal cord and ascend alongside spinal cord, between anterior and posterior roots

       a. Unite to form nerve as they ascend and enter the skull via foramen magnum; wraps margin of foramen magnum to pass through anteromedial part of jugular foramen with CNs IX and X

       b. Supplies 2 voluntary muscles: SCM and trapezius

III. Clinical Considerations

A. Examination of spinal accessory nerve

    1. Examine SCM muscle by asking patient to turn head to 1 side against resistance by examiner's hand; belly of the muscle can be felt to contract firmly if examiner palpates opposite side of neck

    2. Test trapezius muscle by placing both hands on patient's shoulders and palpating muscle on each side between thumb and forefinger; patient is asked to elevate or raise the shoulders against examiner's resistance; there should be equal muscle contraction bilaterally

B. Accessory nerve may be traumatized in skull fractures or by severe enlargement of lymph nodes in neck; in either case, **torticollis** (twisted neck) will result

    1. If nerve is only irritated, torticollis may result in chin being turned to opposite side (due to contraction of SCM on affected side)

    2. If nerve is paralyzed, head will turn toward lesion side, and patient cannot abduct upper limb beyond horizontal position

C. Superficial location of accessory nerve in posterior cervical triangle makes it liable to injury; patient cannot abduct upper limb beyond horizontal, but no torticollis is seen

    1. Paralysis of SCM and superior fibers of trapezius lead to shoulder drooping

    2. Accessory nerve is susceptible to injury during surgical procedures (i.e., lymph node biopsy, cannulation of internal jugular vein, carotid endarterectomy)

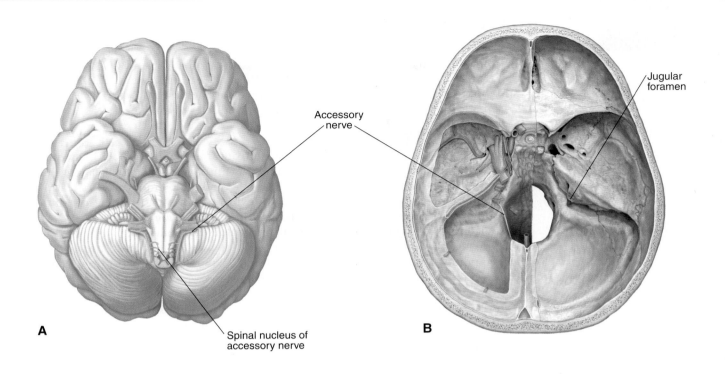

Accessory nerve

Jugular foramen

Spinal nucleus of accessory nerve

A

B

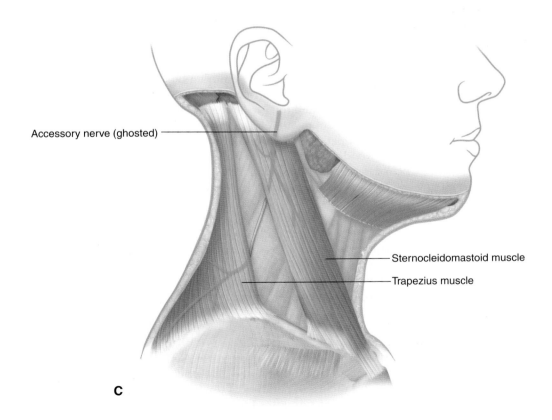

Accessory nerve (ghosted)

Sternocleidomastoid muscle

Trapezius muscle

C

Figure 3.26A–C. Accessory Nerve. **A.** Origin from Brain. **B.** Exit from Skull. **C.** Distribution, Lateral View.

Cranial Nerve XII: Hypoglossal Nerve

I. General Features of Hypoglossal Nerve (CN XII)

A. 3rd most inferiorly coursing CN (after vagus and accessory nerves)

B. Carries somatic motor fibers to intrinsic and extrinsic muscles of tongue

II. Origin, Course, and Branches (Fig. 3.27A–C)

A. Arises from hypoglossal nucleus (medulla) and exits from anterolateral surface of medulla, in anterolateral sulcus between olive and pyramid, by multiple rootlets that pierce dura mater at hypoglossal canal, unite to form nerve, and leave skull to enter carotid sheath

   1. Passes anteroinferiorly lateral to CN X to exit carotid sheath, then continues anteroinferiorly deep to posterior belly of digastric and stylohyoid muscles

   2. Crosses laterally over external carotid artery and is crossed superolaterally by occipital artery

B. Receives communication from cervical nerves C1 and C2 that forms superior root of **ansa cervicalis**, which leaves hypoglossal as it appears below lower border of posterior belly of digastric muscle

C. Passes into submandibular triangle on lateral surface of hyoglossus muscle and enters lowest portion of paralingual space to pass anteromedially into tongue to distribute to all extrinsic (styloglossus, hyoglossus genioglossus) and intrinsic muscles of tongue (Note: palatoglossus muscle is innervated by vagus nerve, because it is primarily soft palate muscle)

D. Branches: none

III. Clinical Considerations

A. Examination of hypoglossal nerve

   1. Inspect tongue with mouth open and tongue lying quietly on floor of mouth to observe involuntary movements (i.e., fasciculations, or small, local involuntary muscular contractions representing discharge fibers innervated by single motor nerve filaments)

      a. Note: protruded tongue always has some involuntary movement

      b. Also note any asymmetry (i.e., scarring or wasting); scarring is commonly seen in patients with generalized seizure disorders

   2. Place wooden tongue depressor, edge upward, in midline of tongue just below lower lip and ask patient to protrude tongue

      a. Normally, tongue is protruded and lies symmetrically on edge of tongue blade

      b. This permits detection of slight tongue deviations not seen if protrusion of tongue without clear midline indication is done

   3. Protruded tongue is examined for scars and condition of its mucous membrane

      a. **Glossitis** seen commonly in patients with vitamin deficiency

      b. **Atrophic mucous membrane** may indicate long-standing pernicious anemia due to vitamin B12 deficiency

   4. Patient is asked to move tongue back and forth rhythmically and as fast as possible

      a. Movement should be smooth and rhythmic

      b. Slowing or dysrhythmia is seen in weakness and in cerebellar dysfunction

B. If nerve is traumatized, paralysis of tongue on affected side occurs

   1. Tongue on that side loses bulk and when protruded turns toward side of lesion due to dragging effect of paralyzed muscles

   2. Moderate dysarthria (disturbance of speech) may also be evident

   3. If lesion is bilateral, patient has problems with swallowing and with speech (Note: all sensations for touch, temperature, and taste are intact)

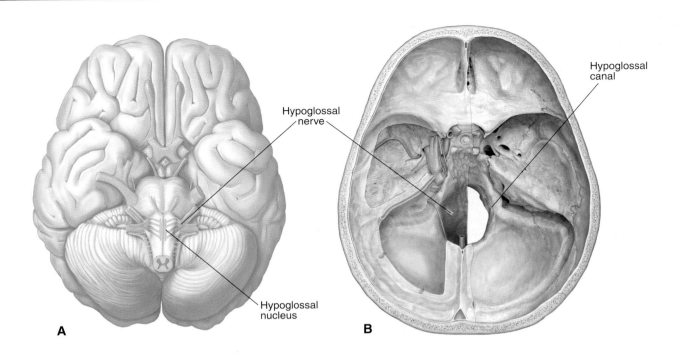

Hypoglossal
nerve

Hypoglossal
nucleus

A

Hypoglossal
canal

B

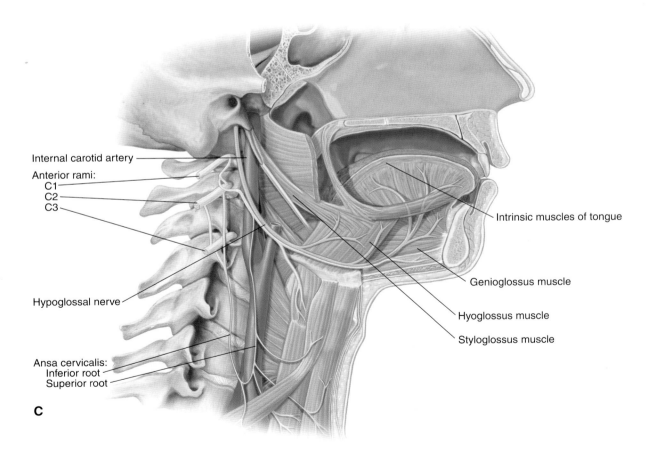

Internal carotid artery

Anterior rami:
C1
C2
C3

Hypoglossal nerve

Ansa cervicalis:
Inferior root
Superior root

C

Intrinsic muscles of tongue

Genioglossus muscle

Hyoglossus muscle

Styloglossus muscle

Figure 3.27A–C. Hypoglossal Nerve. **A.** Origin from Brain. **B.** Exit from Skull. **C.** Distribution, Superior View.

Summary of Arteries of Head and Neck

I. Common Carotid Artery

A. On right: branches from brachiocephalic trunk

B. On left: 2nd branch from aortic arch

C. Branches

    1. Bifurcates at level of superior border of thyroid cartilage

    2. Branches: external and internal carotid artery

II. External Carotid Artery (Fig. 3.28A)

A. Superior thyroid artery

    1. Supplies thyroid gland and larynx

    2. Branch: superior laryngeal artery

B. Lingual artery

    1. Supplies tongue

    2. Branches

        a. Dorsal lingual artery

        b. Deep lingual artery

        c. Sublingual artery

C. Facial artery

    1. Supplies face up to orbit

    2. Branches

        a. Ascending palatine artery

        b. Submental artery

        c. Inferior labial artery

        d. Superior labial artery

        e. Lateral nasal artery

        f. Angular artery

D. Ascending pharyngeal artery

    1. Supplies pharynx

    2. Branches

        a. Pharyngeal branches

        b. Palatine branch

        c. Inferior tympanic branch

        d. Meningeal branch

E. Occipital artery

    1. Supplies muscles of the neck and the posterior aspect of scalp

    2. Branches

        a. SCM branch: passes over hypoglossal nerve

        b. Meningeal branch

        c. Auricular branch

        d. Mastoid branch

        e. Descending branch: to posterior neck muscles

        f. Medial and lateral branches: to scalp

F. Posterior auricular artery

    1. Supplies muscles on base of skull, ear, and small area behind auricle

    2. Branches

        a. Parotid branches

        b. Stylomastoid branch: passes upward in facial canal to tympanic cavity

G. Superficial temporal artery

    1. Supplies auricle, upper parotid gland, masseter origin, temporalis, and lateral scalp

    2. Branches

        a. Transverse facial: forward below zygomatic arch

        b. Anterior auricular branches

        c. Middle temporal artery

        d. Frontal branch

        e. Parietal branch

H. Maxillary
  1. Supplies parotid gland, ear, meninges, muscles of mastication, nasal cavity, nasopharynx, midface, upper and lower teeth and gums, and palate
  2. Branches
      a. Deep auricular artery
      b. Anterior tympanic artery
      c. Middle meningeal artery
      d. Inferior alveolar artery
      e. Masseteric artery
      f. Anterior and posterior deep temporal arteries
      g. Pterygoid branches
      h. Buccal artery
      i. Posterior superior alveolar artery
      j. Infraorbital artery
      k. Pharyngeal artery
      l. Sphenopalatine artery
      m. Descending palatine artery

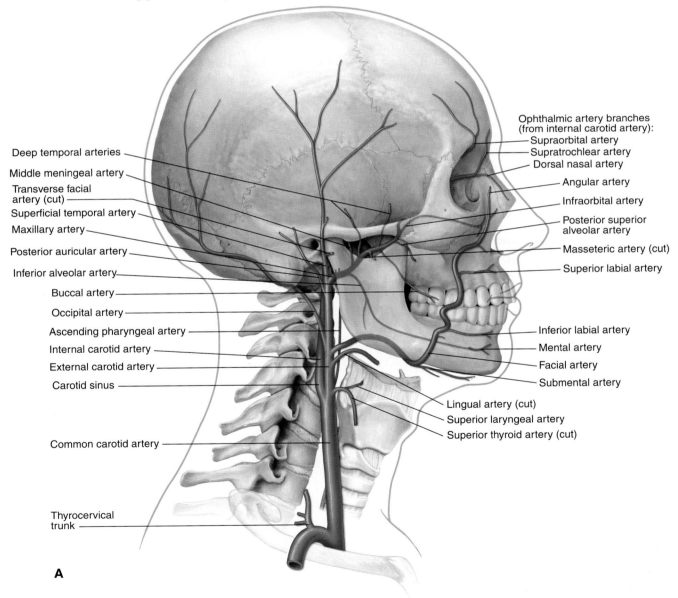

A

Figure 3.28A. Arteries of the Head and Neck, External Carotid Artery, Lateral View.

III. Internal Carotid Artery (Fig. 3.28B,C)

A. Ophthalmic artery
   1. Supplies orbit, forehead, and upper anterior nasal cavity
   2. Branches
      a. Central retinal artery
      b. Meningeal artery
      c. Anterior and posterior ciliary arteries
      d. Lacrimal artery
      e. Supraorbital artery
      f. Posterior ethmoidal artery
      g. Anterior ethmoidal artery
      i. Medial palpebral branches
      j. Dorsal nasal branch
      k. Supratrochlear artery
B. Anterior cerebral artery
   1. Supplies optic nerve and chiasm, medial surface of frontal lobe, corpus callosum
   2. Branches: inferior branches, superior branches, medial striate artery, medial orbitofrontal artery, frontopolar artery, callosomarginal artery, pericallosal artery
C. Middle cerebral artery
   1. Supplies insula, claustrum, nearly all of lateral side of cerebral hemispheres (parts of frontal, parietal, and temporal lobes), lenticular and caudate nuclei, internal capsule
   2. Branches: cortical branches, medial and lateral striate arteries
D. Anterior choroidal artery
   1. Usually directly from internal carotid artery but may branch from middle cerebral artery
   2. Branches: to choroid plexus of lateral and 3rd ventricles, optic tract, tail of caudate, globus pallidus, posterior crus of internal capsule, tuber cinereum, hypothalamus, substantia nigra, red nucleus, and amygdaloid body
E. Posterior communicating artery
   1. Connects internal carotid and posterior cerebral arteries
   2. Branches supply optic tract and chiasm, hypothalamus, cerebral peduncle, thalamus, subthalamus, interpeduncular area, and hippocampal gyrus

III. Subclavian Artery

A. Vertebral artery
   1. Supplies posterior cerebrum, brainstem, and cerebellum
   2. Branches
      a. Posterior spinal arteries
      b. Posterior inferior cerebellar artery
      c. Anterior spinal artery: unite to form single midline vessel
      d. Basilar artery: union of vertebral arteries
         i. Pontine arteries
         ii. Labyrinthine artery
         iii. Anterior inferior cerebellar artery
         iv. Superior cerebellar artery
         v. Posterior cerebral artery
B. Thyrocervical trunk
   1. Supplies thyroid and parathyroid glands, cervical trachea and esophagus, root of the neck
   2. Branches
      a. Inferior thyroid artery
      b. Transverse cervical artery
      c. Suprascapular artery

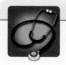

IV. Clinical Considerations

A. Wounds of either face or scalp bleed profusely because of multiple anastomoses, both from side to side and front to back
B. There are anastomoses in head between branches of internal and external carotid arteries, especially through dura mater
C. Branches of posterior superior alveolar supply the gums, molar teeth, and maxillary sinus

D. Branches of infraorbital artery supply orbital structures; maxillary sinus; and premolar, canine, and incisor teeth

E. Descending palatine artery divides into greater and lesser palatine arteries

F. Pharyngeal branch via pharyngeal canal supplies pharynx posterior to auditory tube opening

G. Sphenopalatine artery passes through sphenopalatine foramen and supplies lateral wall and septum of nasal cavity

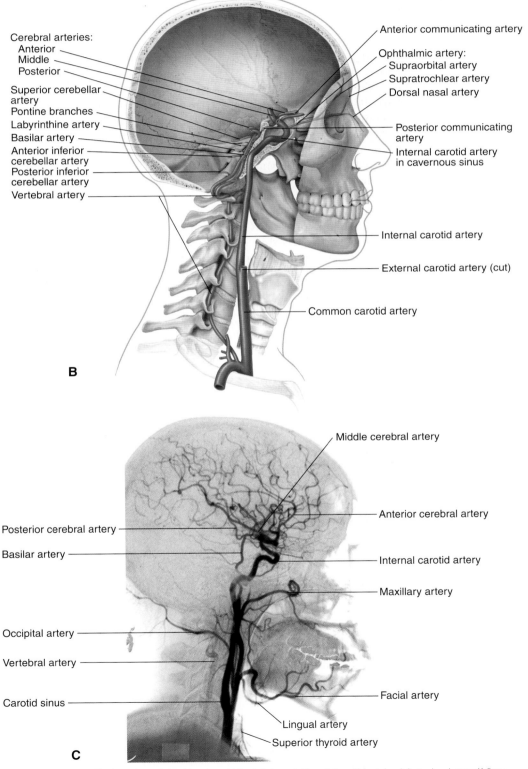

Figure 3.28B,C. B. Arteries of the Head and Neck, Internal Carotid and Vertebral Arteries, Lateral View.
C. Subtraction Angiogram of the Head and Neck, Lateral View.

Summary of Autonomics of Head and Neck

I. Parasympathetics in Head and Neck (Fig. 3.29A)

A. Oculomotor nerve (CN III)

1. Carries presynaptic parasympathetic fibers from Edinger-Westphal nucleus (midbrain tegmentum) via its inferior division to ciliary ganglion, located on lateral surface of optic nerve near apex of orbit

2. Postsynaptic fibers travel in short ciliary nerves, which run parallel with optic nerve to reach and penetrate back of globe

3. Pass through sclera to reach ciliary muscle (for accommodation) and sphincter pupillae muscle

B. Facial nerve (CN VII)

1. Presynaptic parasympathetic fibers arise from lacrimal and superior salivatory nucleus (pons) and leave brain via nervus intermedius to enter internal acoustic meatus

2. Greater petrosal nerve

   a. Branches from geniculate ganglion (sensory) to pass anteromedially to join deep petrosal nerve (postsynaptic sympathetic from internal carotid plexus) to form nerve of pterygoid canal (Vidian's nerve), passing forward to reach pterygopalatine ganglion

   b. Postsynaptic parasympathetic fibers distribute via branches of maxillary nerve (CN V_2) to mucous glands of nasal cavity and palate and via zygomatic branch of V_2 to lacrimal gland in orbit

   c. Deep petrosal nerve fibers pass through pterygopalatine ganglion without synapsing because they are postsynaptic sympathetic fibers

2. Chorda tympani

   a. Additional presynaptic parasympathetic fibers, together with taste fibers, leave facial nerve while it traverses facial canal

   b. Crosses tympanic membrane and exits skull through petrotympanic fissure to join lingual nerve and synapse in submandibular ganglion

   b. Postsynaptic parasympathetic fibers reach submandibular and sublingual glands; taste fibers reach anterior 2/3 of tongue

C. Glossopharyngeal nerve (CN IX)

1. Presynaptic parasympathetic fibers from inferior salivatory nucleus (medulla) form tympanic branch, which passes upward into tympanic cavity to form plexus; forms lesser petrosal nerve which passes across floor of middle cranial fossa to exit skull via foramen ovale and reach otic ganglion

2. Postsynaptic parasympathetic fibers join auriculotemporal nerve (from V_3) to reach parotid gland

D. Vagus nerve (CN X)

1. Presynaptic parasympathetic fibers from dorsal motor nucleus of X (medulla) pass via pharyngeal and laryngeal branches to supply mucous glands of pharynx, larynx, esophagus, and trachea; supplies parasympathetic fibers to viscera of thorax and abdomen

2. Synapses occur within organ wall; postsynaptic fibers are very short

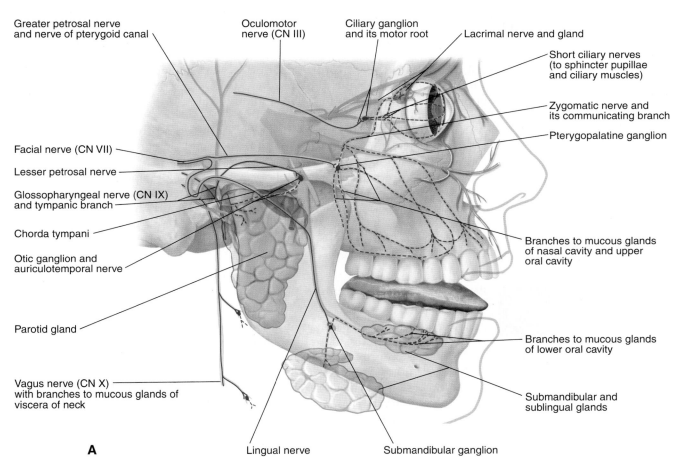

Greater petrosal nerve
and nerve of pterygoid canal

Oculomotor
nerve (CN III)

Ciliary ganglion
and its motor root

Lacrimal nerve and gland

Short ciliary nerves
(to sphincter pupillae
and ciliary muscles)

Zygomatic nerve and
its communicating branch

Pterygopalatine ganglion

Facial nerve (CN VII)

Lesser petrosal nerve

Glossopharyngeal nerve (CN IX)
and tympanic branch

Chorda tympani

Otic ganglion and
auriculotemporal nerve

Branches to mucous glands
of nasal cavity and upper
oral cavity

Parotid gland

Branches to mucous glands
of lower oral cavity

Vagus nerve (CN X)
with branches to mucous glands of
viscera of neck

Submandibular and
sublingual glands

A

Lingual nerve

Submandibular ganglion

Figure 3.29A. Autonomics of the Head and Neck, Parasympathetic Pathways, Lateral View.

II. Sympathetics in Head and Neck (Fig. 3.29B)

A. Presynaptic fibers
   1. From upper 4–5 thoracic sympathetic ganglia
   2. Pass up through sympathetic trunk to synapse in inferior, middle, or superior cervical ganglion

B. Postsynaptic fibers
   1. Gray rami communicantes: reach all cervical spinal nerves for vascular smooth muscle, sweat glands, and arrector pili muscles
      a. Superior cervical ganglion: supplies gray rami to C1–C4
      b. Middle cervical ganglion: supplies gray rami to C5–C6
      c. Inferior cervical ganglion: usually fuses with 1st thoracic ganglion to form stellate ganglion; supplies gray rami to C7–T1
   2. **Cardiac nerves**: descend from each cervical ganglion into chest to reach cardiac plexus
   3. **External carotid nerve**: passes from superior cervical ganglion onto external carotid artery to form perivascular external carotid plexus, supplying blood vessels and skin of face, primarily
   4. **Internal carotid nerve**: passes from superior cervical ganglion onto internal carotid artery to form perivascular internal carotid plexus
      a. Supplies blood vessels of brain, orbit, and forehead
      b. Branches
         i. **Deep petrosal nerve**: joins greater petrosal nerve to form nerve of pterygoid canal and pass through pterygopalatine fossa and ganglion (without synapsing there) to reach blood vessels of deep face
         ii. **Sympathetic root to ciliary ganglion**: passes through superior orbital fissure to traverse ciliary ganglion and short ciliary nerves to reach dilator pupillae muscle and superior tarsal muscle (smooth muscle portion of levator palpebrae superioris)

III. Clinical Considerations

A. **Bell's palsy**
   1. Unilateral facial paralysis of sudden onset
   2. Variable manifestations due to location of facial nerve lesion
      a. Lesion proximal to chorda tympani cause some dryness in mouth and abnormal taste sensation
      b. Lesion proximal to greater petrosal will additionally lack tear production which may cause corneal abrasion

B. **Horner's syndrome**
   1. Interruption of cervical sympathetic trunk
   2. Symptoms include **ptosis** (drooping) of lid (due to loss of smooth muscle portion of levator palpebrae superioris), constricted pupil (**miosis**) due to unopposed action of sphincter pupillae muscle, facial flushing (redness), lack of facial sweating (**anhydrosis**), and increased temperature of the skin due to vasodilation
   3. Lesion may occur in trunk anywhere above T1

C. **Frey's syndrome**
   1. Gustatory sweating: side of patient's face sweats when eating
   2. Occurs after incision in parotid gland; during healing, secretomotor parasympathetic fibers grow out and innervate sweat glands of face

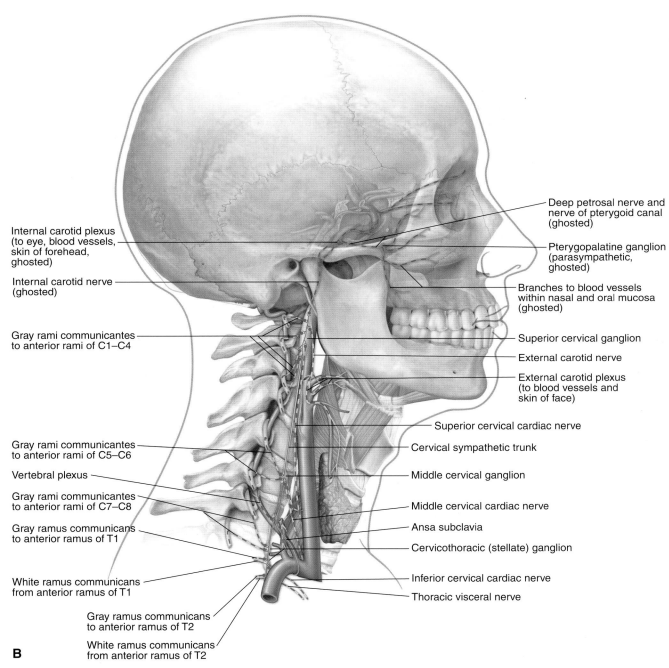

Internal carotid plexus
(to eye, blood vessels,
skin of forehead,
ghosted)

Internal carotid nerve
(ghosted)

Gray rami communicantes
to anterior rami of C1–C4

Gray rami communicantes
to anterior rami of C5–C6

Vertebral plexus

Gray rami communicantes
to anterior rami of C7–C8

Gray ramus communicans
to anterior ramus of T1

White ramus communicans
from anterior ramus of T1

Gray ramus communicans
to anterior ramus of T2

White ramus communicans
from anterior ramus of T2

Deep petrosal nerve and
nerve of pterygoid canal
(ghosted)

Pterygopalatine ganglion
(parasympathetic,
ghosted)

Branches to blood vessels
within nasal and oral mucosa
(ghosted)

Superior cervical ganglion

External carotid nerve

External carotid plexus
(to blood vessels and
skin of face)

Superior cervical cardiac nerve

Cervical sympathetic trunk

Middle cervical ganglion

Middle cervical cardiac nerve

Ansa subclavia

Cervicothoracic (stellate) ganglion

Inferior cervical cardiac nerve

Thoracic visceral nerve

B

Figure 3.29B. Autonomics of the Head and Neck, Sympathetic Pathways, Lateral View.

Note: Page numbers in italics refer to figures